# Current Topics in Pathology
# 95

Springer

*Berlin*
*Heidelberg*
*New York*
*Barcelona*
*Hong Kong*
*London*
*Milan*
*Paris*
*Singapore*
*Tokyo*

S. Love (Ed.)

# Neuropathology

## A Guide for Practising Pathologists

Contributors
M. Black, D. W. Ellison, J. F. Geddes, D. I. Graham, J.-J. Hauw,
M. W. Head, D. A. Hilton, J. W. Ironside, S. Love, J. Lowe, D. Seilhean,
H. V. Vinters, R. O. Weller, H. L. Whitwell, B. S. Wilkins

Springer

Professor Seth Love
Frenchay Hospital
Department of Neuropathology
Bristol BS16 1LE
United Kingdom

With 98 Figures and 19 Tables

ISBN-13:978-3-642-64025-4 Springer-Verlag Berlin Heidelberg New York

Library of Congress Cataloging-in-Publication Data
Neuropathology : a guide for practising pathologists / Seth Love (ed.) ; contributor, H. V. Vinters ... [et al.]. p. ; cm. – (Current topics in pathology ; 95) Includes bibliographical references and index.

ISBN-13:978-3-642-64025-4 e-ISBN-13:978-3-642-59554-7
DOI:10.1007/978-3-642-59554-7

1. Nervous system–Diseases. I. Love, Seth. II. Vinters, Harry V. III. Current topics in pathology ; v. 95. [DNLM: 1. Nervous System Diseases–pathology. WL 140 N4938 2001]. RB1 .E6 vol. 95 [RC347] 616.8'047–dc21



Springer-Verlag Berlin Heidelberg New York
a member of BertelsmannSpringer Science+Business Media GmbH



Production: PRO EDIT GmbH, Heidelberg
Cover design: design & production GmbH, Heidelberg
Typesetting: Fotosatz-Service Köhler GmbH, Würzburg

SPIN 10771310 24/3130/göh – 5 4 3 2 1 0 – Printed on acid-free paper

# Contributors


Black, M. — Department of Forensic Medicine
University of Glasgow,
Glasgow G 12 8QQ, UK

Ellison, D. W. — Cancer Research Unit,
The Medical School,
University of Newcastle,
Newcastle-upon-Tyne NE2 4HH, UK

Geddes, J. F. — Department of Morbid Anatomy,
Royal London Hospital, Whitechapel,
London E1 1BB, UK

Graham, D. I. — Department of Neuropathology,
Institute of Neurological Sciences,
Southern General Hospital,
South Glasgow University Hospitals NHS
Trust, Glasgow G51 4TF, UK

Hauw, J.-J. — Laboratoire de Neuropathologie,
Hôpital Pitié-Salpêtrière,
47 bd. de l'Hôpital,
18259 Paris, France

Head, M. W. — University of Edinburgh CJD
Surveillance Unit,
University of Edinburgh,
Western General Hospital,
Crewe Road, Edinburgh EH4 2XU, UK

Hilton, D. A. — Histopathology Laboratory,
Department of Pathology,
Derriford Hospital, Plymouth PL6 8DH,
UK

Ironside, J. W. — Neuropathology Laboratory,
Western General Hospital, Crewe Road,
Edinburgh EH4 2XU, UK

Love, S. Department of Neuropathology,
Institute of Clinical Neurosciences,
Frenchay Hospital, Bristol BS16 1LE, UK

Lowe, J. Department of Pathology,
University of Nottingham Medical
School, Clifton Boulevard,
Nottingham NG7 2UH, UK

Seilhean, D. Laboratoire de Neuropathologie,
Hôpital Pitié-Salpêtrière,
47 bd. de l'Hôpital, 18259 Paris, France

Vinters, H. V. Department of Pathology and
Laboratory Medicine, Section of
Neuropathology,
Brain Research Institute and
Neuropsychiatric Institute,
UCLA Medical Center, CHS 18-170,
Los Angeles, California 90095-1732, USA

Weller, R. O. Department of Neuropathology,
Mailpoint 813, Level E, South Pathology
Block, Southampton General Hospital,
Tremona Road, Southampton SO16 6YD,
UK

Whitwell, H. L. Department of Pathology,
University of Auckland,
Private bag 92019, Auckland,
New Zealand

Wilkins, B. S. Southampton General Hospital
Department of Pathology,
Mail Point 813, Level E South Block,
Southampton General Hospital,
Southampton SO16 6YD, UK

# Preface

In commissioning this volume of *Current Topics in Pathology*, the editor of the series, Prof. Sir Colin Berry, asked me to produce something "which is aimed at the general pathologist but from the point of view of the neuropathologist who knows what is not being done well". This was easier said than done. Many aspects of neuropathology are encountered only infrequently in general pathology and are best dealt with by referral of material to a specialist unit. Others need more extensive investigation than is practicable in a general pathology setting. Yet neurological disorders in general are common and are encountered by general histopathologists, paediatric and forensic pathologists on a daily basis, particularly in autopsy practice. In inviting contributions to this volume of *Current Topics in Pathology*, I therefore biased the contents towards disorders in which the conduct of the autopsy and the initial approach to neuropathological investigation are of critical importance in making the diagnosis. The authors all have a wealth of experience and expertise and I believe that this is reflected in their approach, which is both personal and practical. Indeed, the emphasis in this book is very much on the provision of practical advice. All of the chapters contain guidelines on the conduct of autopsies as well as information on the macroscopic and basic histological assessment of the nervous system in the relevant disorders. The book includes an appendix with clear diagrams and advice on the sampling of brain tissue for histology and other investigations. The result is a volume of *Current Topics in Pathology* covering a selection of topics in neuropathology that I hope will be of relevance and interest not only to neuropathologists but to those in other branches of histopathology as well.

Spring 2001 SETH LOVE

# Contents

# Autopsy Approach to Infections of the CNS

S. Love



## 1 Introduction

When dealing with infections of the CNS, as with so many other conditions, the key to performing an autopsy that is informative and helpful to clinical colleagues lies in the preparation. This should encompass both a careful review of the clinical notes and investigations, and reflection in advance of the autopsy of the possible pathological processes, their aetiology and pathogenesis. The aim of this chapter is to facilitate the preparation for autopsy investigation of infections of the CNS. Much of the chapter is devoted to considering the likely infective causes of different

Current Topics in Pathology, Vol. 95
S. Love (Ed.): Neuropathology

pathological processes in immunocompetent adults and children, immunosuppressed patients and, where appropriate, in neonates (although the chapter does not cover intrauterine infections). In contrast to most reference books on CNS infections, the present text is subdivided according to the pathological features rather than on an aetiological basis. The emphasis is on the typical macroscopic and microscopic manifestations of infections within broad clinical and pathological categories. The detailed histological and microbiological characterisation of different viruses, bacteria, fungi and parasites is well covered in many large reference books and is beyond the scope of the present text. The chapter includes a short section on acute disseminated encephalomyelitis and concludes with advice as to how to obtain appropriate samples for microbiological analysis.

# 2 Meningitis

## 2.1 Immunocompetent Adults and Children

### 2.1.1 Aseptic Meningitis

The commonest form of meningitis is 'aseptic' meningitis, a term used to describe a short-lived illness with headache, photophobia, neck stiffness and a cerebrospinal fluid (CSF) lymphocytosis, the cause of which is not evident on routine microscopy and culture [39, 68, 81]. Because aseptic meningitis is, almost by definition, benign, this type of meningitis is rarely seen at autopsy and then only if patients die from other complications of the (usually viral) infection, such as myocarditis. The brain appears normal apart from the presence of lymphocytes in the leptomeninges and superficial perivascular spaces. Most cases of aseptic meningitis, especially in children, are caused by non-polio enteroviruses [39, 68, 116, 149]. Mumps virus accounts for some further paediatric cases; the meningitis can precede the parotitis and occasionally occurs without the typical systemic manifestations of infection by this virus. Causes of aseptic meningitis in adults include non-polio enteroviruses, herpes simplex virus type 2 (HSV-2), and human immunodeficiency virus (HIV). The main differential diagnosis is partially treated bacterial meningitis, but this syndrome can result from a wide range of other viral, bacterial, fungal and parasitic infections as well as several non-infective processes [39].

### 2.1.2 Purulent Meningitis

About half of cases of purulent meningitis in immunocompetent adults are due to *Streptococcus pneumoniae* (pneumococcus) [22, 48, 65, 154]. The risk of pneumococcal meningitis is increased in the elderly and debilitated (especially those with a history of alcoholism), in patients who have had a splenectomy and in those with a dural fistula. It may be difficult to find a dural fistula at autopsy, but this should be suspected in patients with meningitis who have a history of head injury or neurosurgery, particularly if there has been more than one episode of meningitis. *Neisseria meningitidis* (meningococcal) meningitis tends to occur in outbreaks that are facilitated by crowded living conditions, such as army barracks and schools, and is an important cause of purulent meningitis in children. *Haemophilus influenzae* is only very rarely responsible for meningitis in adults but is, like *N. meningitidis*, a relatively frequent cause of purulent meningitis in children, especially in those under 2 years of age. Gram-negative bacilli are often responsible

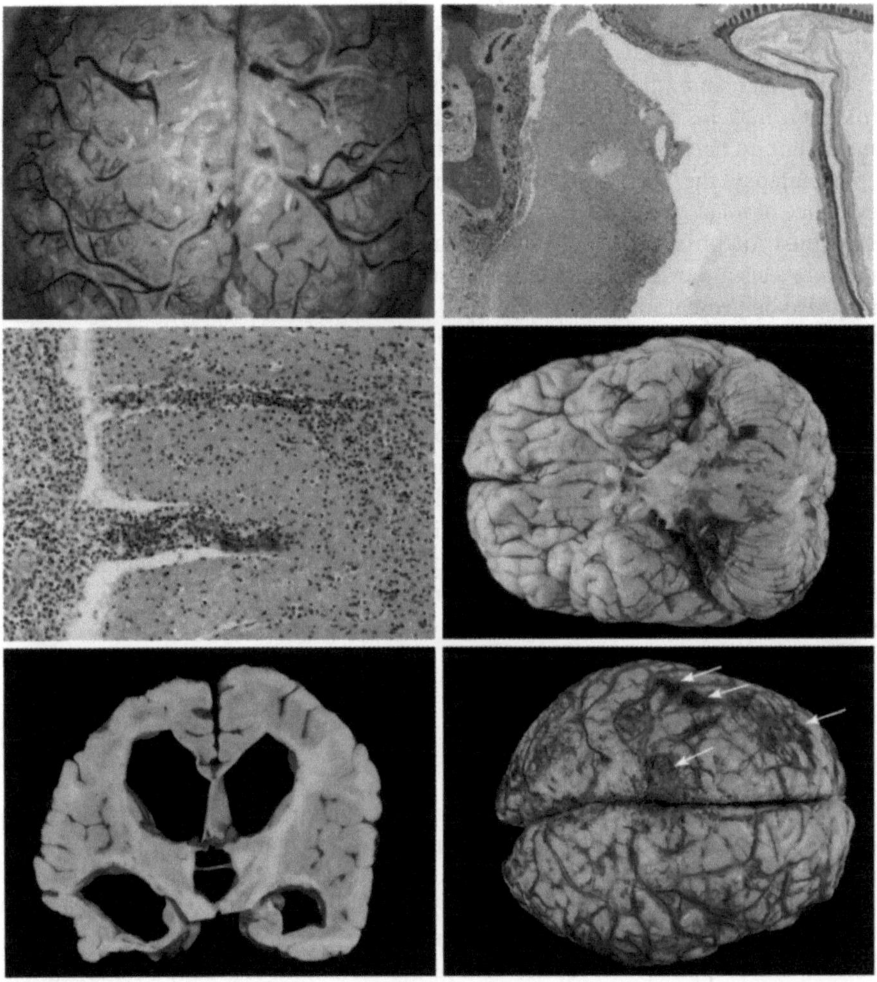

a b c d e f

**Fig. 1 a–f.** Purulent meningitis. **a** Purulent exudate over the vertex of the brain of an infant with pneumococcal meningitis. In this case, the infection had spread from the middle ear (**b**), which is filled with purulent material (tympanic membrane to *right* of figure). Case courtesy of Dr. A. Charles. **c** Histology reveals a purulent exudate in the subarachnoid space and extending along perivascular spaces into the superficial cortex. **d** Exudate over the base of the brain in meningitis complicating neurosurgery. **e** Non-communicating (obstructive) hydrocephalus complicating meningitis. **f** Multiple foci of haemorrhagic discolouration due to infarction (*arrows*) are visible in this case of pneumococcal meningitis for meningitis complicating neurosurgery or head injury. Slime-producing strains of *Staphylococcus epidermidis* are the main cause of meningitis complicating ventricular shunt infection, although *Staphylococcus aureus* or gram-negative bacilli are occasionally responsible.

The clinical presentation of purulent bacterial meningitis is usually with pyrexia, headache, neck stiffness, photophobia, nausea and vomiting, but symptoms and signs of septicaemia and cardiovascular collapse may predominate, particularly in meningococcal infections. About 50% of patients with meningococcal meningitis will have developed a rash, initially maculopapular but later purpuric and often confluent. In children, meningococcal infection is occasionally complicated by Waterhouse-Friderichsen syndrome, comprising septicaemia, shock, acute adrenal haemorrhage and adrenal failure. The presentation of ventriculitis due to shunt infection may be relatively insidious, with malaise, pyrexia, headache and confusion but no neck stiffness or photophobia.

At autopsy, the frontal air sinuses and middle ears should be examined for evidence of local infection (Fig. 1b). The lungs, heart and other tissues should be examined for possible sources of haematogenous infection. Examination of the brain reveals a purulent exudate in the subarachnoid space (Fig. 1c). An exudate may also be present in the ventricles, particularly in patients with meningitis and ventriculitis complicating shunt infection. In *S. pneumoniae* meningitis, the exudate tends to be most prominent over the cerebral convexities, towards the vertex (Fig. 1a). In other types of bacterial meningitis, the exudate is usually, but not always, thickest over the base of the brain (Fig. 1d). The brain is usually swollen, due to oedema and hydrocephalus in variable combination. Mild to moderate hydrocephalus is common (Fig. 1e) and may be either communicating, due to impeded flow of CSF in the subarachnoid space and arachnoid granulations, or non-communicating (obstructive), due to obstruction of the aqueduct or the outflow foramina of the fourth ventricle. Thrombosed cortical blood vessels and foci of infarction may be evident (Fig. 1f).

### 2.1.3 Granulomatous Meningitis

Much the commonest cause of granulomatous meningitis is *Mycobacterium tuberculosis*. Tuberculosis is increasing in incidence in many parts of the world, particularly in Africa and Eastern Europe, where the increase is probably attributable to the high prevalence of HIV infection [125, 126], and the incidence remains high in parts of South-East Asia and some Western Pacific countries [126]. In immunocompetent individuals, tuberculous meningitis is usually a complication of primary mycobacterial infection. In developing countries, in which primary exposure occurs at an early age, tuberculous meningitis is therefore commonest during childhood. In 'developed' countries, primary exposure to patients with active tuberculosis is much rarer and can occur at any age, as a result of which tuberculous meningitis does not show the same predilection for the young. At any age, tuberculous meningitis can complicate the reactivation of dormant infection in patients whose cell-mediated immunity becomes depressed (see below). The incidence of tuberculosis is increasing in urban communities with large numbers of indigent inhabitants and a high prevalence of HIV infection, and in such conditions there is an increased likelihood of exposure, even of immunocompetent individuals. Tuberculous meningitis tends to have an insidious presentation, with pyrexia, headache, malaise and lethargy and, as the disease progresses, neck stiffness, vomiting and the development of cranial nerve palsies and other focal neurological deficits.

Tuberculous meningitis produces a gelatinous or slightly nodular exudate, most pronounced in the Sylvian fissures and over the base of the brain (Fig. 2a) [48, 65]. The exudate can also involve the choroid plexus and ventricular lining. Small tuberculomas may be visible within the exudate and in the superficial brain parenchyma. Mild to moderate hydrocephalus is frequent. Endarteritis is quite a common complication of tuberculous meningitis and causes infarcts, particularly in the cerebral cortex and basal ganglia.

The main non-infective differential diagnosis of tuberculous meningitis is neurosarcoidosis [29, 61, 69, 169]. The CNS is involved in approximately 5% of patients with sarcoidosis, in whom this may be the only site of disease. The base of the brain around the optic chiasm and over the floor of the hypothalamus usually bears the brunt of the granulomatous inflammation, but this can affect the meninges and superficial brain parenchyma anywhere within the cranial cavity or spinal canal, and can also involve the choroid plexus and ventricular lining. The differential diagnosis of granulomatous meningeal inflammation includes several other rare, non-infective disorders – Wegener's disease, idiopathic hypertrophic pachymeningitis and isolated granulomatous angiitis of the CNS.

Rare infective causes of granulomatous meningitis in immunocompetent adults are infections caused by either of the two dimorphic fungi, *Blastomyces dermatitidis* and *Coccidioides immitis* [18, 30, 91, 174]. The former is responsible for North American blastomycosis, endemic in the south-eastern United States, and the latter for coccidioidomycosis, endemic in parts of the south-western United States and Central and South America. These fungi cause granulomatous inflammation of the meninges and brain parenchyma. The parenchymal disease usually takes the form of multiple small granulomas but purulent inflammation with abscess formation can occur [11]. The portal of entry of both of these fungi is the respiratory tract, and CNS involvement is usually a sequel of pulmonary disease, which should be sought at autopsy. Meningitis due to the yeast, *Cryptococcus neoformans*, can occur in the absence of immunosuppression but is far more often a complication of depressed cell-mediated immunity, malignancy or general inanition and is therefore discussed below (in Sect. 2.2).

Meningovascular syphilis is now rarely seen but in recent years the incidence of early syphilis has risen in certain high-risk groups such as prostitutes and their clients, especially in sub-Saharan Africa, South-East Asia and Eastern Europe [44, 47, 80, 100, 124, 136, 138, 152, 177]. The frequency of meningovascular syphilis and other tertiary manifestations of this disease may also have increased within these groups, particularly in patients with concomitant HIV infection (see Sects. 2.2 and 5.1.2). Meningovascular syphilis comprises a combination of (1) thickened fibrotic leptomeninges that are infiltrated by lymphocytes and plasma cells and may contain miliary gummas, and (2) multifocal intracranial arteritis, in which affected arteries and arterioles are infiltrated by mononuclear inflammatory cells and develop marked collagenous intimal thickening that may completely occlude the lumen [48, 63, 65]. The arteritis may cause ischaemic damage, including frank infarcts.

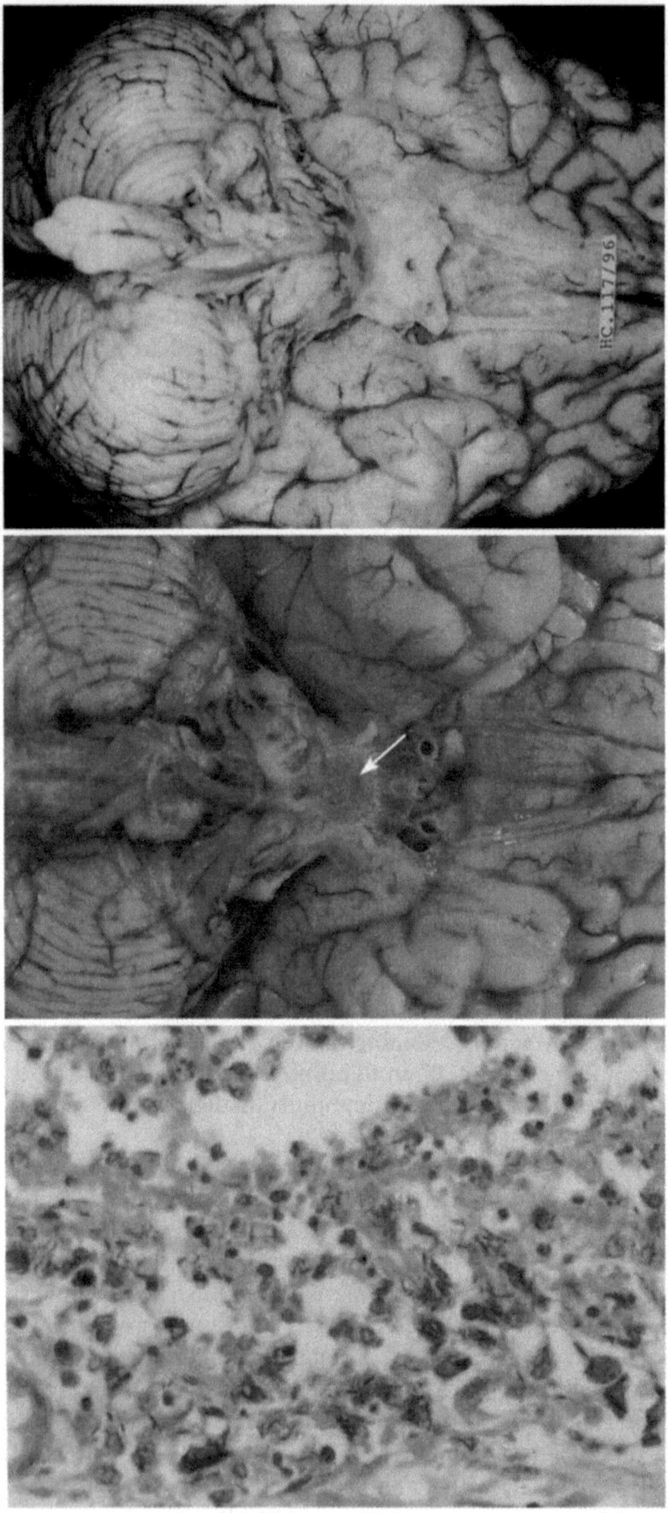


a

b

c

## 2.2 Immunosuppressed Patients

As already noted, the risk of pneumococcal meningitis is increased by debilitation and splenectomy. The risk of both pneumococcal and *H. influenzae* infections is also increased in hereditary splenic hypoplasia [87] and a range of other, rare immunodeficiency states. Patients with deficiencies in the 'early' complement proteins, C1, C4 and C2, are at risk of pneumococcal infections, including meningitis [148, 176] and those with C3 deficiency tend to develop recurrent, severe pneumococcal and meningococcal infections [129, 148]. Recurrent meningococcal infections are also associated with 'late' complement protein deficiencies, involving C6–9, but these infections tend to have a low mortality [88, 148, 155, 204]. Inherited deficiency of properdin predisposes to meningococcal infections that have a high mortality [148, 155]. Other inherited immunodeficiency diseases that predispose to purulent bacterial meningitis include X-linked agammaglobulinaemia [82] and glucose-6-phosphate dehydrogenase deficiency [105]. Acquired disorders of humoral immunity, such as granulocytic leukaemia and granulocytopoenia, also predispose to purulent meningitis. This is most often bacterial, due to pneumococcus, gram-negative bacilli (especially *Pseudomonas aeruginosa*) or occasionally *Listeria monocytogenes.* Rarely, *Candida* species are responsible.

Patients with depressed cell-mediated immunity (especially those with AIDS, but also organ transplant recipients, patients with lymphomas and lymphocytic leukaemias and those with rarer immunosuppressive disorders) are at risk of tuberculous meningitis. This is due to reactivation of infection in primary tubercles, either within the brain itself (in so-called Rich's foci) or in other tissues, in which case the CNS is infected during subsequent haematogenous dissemination. In severely immunosuppressed patients, tuberculous meningitis is characterised by the presence of abundant mycobacteria and an absence or paucity of granulomas (Fig. 2c) [48].

There is some evidence of an increased prevalence of meningovascular and other forms of neurosyphilis in HIV-infected patients [14, 17, 54, 72, 160]. HIV infection may accelerate the progression to tertiary syphilis and increase the likelihood of CNS involvement, particularly in the form of meningovascular disease, although this is more contentious [14, 85, 132, 160]. Meningovascular syphilis manifests pathologically with fibrous thickening and chronic lymphocytic and plasmacytic inflammation of the meninges over the brain or spinal cord, and concentric collagenous thickening and inflammation of the intima of arteries and arterioles, leading to foci of ischaemic damage (see Sect. 5.1.2).

Depressed cell-mediated immunity increases the risk of fungal meningitis due to *Cryptococcus neoformans* or *Histoplasma capsulatum* [40, 99, 112, 168, 183, 191,

**Fig. 2a–c.** Tuberculous meningitis and neurosarcoidosis. **a** Nodular exudate (*arrow*) over the base of the brain in tuberculous meningitis. Original figure courtesy of Prof. L. Chimelli. Reproduced with permission, from [48]. **b** Granulomatous exudate in neurosarcoidosis. The basal meninges are thickened and a yellowish grey exudate (*arrow*) surrounds the optic nerves and pituitary stalk. **c** Numerous acid-fast mycobacteria in an AIDS patient with tuberculous meningitis. Original figure courtesy of Prof. L. Chimelli. Reproduced with permission, from [48]

192]. The abnormalities on external examination of the brain in cryptococcal meningitis tend to be mild. The surface of the brain may appear slimy and the leptomeninges thickened. Sectioning of the brain shows perivascular spaces in the cortex and basal ganglia to be expanded by numerous thickly encapsulated yeasts to form multiple small cystic spaces, likened to soap bubbles (Fig. 3a). The cryptococcal yeasts may be mistaken for corpora amylacea on casual microscopic examination (Fig. 3b). Involvement of the CNS by histoplasmosis is usually a

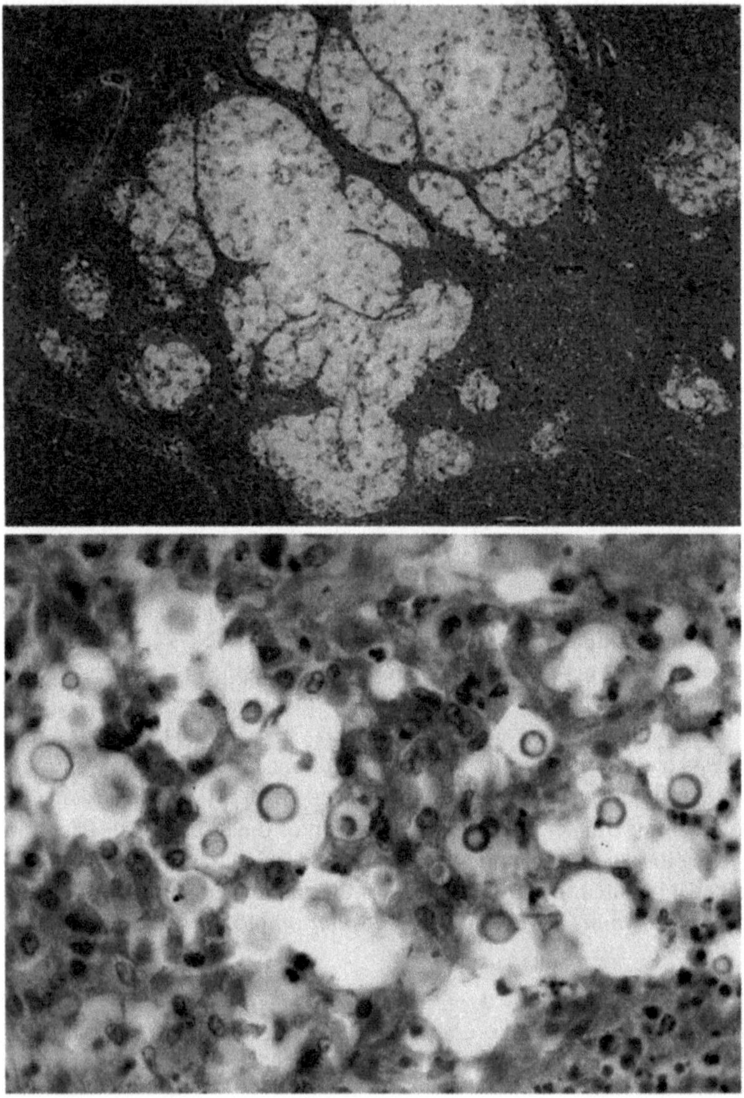

a

b

**Fig. 3a, b.** Cryptococcal meningitis. **a** Expanded perivascular spaces in the basal ganglia contain numerous yeasts. **b** Meningeal inflammatory exudate within which are scattered, spherical yeasts resembling corpora amylacea manifestation of disseminated fungal infection. *Histoplasma* causes a granulomatous meningitis resembling that of tuberculous infection. A gelatinous or nodular, yellowish grey exudate is usually visible over the base of the brain and small granulomas or abscesses are often present in the brain parenchyma. The yeasts measure only 2–5 µm in diameter and are difficult to see in haematoxylin- and eosin-stained sections but, like other fungi, are readily demonstrated by PAS staining or methenamine silver impregnation. Both acquired defects in cell-mediated immunity and certain rare inherited immunodeficiency disorders predispose to systemic candidal infections, including meningitis [60, 98]. However, in *Candida* infections of the CNS, parenchymal brain lesions usually predominate (see below).

Free-living amoebae of the genera *Acanthamoeba* and *Balamuthia* are an occasional cause of granulomatous meningoencephalitis in patients who are immunosuppressed or severely debilitated [48, 109, 153]. The meningeal inflammation is patchy, the distribution of meningeal exudate being related to necrotic lesions in the underlying brain parenchyma. Granulomatous meningoencephalitis is described in more detail in Sect. 3.2.

## 2.3 Neonates

The commonest causes of meningitis in neonates are bacterial: group B streptococci and *Escherichia coli* [56, 73, 119, 143, 171, 186]. Low birth weight, prolonged rupture of amniotic membranes and puerperal sepsis are the major risk factors. Group B streptococci are readily spread by contact within hospital wards, leading to local outbreaks of this type of neonatal meningitis. Other bacteria that are, less often, responsible for meningitis in neonates include *Listeria monocytogenes*, *S. aureus*, *Citrobacter*, *Klebsiella* and *Enterobacter* species, *Pseudomonas aeruginosa* and other gram-negative bacilli.

The initial clinical signs of neonatal meningitis are usually non-specific and include poor feeding, diarrhoea and vomiting, irritability or lethargy. The development of neck stiffness, bulging of the fontanelle and signs of shock are late manifestations. At autopsy, the brain appears swollen and the leptomeninges markedly congested. A purulent subarachnoid exudate is usually visible, particularly over the base of the brain (Fig. 4a). A particularly frequent finding in this age group is the presence of haemorrhagic infarcts, associated with thrombosis of superficial veins and arteries (Fig. 4b) [48]. Another occasional finding is the presence of coexistent cerebral abscesses, especially in gram-negative bacterial infections.

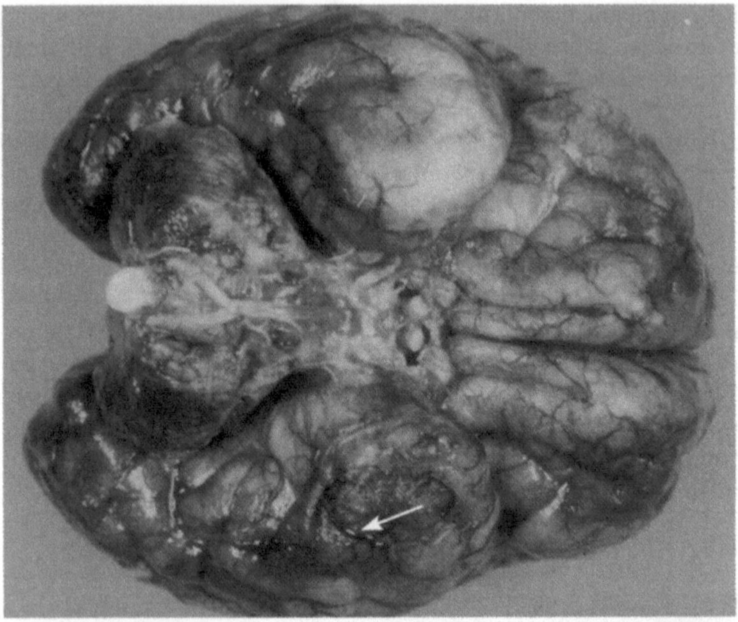

a

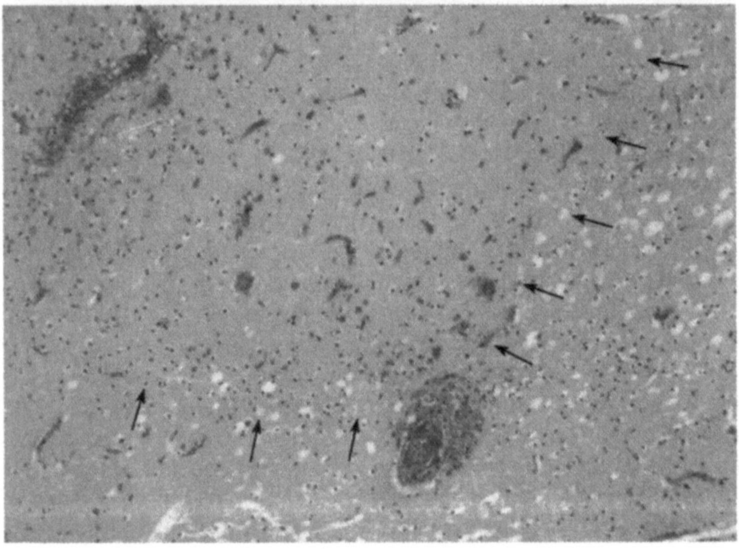

b

**Fig. 4a, b.** Neonatal meningitis. **a** External examination of the brain in this case of group B streptococcal meningitis reveals a scanty basal purulent exudate, marked leptomeningeal congestion and focal venous thrombosis (*arrow*) with infarction of the underlying temporal cortex. Original figure courtesy of Dr. H. Porter. Reproduced with permission, from [48]. **b** Thrombosis of superficial cortical blood vessels with acute infarction of the adjacent cortex (*arrows*)

# 3 Abscesses, Empyemas and Parenchymal Granulomas

## 3.1 Immunocompetent Adults and Children

### 3.1.1 Brain Abscess

Approximately half are due to local spread of infection from a paranasal sinus, middle ear or dental root [19, 46, 147, 162, 199]. The pathogen most often isolated from these brain abscesses is *Streptococcus milleri*. Bacteria less frequently isolated include a wide range of aerobic and anaerobic streptococci, staphylococci and gram-negative bacilli. The resulting abscess is usually solitary, the location varying according to the source of infection. When the source is an infection of a paranasal sinus, the abscess involves the adjacent part of the frontal lobe. Abscesses associated with middle ear infections tend to involve the temporal lobe or anterior part of the parietal lobe but may occasionally occur in the cerebellum. Cerebral abscesses complicating dental root infections usually involve the frontal lobes; occasionally responsible in such cases is *Actinomyces israelii*, a filamentous gram-positive bacterium that tends to cause multiloculated cerebral abscesses.

Haematogenous sources of infection in adults include bronchiectasis, lung abscess and endocarditis. In children, congenital heart disease or pulmonary arteriovenous malformation with right-to-left shunting carries a substantial risk of development of brain abscesses (Fig. 5a), presumably because of the combination of relative hypoxaemia, bypass of the pulmonary capillary bed, and increased blood viscosity due to polycythaemia. Patients with haematogenously derived infection may develop multiple brain abscesses. Although typically these occur at the junction of cerebral cortex and white matter (Fig. 5b), in some cases microabscesses are widely scattered throughout the brain. The most frequent pathogens are *Streptococcus viridans* and microaerophilic or anaerobic streptococci. Rare, non-bacterial causes of brain abscesses in immunocompetent patients include *Entamoeba histolytica*, *C. neoformans* (cryptococcomas), *C. immitis* and *B. dermatitidis* (for further information about these last two pathogens see also Sect. 2.1.3). Amoebic brain abscesses occur only in patients who already have intestinal and liver or pulmonary amoebiasis. Cryptococcomas are described in Sect. 3.1.4.

Irrespective of the underlying aetiology, virtually all patients will develop headache and pyrexia and, depending on the size and site of the abscess or abscesses, evidence of raised intracranial pressure and focal neurological deficits. Other clinical manifestations will vary according to the predisposing conditions, the source of sepsis and the presence of associated pathology, such as embolic infarcts in patients with endocarditis.

The macroscopic and microscopic appearances of abscesses vary according to their age [48, 65, 199]. During the first week or so, when the histology is that of focal suppurative encephalitis and the abnormalities are often poorly circumscribed, the macroscopic changes may be limited to focal brain swelling and congestion. The early microabscesses associated with haematogenous infection are often centred on small blood vessels showing fibrinoid necrosis; macroscopically, these appear as small haemorrhages or foci of haemorrhagic softening [131]. Older abscesses will

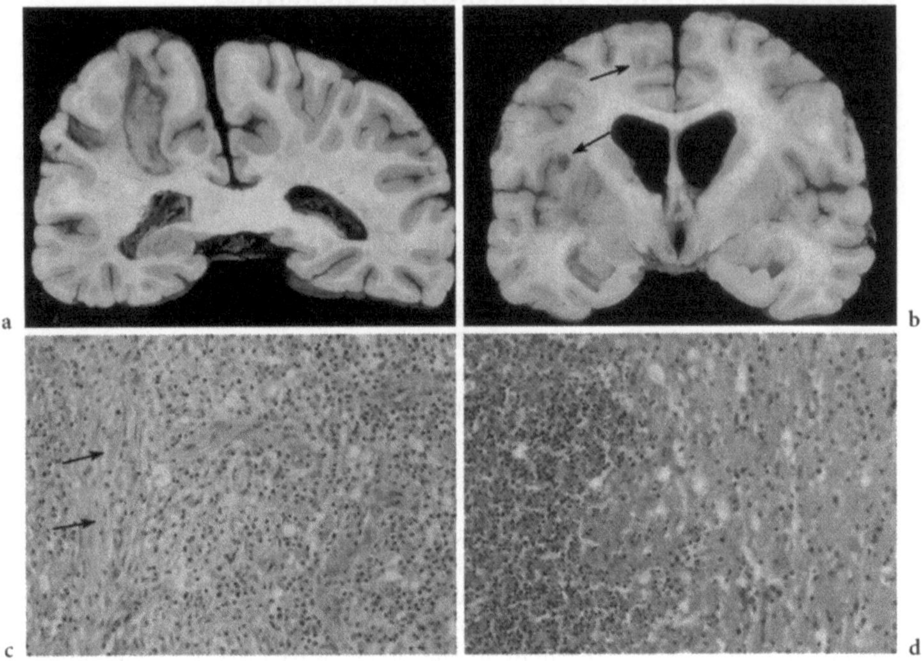

**Fig. 5a–d.** Brain abscess. **a** Large abscess in parietal lobe of a patient with a complex cardiac malformation and right-to-left shunting. **b** Multiple small abscess (*arrows*) at the junction of cortex and white matter in a patient with septicaemia due to *S. aureus*. **c, d** Sections through the superficial (**c**) and deep (**d**) parts of a cerebral abscess. Note the proliferation of fibroblasts and deposition of collagen (*arrows*) in **c** and their absence from the deep margin of the abscess

have collagenous capsules of variable thickness and a well-defined core of purulent material. The capsule tends to be thicker on the superficial aspect of the abscess (Fig. 5c) than on its deep aspect (Fig. 5d). If cutting into an abscess releases a foul odour (usually detectable even after fixation of the brain), anaerobic infection is likely. Amoebic brain abscesses have irregular necrotic cores that are surrounded by reactive brain tissue without collagenous encapsulation [48, 109]. The trophozoites, which are often mistaken for macrophages, have a round vesicular nucleus with a central karyosome and can usually be found in the 'wall' of the abscess.

### 3.1.2 Subdural Empyema

The antecedents of subdural empyemas are similar to those of brain abscesses (local infections, trauma, neurosurgery and systemic foci of purulent infection) and likewise the range of pathogens [45, 93, 199]. In children, the development of a subdural empyema may complicate purulent meningitis. The macroscopic and microscopic features are simply of pus in the subdural space, usually but not always in the supratentorial compartment. The pus may be encapsulated by granulation tissue of variable thickness.

### 3.1.3 Extradural Empyema

This usually occurs within the spinal canal. The source of infection is often local – adjacent vertebral osteomyelitis or a retropharyngeal abscess – but haematogenous spread may occur from distant foci of purulent infection [58]. *S. aureus* is the bacterium usually isolated, gram-negative bacilli much less frequently.

### 3.1.4 Parenchymal Granulomas

The differential diagnosis of parenchymal brain granulomas includes tuberculosis, syphilis, Whipple's disease, fungal infections and parasitic diseases.

Tuberculomas are still relatively common in parts of the world with a high prevalence of tuberculosis, particularly in much of Africa, South-East Asia and some Western Pacific countries [125, 126]. They most often occur in children, in whom the tuberculomas tend to be infratentorial: in the cerebellum or pons. In adults, tuberculomas usually occur above the tentorium [63]. Their appearances are similar to those of tuberculomas elsewhere in the body, with central caseous necrosis surrounded by a granulomatous inflammatory reaction that includes Langhans-type giant cells, and a surrounding zone of collagenous fibrosis Fig. 6).

Syphilitic gummas are now rare, although as noted in Sect. 2.1.3, this situation may change, as the incidence of syphilis increases in some Eastern European,

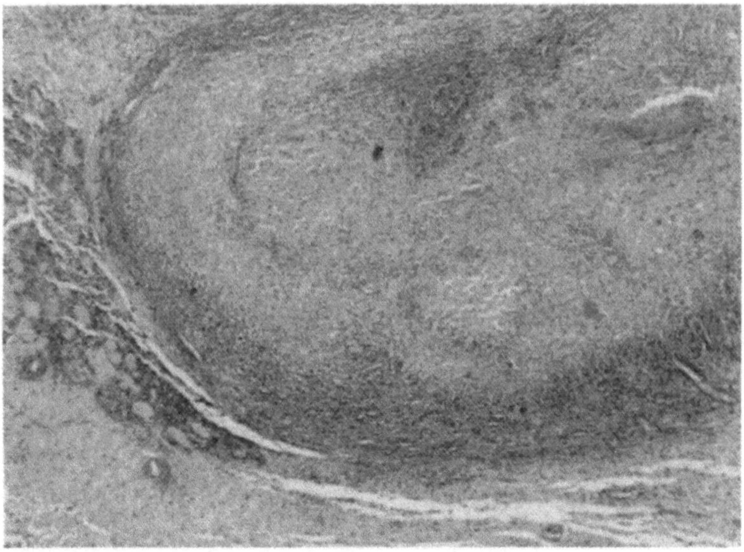

**Fig. 6.** Cerebral tuberculoma. The section includes part of a tuberculoma and the adjacent brain tissue. There is a central caseous necrosis surrounded by a rim of epithelioid macrophages and Langhans-type giant cells, and an outer zone of lymphocytes, fibroblasts and collagen. The collagen fibres appear dark in this haematoxylin/van Gieson preparation

South-East Asian and sub-Saharan African countries, especially in high-risk groups such as prostitutes and their partners [44, 47, 59, 80, 95, 100, 124, 136, 138, 152, 165, 177].

Whipple's disease is caused by a gram-positive bacillus, *Tropheryma whippelii*, that accumulates in large numbers within macrophages in affected tissues. The small intestine is the main site of disease in most patients, but other tissues may be involved, including the CNS [137, 139, 159, 198]. The manifestations of CNS disease are variable and can include ophthalmoplegia, oculomasticatory myorhythmia, facial or ocular myoclonus, sleep and eating disturbances, confusion and dementia [3, 43, 111, 141, 187, 203]. Macroscopic examination of the brain may reveal foci of granular yellow discolouration, especially in the thalamus, hypothalamus and around the aqueduct. Microscopy shows these foci to contain clusters of macrophages within which is intensely PAS-positive, diastase-resistant material. The bacilli may be difficult to demonstrate with a Gram stain but can be impregnated with methenamine silver.

Isolated parenchymal or meningeal fungal granulomas are a very infrequent finding in immunocompetent patients although multiple small granulomas or abscesses are a feature of *Blastomyces dermatitidis* and *Coccidioides immitis* meningitis. Cryptococcomas are an unusual manifestation of *C. neoformans* infection but, when they do develop, tend to affect patients with preserved immune function. The appearance of cryptococcomas is variable: some are densely fibrotic lesions with granulomatous inflammation, others are large gelatinous lesions full of yeasts, or they may resemble bacterial abscesses [30, 48, 153].

Symptomatic CNS involvement in schistosomiasis is relatively rare and occurs in patients in whom large, discrete deposits of ova within the brain or spinal canal elicit a focal granulomatous reaction. These deposits of large numbers of ova are thought to result from anomalous migration of adult worms to sites within or close to the CNS [134]. Patients develop clinical features of an intracranial space-occupying lesion or of a painful radiculopathy and myelopathy that may progress within days to paraplegia. More common is the presence of sparsely scattered and usually asymptomatic granulomas that result from retrograde embolisation of ova through the pelvic veins and valveless vertebral venous plexus in patients with hepatointestinal schistosomiasis and portal hypertension or with severe urinary schistosomiasis. In such cases *S. haematobium* and *S. mansoni* ova are most likely to lodge within the meninges surrounding the lumbosacral spinal cord but *S. japonicum* ova may lodge within the brain. The sparsely scattered granulomas that develop in relation to the ova are usually an incidental finding at autopsy but may be associated with seizures or, rarely, focal haemorrhage [134]. The occurrence of granulomatous inflammation in relation to parasitic cysts is considered in Sect. 4.

### 3.2 Immunosuppressed Patients

In addition to those already discussed, a wide range of bacteria, fungi and protozoa can cause brain abscesses or, at least, focal necrotic lesions, in patients who are immunosuppressed. The potential bacterial pathogens include *Nocardia asteroides*, *Listeria monocytogenes*, a range of gram-negative bacilli and *M. tuberculosis*. The principal parasite to consider in this context is *Toxoplasma gondii*. The range of fungi includes *Aspergillus fumigatus* or *flavus*, fungi in the family Mucoraceae that cause cerebral mucormycosis, and *Candida* species. The rhinocerebral form of mucormycosis differs somewhat from the other opportunist fungal infections in its frequent association with poorly controlled diabetes mellitus and ketoacidosis; in contrast, the disseminated cerebral mucormycosis that results from haematogenous brain infection occurs in the context of immunosuppression, intravenous drug abuse or in children with severe diarrhoea and dehydration [30, 48, 153].

a
b
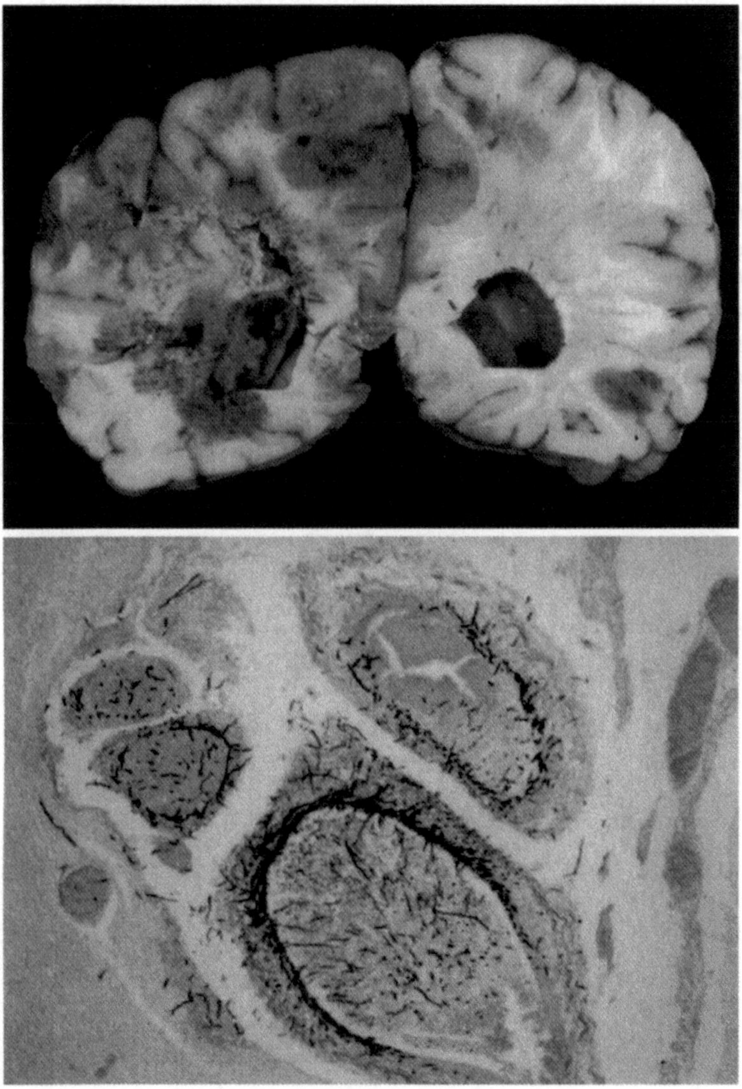

**Fig. 7 a, b.** Cerebral aspergillosis. **a** Extensive haemorrhagic necrosis in an immunosuppressed patient with cerebral aspergillosis. **b** Grocott silver impregnation reveals extensive invasion of blood vessels and vessel walls by the fungal hyphae

The pathological characteristics of these infections are quite varied. The bacterial infections tend to produce typical abscesses. In patients with depressed cell-mediated immunity, even *M. tuberculosis* may cause purulent infection and brain abscess formation (this is well documented in patients with AIDS). *Aspergillus* species and the various fungi responsible for rhinocerebral mucormycosis (of which species of *Rhizopus* are mostly responsible) invade the walls of cerebral blood vessels to cause vessel necrosis and thrombosis, and haemorrhagic necrosis of brain tissue. In the case of *Aspergillus* infections, these are generally multiple and scattered throughout the brain (Fig. 7a, b), as a result of haematogenous dissemination of the infection, but some patients develop localised cerebral infections due to direct spread of *Aspergillus* (e.g. from an infected paranasal sinus or complicating local trauma) [16, 48, 153, 189, 200]. In rhinocerebral mucormycosis, the foci of haemorrhagic necrosis are concentrated in the frontal region (Fig. 8), but thrombosed blood vessels and haemorrhagic necrotic tissue are also present in the orbit and paranasal sinuses [30, 48]. In disseminated cerebral mucormycosis, multiple haemorrhagic, necrotic lesions are present and can involve any part of the brain. Cerebral candidiasis is usually a late manifestation of widespread systemic disease. The yeasts and pseudohyphae of *Candida albicans* tend to occlude small blood vessels within the brain to produce multiple lesions that are smaller than those caused by the filamentous fungi described above and may difficult to resolve macroscopically. The lesions may initially be haemorrhagic or simply necrotic, and evolve into small abscesses or granulomas [30, 48, 101, 130].

Symptomatic cerebral toxoplasmosis was relatively uncommon before the advent of AIDS but did occasionally affect immunocompetent patients or those

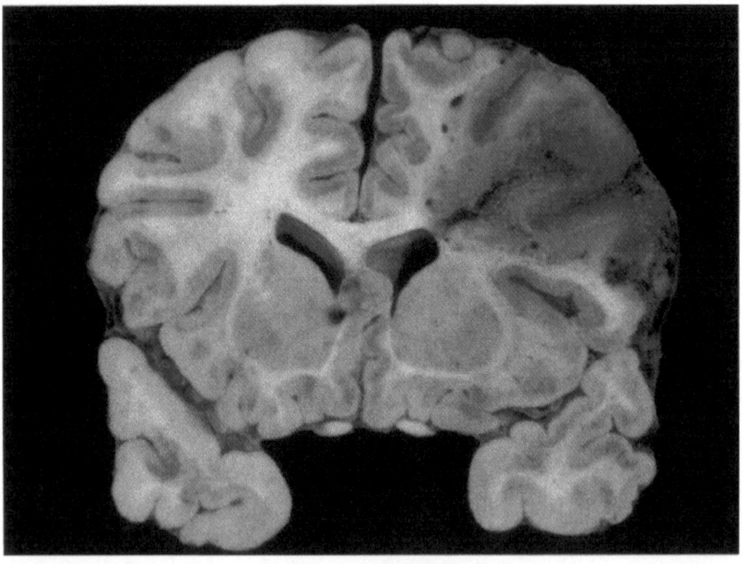

**Fig. 8.** Rhinocerebral mucormycosis. Extensive haemorrhagic necrosis in the right frontal lobe. Necrotic tissue had previously been resected from the anterior part of the frontal lobe in this patient, who was also receiving antifungal therapy, but the infection had continued to spread posteriorly

with other causes for immunosuppression. Toxoplasmosis is one of the commonest causes of an intracranial space-occupying lesion in patients with AIDS. In most cases, this probably reflects reactivation of dormant disease. The clinical manifestations are those of any space-occupying lesion within the brain. The lesions may be solitary but more often examination of brain slices reveals multiple foci of coagulative or haemorrhagic necrosis surrounded by a mixed or mononuclear cell inflammatory infiltrate (Fig. 9a, b) [48, 52, 71, 153, 170]. The basal ganglia and cerebral white matter are often involved but the lesions can occur in any part of the brain. Older lesions appear cavitated, due to resorption of the necrotic material. In dormant infections, the protozoal trophozoites are confined to large cysts that have a double-layered, slightly refractile wall and measure up to about 100 µm in diameter. Active lesions contain large numbers of extracellular trophozoites, and intracellular clusters of oval or crescent-shaped trophozoites within phagocytic vacuoles and larger membrane-bound pseudocysts (Fig. 9c). The extracellular trophozoites can be confused with nuclear debris or small foci of mineralisation but are readily demonstrated immunohistochemically (Fig. 9d).

Granulomatous amoebic encephalitis is a disorder of patients who are immunosuppressed or severely debilitated [109]. It is caused by free-living amoebae of the genera *Acanthamoeba* and *Balamuthia*. The amoebae reach the CNS

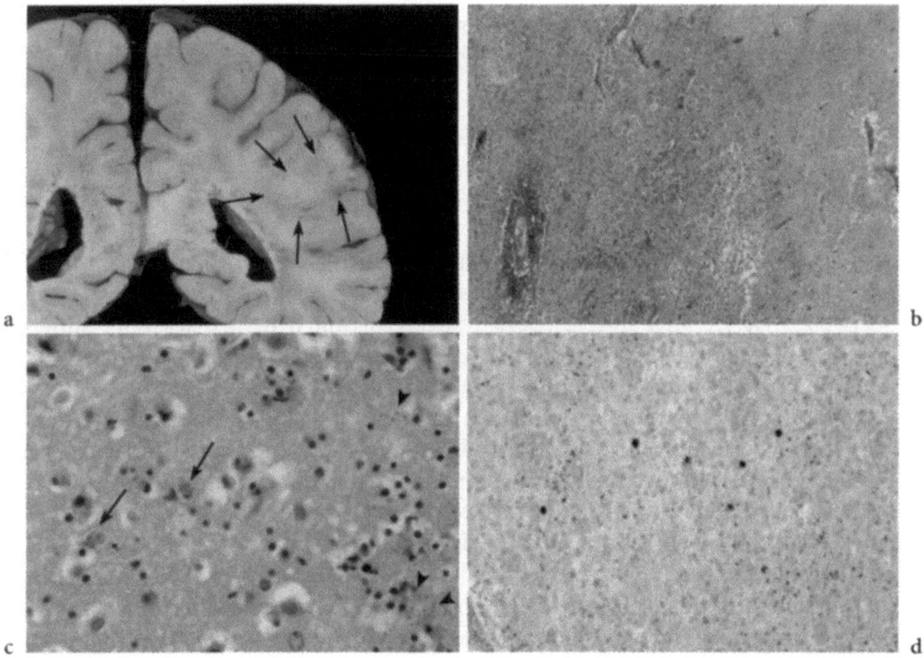

**Fig. 9a–d.** Cerebral toxoplasmosis in a patient with systemic lymphoma. **a** Well-circumscribed focus of coagulative necrosis in the right parietal lobe (*arrows*). **b** Histology shows a chronic inflammatory infiltrate in brain tissue adjacent to the necrosis. **c** At higher magnification, one can discern *Toxoplasma* trophozoites in pseudocysts (*arrows*) and extracellularly (*arrowheads*). **d** The extracellular trophozoites and larger pseudocysts are well demonstrated immunohistochemically

haematogenously, in most cases from a focus of infection in the lungs or skin, and produce multiple foci of softening and necrosis that may be haemorrhagic. Patients develop non-specific features of encephalitis, often associated with seizures, focal neurological deficits and cranial nerve palsies. The disease progresses over weeks or months and is usually fatal. At autopsy, the brain is swollen and includes scattered foci of softening and haemorrhagic necrosis [48, 109, 153]. Microscopy reveals a chronic inflammatory infiltrate that may be granulomatous and is most intense around blood vessels and in the meninges overlying necrotic lesions. Amoebic trophozoites and cysts are present in and around the walls of blood vessels. The amoebae have a large vesicular nucleus with a prominent central nucleolus. The cysts have a thick, double-layered wall.

As noted in Sect. 5.1.2, acute infection by *T. cruzi* (American trypanosomiasis, Chagas disease) may cause a low grade encephalitis but the brunt of the disease involves the peripheral autonomic nervous system. However, immunosuppressed patients may develop multifocal granulomatous or necrotising lesions in the CNS, probably due to reactivation of dormant infection [31, 48]. These lesions contain numerous intracellular amastigote parasites.

### 3.3 Neonates

In neonates, brain abscesses are an occasional complication of purulent meningitis [166]. The pathogens most frequently responsible are *Citrobacter diversus* and *Proteus mirabilis*.

## 4 Parasitic Cysts

This section covers cysticercosis and hydatid disease, the two main causes of parasitic cysts of the CNS. Other parasitic diseases of the CNS are covered in Sects. 2.2, 3.1.4, 3.2, 5.1.1 and 5.2). Both cysticercosis and hydatid disease are caused by cestodes, *Taenia solium* (the pork tape worm) and *Echinococcus granulosus* (or, less commonly, *E. multilocularis*) respectively [133, 173].

Cysticercosis is particularly common in South and Central America, parts of Asia and Africa, and occurs with moderate frequency in Spain, Portugal and Eastern Europe. Man is usually the definitive host and acquires the infection by ingesting inadequately cooked pork containing viable cysticerci. The larvae emerge and attach to the intestinal wall by means of their scolices. The larvae develop into mature tapeworms within the small intestine and shed proglottids that contain the parasitic ova, in the faeces. The normal intermediate hosts are pigs, which eat the ova. The oncospheres (ova from which the coat has been digested) penetrate the pig's intestinal mucosa and are disseminated through the blood stream to muscle and other tissues (including the CNS), where encystment occurs. Man may become an intermediate host by ingestion of food contaminated with ova excreted by someone else (heteroinfection) or, in the case of carriers of the adult tapeworm (i.e. definitive hosts), by faeco-oral autoinfection. It is, in addition, possible that reverse peristalsis of ova may account for some cases of autoinfection.

The clinical manifestations of CNS cysticercosis depend on the number and distribution of cysts and the severity of associated inflammation [133]. The disease is often asymptomatic. Manifestations of symptomatic CNS involvement include focal or generalised seizures, headache, vomiting, papilloedema, vertigo, exacerbation of symptoms or even loss of consciousness precipitated by sudden movements of the head, focal neurological deficits (occasionally due to spinal disease), dementia or sudden death.

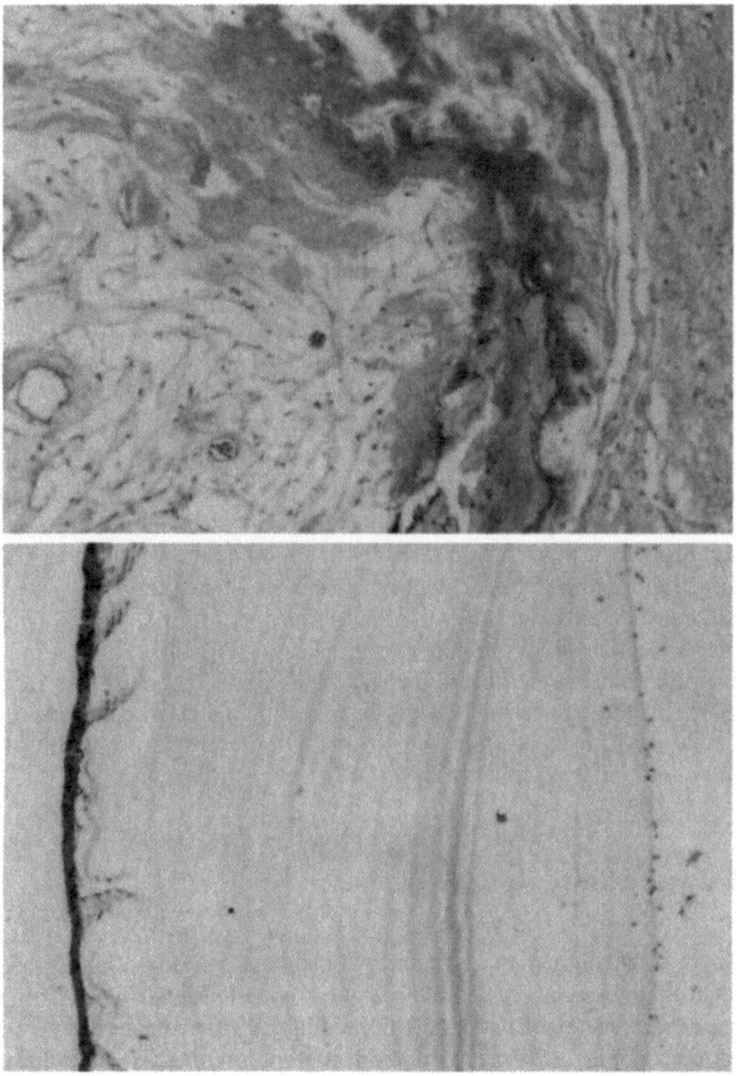

**Fig. 10 a, b.** Parasitic cysts within the brain. **a** Section through part of a long-dead cysticercus, replaced by collagenous, partly calcified tissue. **b** Wall of hydatid cyst. A thick laminated cuticle and a thin inner germinal layer are visible in this section. Reproduced with permission, from [48]

Autopsy examination reveals cysts in the brain parenchyma, leptomeninges or ventricles [48, 133, 153]. The viable cysts measure 1–2 cm in diameter and contain a single scolex. Those in the meninges or ventricles are translucent and may form grape-like clusters. The cyst wall has three layers: an outer cuticular layer with multiple small protrusions (microtricha), a middle cellular layer and an inner reticular layer. Suckers and hooklets may be visible in the enclosed scolex. There is little inflammatory reaction around viable cysts. Upon death of the parasite, the cysticercus undergoes necrosis and elicits a mixed inflammatory reaction that includes neutrophils, eosinophils, lymphocytes, macrophages and multinucleated giant cells. The inflammatory process may involve adjacent blood vessels with resulting thrombosis and infarction, and the meninges, with consequent fibrosis and chronic hydrocephalus. In time, the parasitic cysts are replaced by nodules of fibrous, partly calcified material (Fig. 10a).

Hydatid disease is most frequent in sheep-rearing countries, in South America, Australia, New Zealand, the Mediterranean region and the Middle East [48, 153, 173]. In the UK, most cases occur in Wales and the Shetland Islands. The dog is the definitive host and acquires the infection by ingesting mutton containing viable hydatid cysts. The larval scolices attach to the intestinal wall, the worm matures and sheds ova in the faeces of the dog. The intermediate hosts are sheep or man, that eat the ova, from which the hatched embryos emerge, penetrate the intestinal mucosa and are disseminated through the blood stream to liver, lungs and other tissues (including the CNS). There, encystment occurs.

Hydatid disease is most common in children. CNS involvement usually manifests with focal neurological symptoms and signs but seizures or features of raised intracranial pressure may occur. Within the CNS, the cysts of *E. granulosus* are usually solitary, spherical and uniloculate, and are most often located within the cerebrum, in the perfusion territory of the middle cerebral artery. They contain clear fluid and a granular deposit of scolices ('hydatid sand'). The cyst wall has three layers: an outer adventitial layer (of host origin), a thick, laminated, PAS-positive cuticle and a thin inner germinal layer (Fig. 10b). Suckers and double rows of hooklets may be visible in the enclosed scolices. There is scant reaction around viable hydatid cysts, which may enlarge to a diameter of several centimetres. Dead cysts may provoke a granulomatous reaction with giant cells but the degree of inflammation is usually mild.

## 5 Encephalitis

There is usually perivascular and parenchymal inflammation in the brain tissue adjacent to brain abscesses and granulomas, and perivascular inflammation in the superficial cortex of patients with meningitis. However, in this section, the term encephalitis is used in a restricted sense, to describe diseases with more diffuse parenchymal brain inflammation. It should be noted that the pathological distinction between some forms of necrotising encephalitis covered in this section and some of the focal or multifocal inflammatory necrotic lesions described above is not always clear-cut. This is particularly so in patients with depressed immunity, in whom the inflammatory response and pattern of tissue damage may be atypical.

The terms panencephalitis or panmyelitis are used to describe diffuse inflammation affecting both grey and white matter in at least part of the brain or spinal cord. The terms polioencephalitis and poliomyelitis describe inflammation that is largely restricted to the grey matter of the brain and spinal cord. In this section, the label 'viral diseases of the white matter' is used in preference to leukoencephalitis because of the limited degree of inflammation in some of the viral infections in which there are selective white matter abnormalities, and the fact that none of the bacterial, fungal or parasitic infections causes this restricted distribution of disease.

## 5.1 Immunocompetent Adults and Children

### 5.1.1 Necrotising Panencephalitis or Panmyelitis

The commonest cause of sporadic necrotising encephalitis in children and adults is herpes simplex virus type 1 (HSV-1) [81, 194]. Patients present with fever, headache and confusion, and focal neurological signs of temporal and frontal lobe damage [86, 164, 195]. The focal signs can include dysphasia, hemiparesis, ataxia and focal seizures. The CSF usually shows a moderate lymphocytosis and focal temporal lobe abnormalities are demonstrable in CT scans, MR images and EEGs. Typically, autopsy reveals bilateral, asymmetrical haemorrhagic necrosis involving the anterior part of the temporal lobes (Fig. 11 a), the posterior inferior part of the frontal lobes, the insulae and cingulate gyri, and microscopy reveals a meningeal and perivascular infiltrate of lymphocytes, sheets of foamy macrophages (Fig. 11 b) and, at the edge of the regions of necrosis, eosinophilic nuclear and cytoplasmic viral inclusions [2, 48, 51, 102]. In early disease, however, the brain may simply have slightly swollen and congested temporal lobes or may even appear macroscopically normal, and microscopy may reveal no inclusions and little or no parenchymal inflammation. However, immunohistochemistry at this early stage discloses abundant viral antigen in the regions of predilection noted above. Viral antigen can be detected for about 3 weeks (Fig. 11 c) [50]. In patients dying some weeks after the onset of herpes encephalitis, affected parts of the brain may have become cavitated and atrophic [128].

Few of the other viral encephalitides that affect immunocompetent individuals are necrotising. Necrotic lesions occur in the dorsomedial pons and medulla of some children with poliovirus or enterovirus 71 infection [10, 103]; this was a prominent feature of the neurological involvement in recent Malaysian and Taiwanese epidemics of enterovirus 71 infection [74, 103] in which children developed myoclonus and acute cardiorespiratory collapse, the latter probably due to damage to the vasomotor centres in the brain stem. Occasionally, arbovirus encephalitides, Japanese encephalitis and tick-borne encephalitis in particular, are associated with parenchymal haemorrhage or necrosis [76, 115]. B virus (Herpesvirus simiae) is a very rare cause of human encephalomyelitis – the virus is endemic in certain Old World primates, particularly of the genus *Macaca*, that are used as laboratory animals or occasionally kept as pets – and when transmitted to

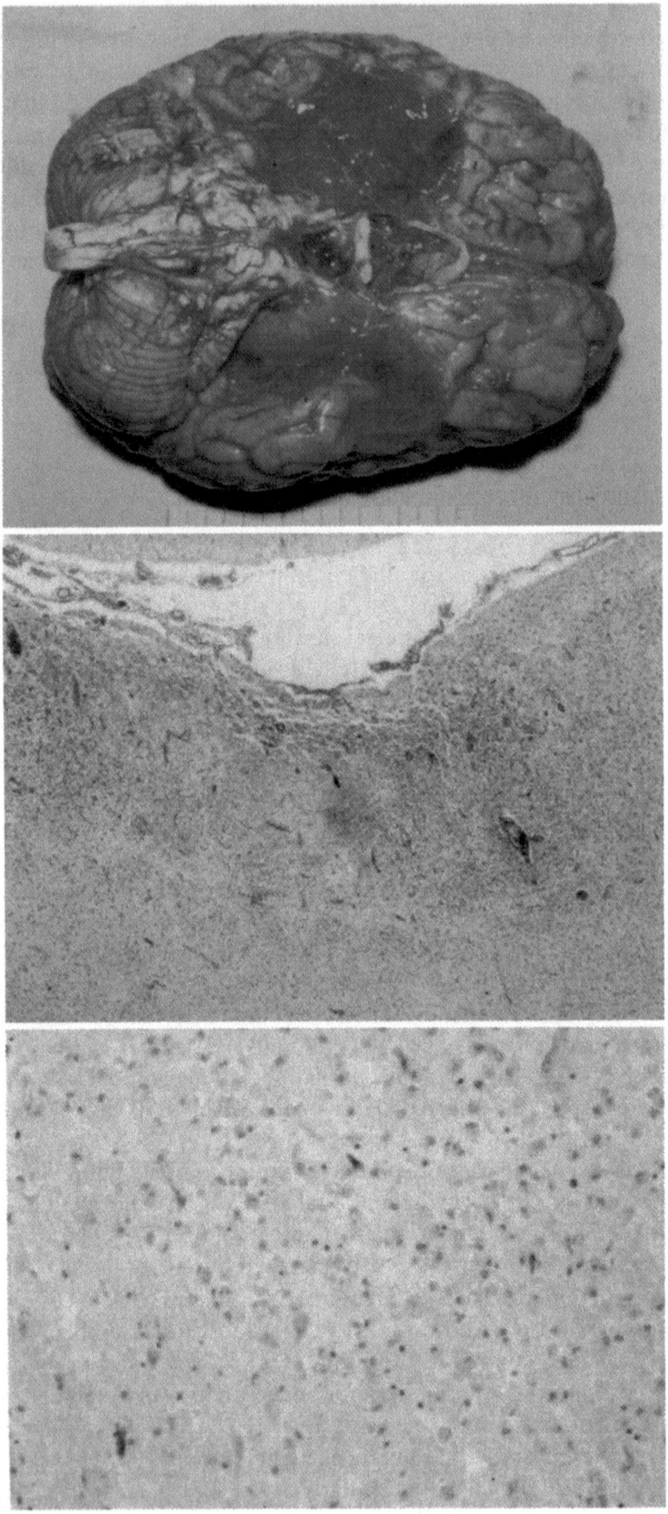

a b c

humans through bites or scratches can cause widespread necrotising panencephalomyelitis [25–27, 194].

A recent outbreak of encephalitis in Malaysia and Singapore was caused by a novel paramyxovirus, Nipah virus, probably transmitted to humans from pigs. Autopsy examination of three cases revealed vasculitis involving arterioles, capillaries and venules, with associated thrombosis and infarction, particularly in the CNS [37]. Eosinophilic inclusion bodies were present in neurons adjacent to vasculitic blood vessels.

Varicella-zoster virus (VZV) is a rare cause of CNS disease in immunocompetent individuals. Approximately 1 in 4,000 cases of chicken pox develops 'cerebellitis' – a short-lived, benign ataxic illness. Less-frequent complications of chicken pox include meningoencephalitis and post-infectious acute disseminated encephalomyelitis (see Sect. 6). A rare manifestation of VZV infection (some patients have concurrent ophthalmic zoster) is cerebral infarction due to vasculitis, usually involving the ipsilateral internal carotid artery or another major intracranial artery [48, 90]. Other CNS manifestations of VZV infection are largely restricted to patients with depressed cell-mediated immunity and are covered in Sect. 5.2.

The development of purulent brain abscesses is preceded by a 2–3 day period of focal cerebritis or cerebellitis that is poorly circumscribed macroscopically and may on microscopy cause confusion with necrotising encephalitides, although the restricted distribution of inflammation, its purulent nature and the presence of related pathology outside of the CNS (e.g. in the middle ear or lungs) should enable the correct diagnosis to be made. Early encapsulation is much better demonstrated by reticulin impregnation than with haematoxylin and eosin or trichrome stains.

Primary amoebic meningoencephalitis is an uncommon disorder caused by *Naegleria fowleri* [48, 109, 153]. This usually affects previously healthy children or adults, who acquire the infection whilst swimming or diving in fresh water. The amoebae spread to the CNS through the cribriform plate and cause a fulminant encephalitis with scanty inflammation but extensive haemorrhagic necrosis of the olfactory bulbs and tracts, the orbital region of the frontal lobes and the adjacent part of the temporal lobes, in a distribution resembling that of herpes encephalitis. Progression from the initial meningitic symptoms to coma and death takes 2–3 days. The motile amoebae are visible on examination of fresh CSF under a coverslip, with phase contrast or dark field illumination, or simply after lowering the sub-stage condenser [109]. In histological sections, the amoebae are clustered in perivascular spaces in and adjacent to the necrotic brain parenchyma. The nuclear staining in these regions may be poor and the amoebae are occasionally confused with macrophages. Unlike macrophages, however, the amoebae have a vesicular nucleus that contains a large central karyosome.

**Fig. 11a–c.** Herpes encephalitis. **a** Examination of the under-surface of the brain reveals bilateral haemorrhagic necrosis of the anterior and medial parts of the temporal lobes. Reproduced with permission, from [48]. **b** Section of temporal lobe, stained with luxol fast blue and cresyl violet. A dense infiltrate of inflammatory cells extends from the leptomeninges, through the cortex and into the white matter. **c** Two weeks after the start of the encephalitis, viral antigen is still immunohistochemically detectable in a few degenerate-looking neurons towards the edge of the inflammatory infiltrate

The CNS findings in cerebral malaria can include the presence of ring haemorrhages around necrotic small blood vessels. Apart from these lesions, however, necrosis is not a feature, and the disorder is considered more fully in Sect. 5.1.2.

The differential diagnosis of necrotising panencephalitis includes non-infective disorders, such as ischaemic and hypoxic lesions, vasculitides, drugs, toxins and metabolic disorders. Necrotising myelopathy may be a paraneoplastic manifestation of systemic carcinoma, although in some instances the myelopathy is probably due to reactivation of latent HSV-2 infection.

### 5.1.2 Non-necrotising Panencephalitis or Panmyelitis

Although necrosis of infected brain tissue is a characteristic feature of established herpes simplex encephalitis (Sect. 5.1.1, but see also Sect. 5.2), the brain may initially show only mild congestion and swelling of the temporal lobes, with scanty inflammation. Viral antigen is, however, usually abundant at this early stage so that the diagnosis can readily be made with the help of immunohistochemistry.

Several arboviruses (RNA viruses transmitted by mosquitoes, ticks or other arthropod vectors) can cause acute panencephalitis or encephalomyelitis [15, 23, 28, 38, 49, 57, 83, 92, 94, 96, 97, 114, 135, 140, 146, 172, 181, 193]. These have restricted geographical distributions that reflect those of the vectors and of the natural bird or animal hosts (Table 1). The clinical manifestations are relatively non-specific and include pyrexia, malaise, myalgias, headache, vomiting and focal neurological deficits. Japanese encephalitis (and rarely other arboviruses such as those of the tick-borne encephalitis complex) may cause a poliomyelitis- or polioencephalomyelitis-like illness with flaccid or spastic paralysis [96, 113, 115, 135, 167]. The arbovirus encephalitides are usually non-necrotising (although foci of necrosis or haemorrhage can occur, especially in Japanese encephalitis). The brain may be swollen and congested but more often appears macroscopically normal. Microscopy reveals perivascular and parenchymal infiltrates of chronic inflammatory

**Table 1.** Geographical distribution of the arboviruses that most often cause human encephalitis

| Arbovirus | Main geographical distribution |
|---|---|
| Eastern equine encephalitis virus | Eastern and Gulf coast states of USA, Caribbean, South America |
| Western equine encephalitis virus | Western and Midwestern USA |
| Venezuelan equine encephalitis virus | South and Central America, south-western USA |
| St. Louis encephalitis virus | Endemic throughout the Americas |
| Japanese encephalitis virus | South-East Asia |
| Murray Valley encephalitis virus | South-western Australia, New Guinea |
| Powassan encephalitis virus | Canada, northern USA, Russia |
| Russian spring-summer encephalitis virus | Russia, East Asia |
| La Crosse virus | Midwestern USA |
| Tahna virus | Czech Republic, Slovakia |
| Jamestown Canyon virus | North-western and central USA |

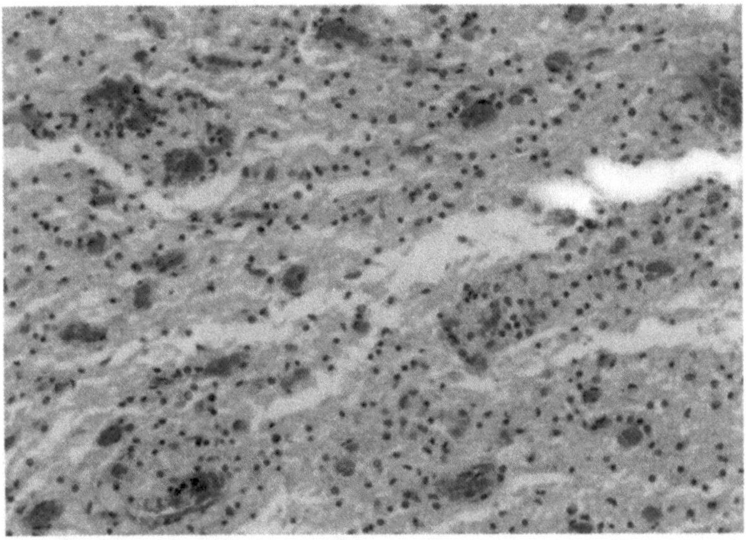

**Fig. 12.** Japanese encephalitis virus infection. Chronic perivascular and parenchymal inflammation in the cervical cord. Section courtesy of Prof. F. Scaravilli

cells in the grey and white matter with neuronophagia and microglial nodules (for further description of these see Sect. 5.1.3) [48, 51, 102]. The deep grey nuclei and brain stem tend to be most severely affected. Viral inclusions are not visible on light microscopy. Japanese encephalitis may cause severe inflammation of the grey matter in the brain stem and spinal cord (Fig. 12).

HIV is, of course, a major cause of immunosuppression but is itself an infection of individuals who are, for the most part, immunocompetent. Much of the CNS pathology in AIDS is secondary to immunosuppression and systemic disease, but some of the neuropathological abnormalities are directly attributable to HIV, which can cause several patterns of chronic encephalitis and a range of relatively subtle cognitive and motor deficits. In the absence of secondary abnormalities due to opportunistic infection or neoplasia, the brain often appears macroscopically normal although slicing after fixation may reveal ill-defined grey discolouration of the white matter. The white matter tends also to bear the brunt of obvious histological abnormalities, that can include, in various combinations, diffuse gliosis and poor staining of myelin, the changes of multinucleated giant cell encephalitis, and vacuolar myelopathy (see Sect. 5.1.4). However, patients may also develop, often in combination with other white matter abnormalities described in Sect. 5.1.4, a low-grade non-necrotising panencephalitis, with perivascular cuffing by lymphocytes and scattered microglial nodules (Fig. 13) [6, 13, 20, 21, 62, 163, 188]. The distinction between HIV encephalitis and opportunistic infection by cytomegalovirus (CMV), in particular, can be difficult and depends on the identification of typical HIV-related multinucleated giant cells or HIV antigen on the one hand, and cytomegalic inclusion cells or CMV antigen on the other. The two infections often co-exist.

Other viral causes of subacute or chronic panencephalitis or panmyelitis include measles virus, human T-cell lymphotropic virus type I (HTLV-I) and rubella.

a b c d e f

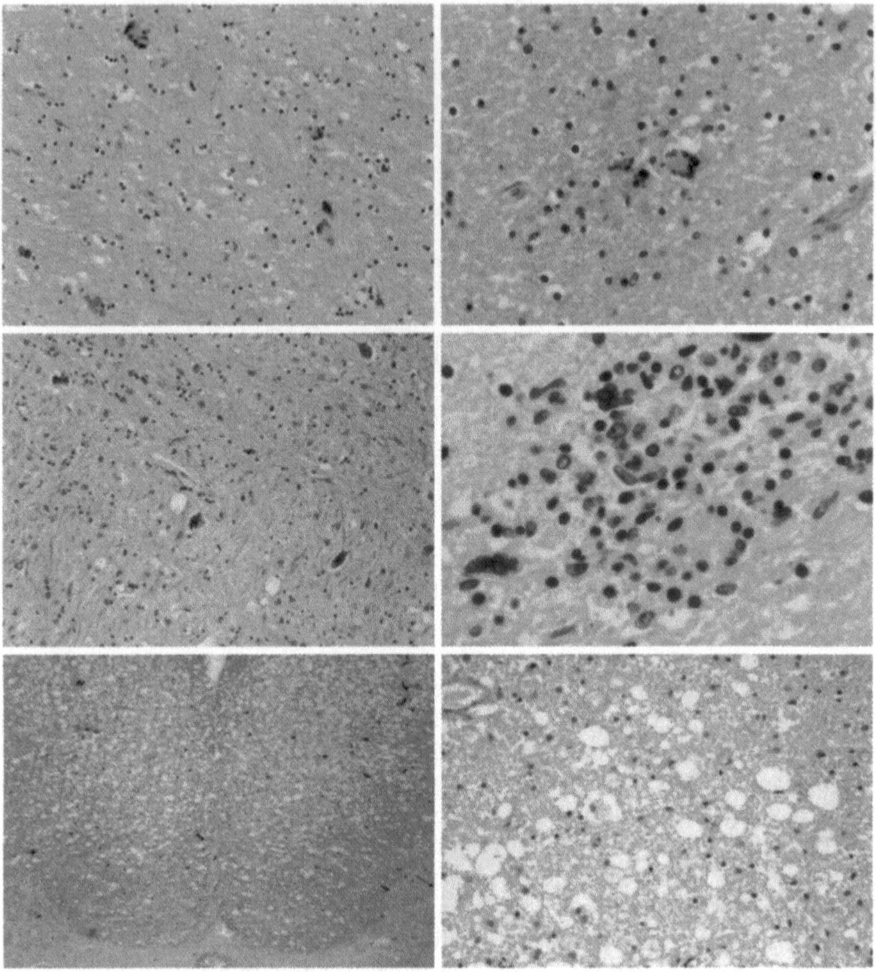

**Fig. 13 a–f.** HIV encephalitis and vacuolar myelopathy. Characteristic of HIV encephalitis is the presence of multinucleated giant cells, predominantly in the cerebral white matter (**a**, **b**) and deep grey nuclei (**c**). The white matter often appears hypercellular due to the presence of astrocytes and activated microglia. Microglial nodules may be present in the grey or white matter, and may include multinucleated giant cells (**d**). Vacuolar myelopathy is characterised by intramyelinic vacuolation and later degeneration of spinal white matter. The vacuolation affects the posterior columns (**e**), as illustrated in this section stained with solochrome cyanin, and the lateral columns. **f** Similar white matter vacuolation is occasionally seen in the cerebral hemispheres. **c** and **d** courtesy of Prof. C. A. Wiley

Between 0.4 and 9.7 per million infections of immunocompetent individuals with wild-type measles virus are complicated, several years later, by the development of subacute sclerosing panencephalitis (SSPE) [24, 53, 108, 117]. The disease usually presents between 5 and 15 years of age and is commoner in patients whose initial measles infection occurred before the age of two. The risk is reduced 10- to 20-fold by measles vaccination. Over a period of 6–12 months, patients progress from mild intellectual impairment and behavioural abnormalities through rapidly progressive dementia to eventual stupor, in which state patients may remain for several years, with occasional periods of apparent clinical improvement or stabilisation [79]. The stage of accelerated intellectual decline is usually associated with the development of motor disturbances - particularly of repetitive, symmetrical myoclonus. Fifty percent or more of patients develop visual disturbances due to a macular chorioretinitis. Neuropathological examination reveals a widespread, chronic panencephalitis (Fig. 14), with striking microglial hyperplasia, astrocytic gliosis, loss of neurons,

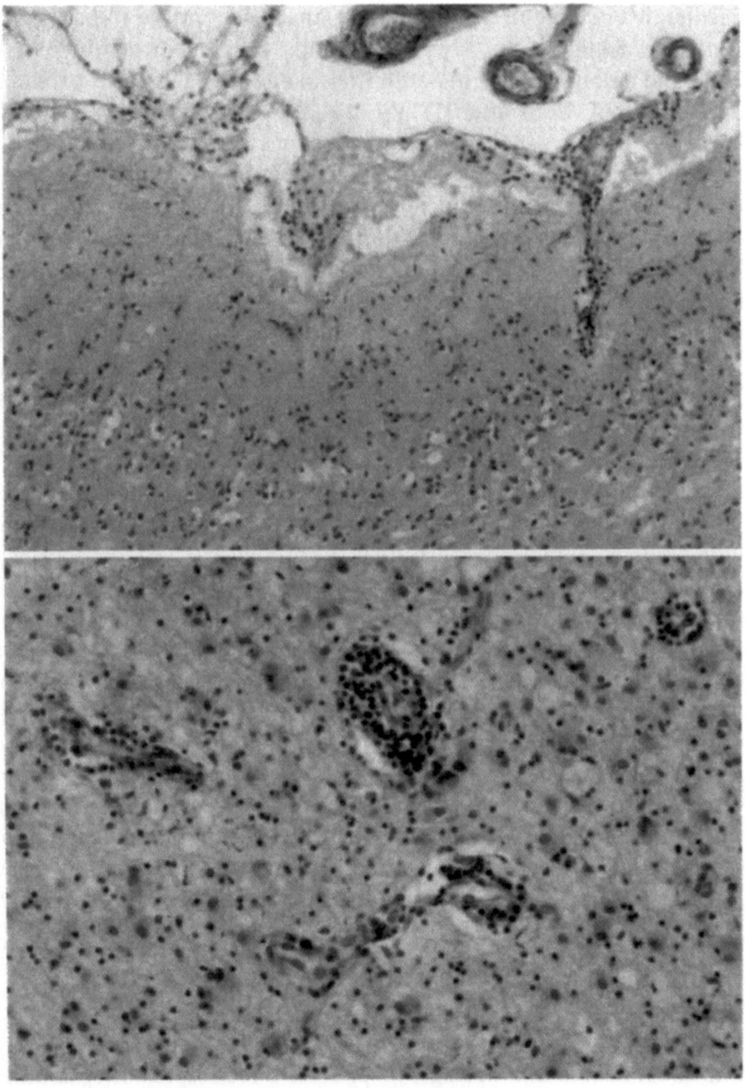

a

b

**Fig. 14a, b.** Subacute sclerosing panencephalitis. Sections of cerebral cortex (**a**) and white matter (**b**) illustrate the typical widespread inflammation, neuronal loss and gliosis occasional neuronophagia and, in most cases, sparse intranuclear inclusions, most readily detected immunohistochemically [48, 51]. In longer surviving patients, neurofibrillary tangles develop, in a distribution similar to that of tangles in Alzheimer's disease (i.e. involving the hippocampus and cerebral cortex, the nucleus basalis of Meynert, the hypothalamus and the brain stem raphe nuclei) [106, 107].

HTLV-I is responsible for several diseases, the most notable being adult T-cell leukaemia/lymphoma and tropical spastic paraparesis (TSP, also called HTLV-I-associated myelopathy or HAM). HTLV-I has also been associated with a range of other, mostly inflammatory, diseases including polymyositis, dermatomyositis and peripheral neuropathy [185, 190]. HTLV-I infection, which is transmitted through breast milk, sexual intercourse, blood transfusion or the sharing of contaminated needles, is endemic in south-western Japan, the Caribbean basin, parts of South America, Melanesia, the Seychelles Islands, parts of Africa (including clusters in Zaire and amongst Zulus in South Africa) and probably parts of India. The risk of developing HAM/TSP after HTLV-I infection is small – approximately 0.25% over a lifetime of 75 years [84]. The age of onset of HAM/TSP is very variable but ranges from 35 to 50 years in most cases. Patients develop progressive spastic paraparesis, usually associated with sphincter disturbances [8, 9, 118, 142]. Backache is common. Most patients are chair-bound within 10 years. At autopsy, the brain is largely spared. The spinal meninges may appear thickened and the cord atrophic, particularly in the lower thoracic region. Microscopy reveals an infiltrate of lymphocytes and macrophages in the spinal grey and white matter, especially in the lower thoracic region [48, 51, 77, 78, 102]. Small blood vessels in the spinal parenchyma usually have thickened, hyaline walls. Progression of disease leads to degeneration and gliosis of the long tracts in the spinal cord, the lateral columns being most severely involved.

The pathological findings in rubella encephalitis in the neonatal period are described in Sect. 5.3. Very rarely, congenital or early childhood rubella is complicated by the development, several years later, of a chronic panencephalitis [178–180]. A characteristic feature is the presence of periodic acid-Schiff-positive, mineralised material within and adjacent to the walls of blood vessels in the white matter of the cerebrum and cerebellum.

A bacterial cause of panencephalitis or panmyelitis is *Treponema pallidum*. Syphilitic disease of the CNS takes several forms, most of which occur during tertiary disease. These include meningovascular syphilis, general paresis and tabes dorsalis. The pathological features of meningovascular syphilis are discussed in Sect. 2.1.3. Both general paresis and tabes dorsalis are late manifestations of tertiary disease, occurring up to 20 years after the initial infection. Untreated general paresis causes insidiously progressive impairment of attention and cognition, psychiatric disturbances, seizures, motor dysfunction and incontinence. Autopsy reveals moderate brain atrophy, fibrotic meninges, scanty meningeal and parenchymal inflammation, gliosis and striking proliferation of rod-shaped microglia (Fig. 15a, b) [63,

**Fig. 15a–c.** General paresis of the insane (GPI) and tabes dorsalis: late tertiary manifestations of *T. pallidum* infection. **a** In GPI there is usually patchy perivascular and meningeal inflammation. **b** A characteristic finding is the presence of rod-shaped microglia, demonstrated here by Hortega silver impregnation. **c** Tabes dorsalis causes posterior column degeneration, particularly of the gracile funiculi (containing fibres originating from the lumbar dorsal root ganglia), as shown (*arrow*) in this Loyez-stained section of upper cervical cord

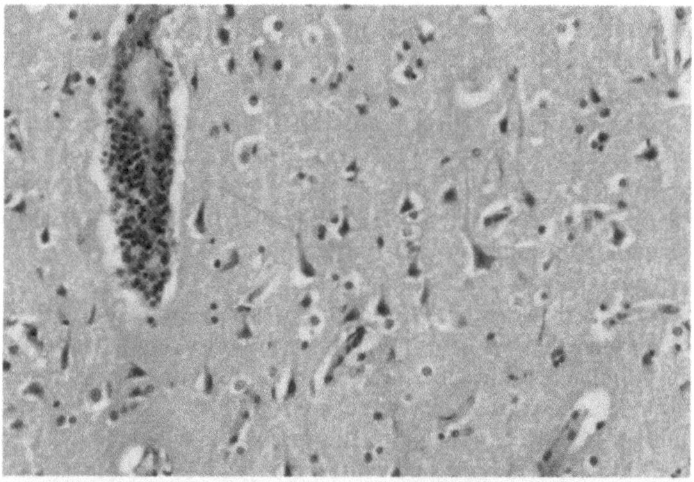

a

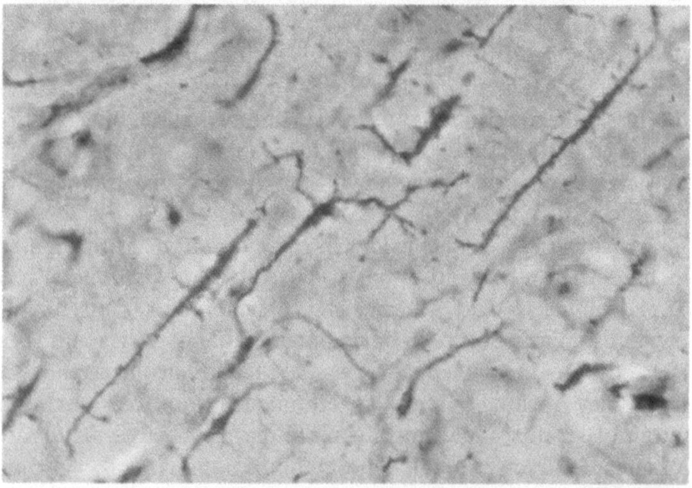

b

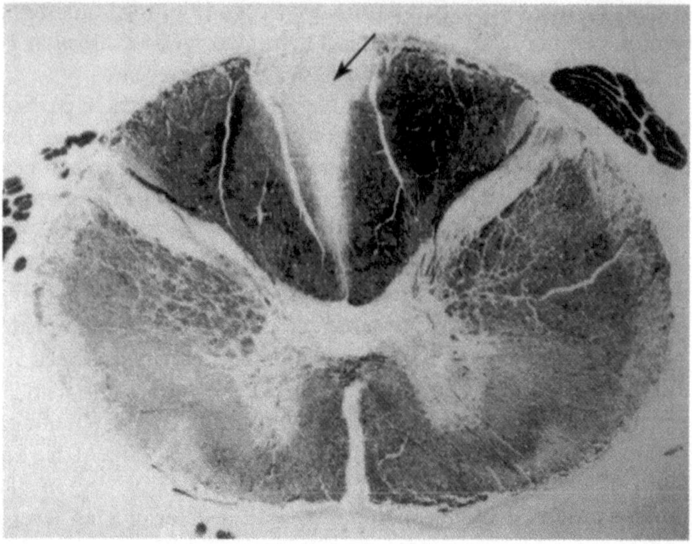

c

65]. Spirochaetes are rarely demonstrable. In tabes dorsalis, patients develop 'lightning pains', paraesthesiae and progressive loss of perception of pain and proprioception, predominantly in the lower limbs. Autopsy reveals fibrosis and mild inflammation of the spinal leptomeninges, dorsal root ganglion cell loss, proliferation of dorsal root ganglion satellite cells, the formation of nodules of Nageotte (clusters of dorsal root ganglion satellite cells, marking the sites of ganglion cell degeneration) and posterior column degeneration [63, 65] (Fig. 15c). The changes are most marked in the lumbar region of the cord.

Lyme disease, due to *Borrelia burgdorferi*, is another, rare, bacterial cause of chronic CNS disease with clinical features of encephalomyelitis. The scant available data from autopsy studies suggest that the extent of CNS inflammation is, however, very limited. Chronic perivascular inflammation and axonal degeneration have been demonstrated in peripheral nerves [175].

Rickettsial infections may cause perivascular lymphocytic cuffing and microglial nodules in the grey and white matter, with or without vascular thrombosis and haemorrhages [48]. Non-infective processes to consider in cases of non-necrotising panencephalitis or panmyelitis include reactive inflammation in relation to hypoxic, ischaemic or toxic brain damage; paraneoplastic encephalitis and myelitis, which predominantly affects the grey matter but can also involve the white matter and Rasmussen's encephalitis, an idiopathic disorder characterised by intractable epilepsy associated with progressive, predominantly unilateral chronic encephalitis.

Parasitic diseases to consider in cases of non-necrotising meningoencephalitis include African trypanosomiasis, caused by *Trypanosoma brucei rhodesiense* and *T. b. gambiense*, and American trypanosomiasis, caused by *T. cruzi*. African trypanosomiasis occurs in parts of sub-Saharan Africa and is transmitted by the tsetse fly. Meningoencephalitis is a late feature of the disease. Clinical manifestations may include lassitude, somnolence (or occasionally insomnia), extrapyramidal features (parkinsonism, chorea), psychiatric disturbances, paralysis and seizures. Histology reveals leptomeningeal, perivascular and parenchymal infiltration by mononuclear inflammatory cells (Fig. 16a), microglial activation, formation of microglial nodules and astrocytic gliosis. Morular cells (plasma cells containing clusters of Russell bodies) are characteristic.

American trypanosomiasis (Chagas disease) occurs in parts of South and Central America. The parasite is transmitted by the reduviid bug. Encephalitis may be a feature of the acute infection, and in cases coming to autopsy at this stage the brain contains scattered microglial nodules and amastigote forms of the parasite within glial cells (Fig. 16b) or at the centre of the nodules [31, 48, 153]. Encephalitis is not a prominent feature of chronic infection, in which complications of autonomic disease and destruction predominate (megaoesophagus, megacolon, cardiomyopathy). Reactivation of *T. cruzi* infection in immunosuppressed patients causes a multifocal necrotising encephalitis, described in Sect. 5.2.

Cerebral malaria complicates 1%–10% of infections with *Plasmodium falciparum*, transmitted by the *Anopheles* mosquito. This is a major cause of morbidity and mortality in tropical and subtropical parts of Asia, Africa and South America and can also affect travellers from or through those regions. Patients develop a rapidly progressive encephalopathy, with a deteriorating level of consciousness and seizures. On macroscopic examination, the brain may show no more than

a

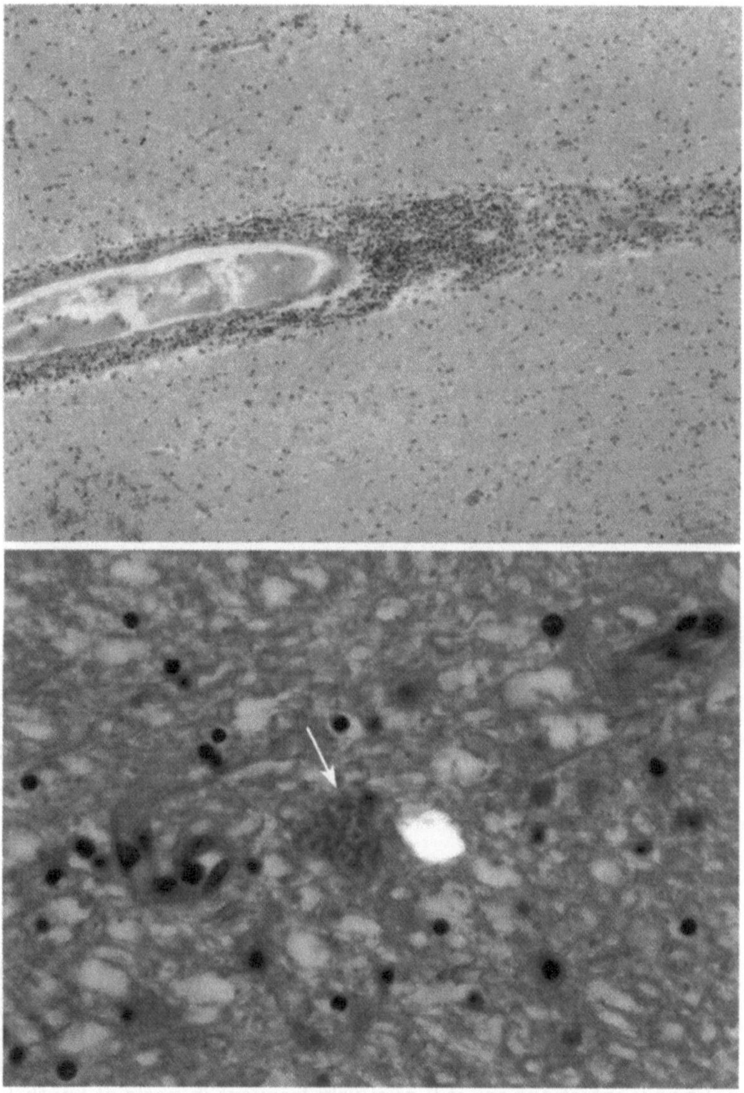

b

**Fig. 16a, b.** Trypanosomiasis. **a** Meningoencephalitis is a late feature of African trypanosomiasis and causes leptomeningeal, perivascular and parenchymal infiltration by mononuclear inflammatory cells. Courtesy of Prof. J.H. Adams. **b** Amastigote forms of *T. cruzi* within a glial cell (*arrow*) in acute Chagas disease (American trypanosomiasis). Reproduced with permission, from [48]

congestion and swelling but in most cases numerous petechial haemorrhages and scattered ring haemorrhages are visible, predominantly in the white matter [48, 153, 184]. Microscopy shows sequestration of red blood cells in engorged capillaries and venules. Within many of the red blood cells are malaria parasites or granules of malarial pigment. Petechial haemorrhages are most numerous in regions of sequestration [184]. The larger ring haemorrhages are centred on

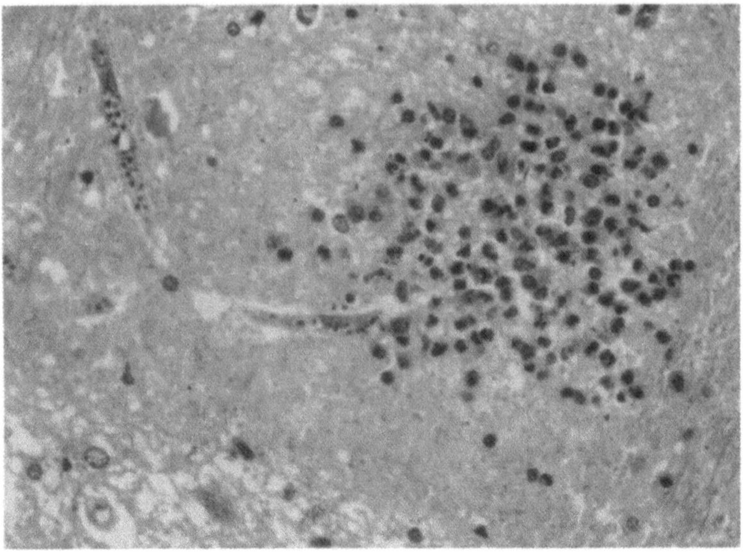

**Fig. 17.** Cerebral malaria. The section shows a Dürck granuloma adjacent to a capillary containing parasitised red blood cells and red cells with brown malarial pigment

necrotic blood vessels. Inflammation is usually very scanty. There may mononuclear inflammatory infiltrates in the leptomeninges and parenchyma and compact aggregates of neutrophils, lymphocytes, macrophages and astrocytes (Dürck granulomas) related to the resorption of ring haemorrhages (Fig. 17).

### 5.1.3 Polioencephalitis and Poliomyelitis

These terms refer to selective inflammation of the grey matter in the brain (polioencephalitis) or spinal cord (poliomyelitis). Most often responsible are viruses of the genus *Enterovirus*, which includes the polioviruses, group A and group B coxsackieviruses, echoviruses and enteroviruses [81, 122, 149]. Paralytic poliovirus infections are still relatively frequent in parts of South-East Asia and West Africa but in most parts of the world, because of the success of vaccination programmes, polioencephalitis and poliomyelitis are usually caused by the rare reversion to neurovirulence of attenuated vaccine-related strains of poliovirus or by other non-polio enteroviruses such as enteroviruses 70 and 71 (more frequently responsible for acute haemorrhagic conjunctivitis, and hand-foot-and-mouth disease or herpangina, respectively), echovirus 30 and several of the coxsackieviruses. Children and infants are much more susceptible than adults.

The illness associated with poliovirus and non-polio enteroviral encephalitis and myelitis is, typically, biphasic. The initial intestinal infection and primary viraemia are often accompanied by mild, non-specific symptoms such as sore throat, gastrointestinal upset, mild pyrexia and headache. Patients may also develop the typical cutaneous and mucosal lesions of hand-foot-and-mouth disease or herpangina. The development of paralysis is often heralded by muscle pain or stiffness. Bulbar involvement occurs in 10%–15% of patients (but a much higher proportion in recent epidemics of enterovirus 71 infection) and can cause myoclonus, cranial nerve palsies, cardiac arrhythmias and disturbances of respiration [74, 103].

Autopsy examination in the acute phase reveals a chronic inflammatory infiltrate in the affected regions of grey matter. The disease shows a predilection for the spinal grey matter, motor nuclei in the medulla and pons, reticular formation, deep cerebellar nuclei and primary motor cortex. Within the inflamed grey matter, lymphocytes and microglia tend to accumulate around dying neurons, a process termed neuronophagia (Fig. 18). The inflammation is not generally necrotising but as noted in Sect. 5.1.1, enterovirus 71 infection may produce destructive lesions with foci of cavitation in the brain stem. Clusters of microglia (microglial nodules) persist for days to weeks after the neurons have been phagocytosed. In long-term survivors of poliomyelitis, the affected regions of grey matter are usually severely depleted of neurons, with loss of nerve fibres from the anterior roots and atrophy of the corresponding muscles. There may be scanty residual inflammation.

Rabies has been eradicated from several island countries or states, including Britain, Ireland, Japan, Australia, New Zealand, Iceland and Hawaii, and is now uncommon in most other parts of the world, apart from Asia, where there are still approximately 35,000 deaths from rabies each year, most of those in India [201, 202]. In the majority of cases the disease is acquired through the bite of a rabid dog. In parts of Europe and North America, where government programs have largely eliminated stray dogs and vaccination has limited or eradicated rabies in domestic pets, wild animals are usually responsible for transmitting the disease – bats, rac-

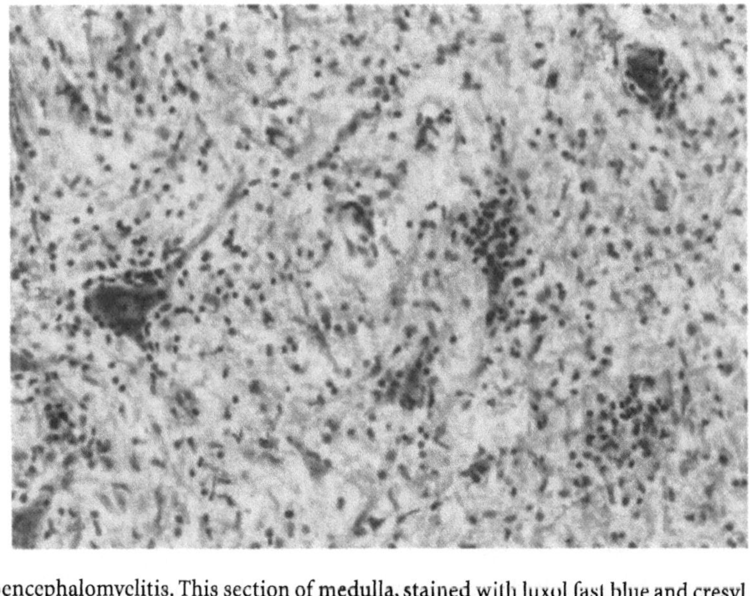

**Fig. 18.** Polioencephalomyelitis. This section of medulla, stained with luxol fast blue and cresyl violet, illustrates neuronophagia – the dense accumulation of lymphocytes and microglia around dying motor neurons

coons, skunks and coyotes (in North America), foxes (particularly in Europe but also in parts of North America, Africa and the Middle East), wolves (in Asia and parts of Europe), jackals (in Africa) and mongooses (in Africa and parts of Asia). The latent period is usually 30–90 days, but can range from only a few days to over 1 year [70, 121, 182]. After a prodromal period of 'flu-like symptoms, lasting several days, the acute neurological disease usually takes the form of 'furious' (encephalitic) rabies, characterised by insomnia, agitation and aggressive behaviour (which can include biting), hypersalivation, pupillary dilatation, piloerection, hallucinations, hydrophobia, dysphagia, dysarthria and nystagmus. A small proportion of patients develops 'dumb' (paralytic) rabies, which can include paralysis of one or more limbs, or ascending paralysis simulating Guillain-Barré syndrome. The two forms of rabies may overlap. Terminal manifestations include inappropriate ADH secretion, diabetes insipidus, haematemesis, cardiac and respiratory failure. Death usually occurs within 1–2 weeks.

In rabies, the brain and spinal cord usually appear macroscopically normal. The histological features are of a polioencephalomyelitis that predominantly affects the hippocampus, medial temporal neocortex and cerebellum, but can involve the spinal cord, brain stem and other parts of the cerebral cortex [70, 121, 182]. Infected neurons may contain distinctive eosinophilic cytoplasmic inclusions bodies (Negri bodies) (Fig. 19). There is usually evidence of neuronophagia, but inflammation may be very scanty. In the late stages of disease, the virus spreads centrifugally to peripheral tissues and can be identified antemortem in corneal cells and cutaneous nerve fibres.

Detailed assessment of the cerebral grey matter in patients with HIV infection may reveal mild, diffuse gliosis and microglial activation – a pattern of disease clas-

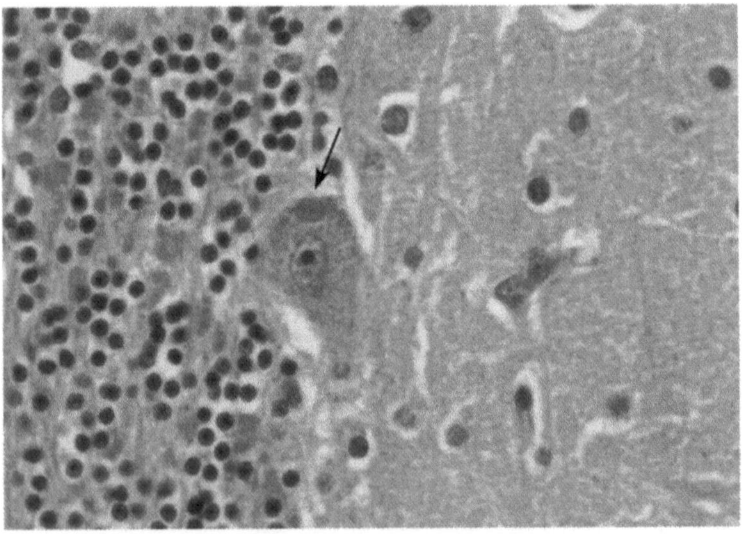

**Fig. 19.** Rabies. The Purkinje cell contains a Negri body (*arrow*) – a well-circumscribed, eosinophilic, cytoplasmic inclusion. Note the lack of adjacent inflammation. Courtesy of Prof. L. Chimelli

sified as diffuse poliodystrophy [21]. The changes may occasionally be marked and associated with obvious neuronal loss and cerebral atrophy. Multinucleated giant cells and other HIV-infected cells may or may not be present in the affected grey matter.

Rarely, arboviral infection, particularly that caused by Japanese encephalitis virus or the tick-borne encephalitis complex, can cause paralytic polioencephalomyelitis. Neuropathological examination in these cases shows severe inflammation of the grey matter in the brain stem and spinal cord. The pathological findings in arboviral encephalitides are considered in more detail in Sect. 5.1.2.

### 5.1.4 Viral Disease of the White Matter

Progressive multifocal leukoencephalopathy (PML), caused by a papovavirus, JC virus, is usually a disease of patients with depressed cell-mediated immunity and is considered in Sect. 5.2. HIV infection, a cause of depressed cell-mediated immunity (and an infection that therefore predisposes to PML) can itself cause several patterns of white matter disease. These include multinucleated giant cell encephalitis (see also Sect. 5.1.2), vacuolar myelopathy, cerebral leukoencephalopathy and necrotising leukoencephalopathy [20, 21, 62, 89, 156, 158, 188].

Vacuolar myelopathy, affects up to 25% of patients with AIDS and causes spastic paraparesis, ataxia and incontinence. Autopsy examination of the spinal cord reveals vacuolation of spinal white matter in the posterior and lateral spinal columns (Fig. 13e). This leads to breakdown of myelin and degeneration of axons. These changes are not specifically associated with productive HIV infection in the affected parts of the cord, and so giant cells and viral antigen are not usually demonstrable. The pathological findings resemble those of subacute combined degeneration due to vitamin $B_{12}$ deficiency. The cerebral leukoencephalopathy of HIV infection is characterised by diffuse gliosis and pallor of myelin staining, with or without associated giant cell encephalitis. Less commonly, the cerebral white matter may show vacuolation similar to that in vacuolar myelopathy (Fig. 13f). Necrotising leukoencephalopathy is a rare manifestation of AIDS; the cerebral white matter shows patchy necrosis, reactive gliosis and dystrophic calcification.

The differential diagnosis of diffuse or necrotising leukoencephalopathy is wide and includes ischaemia, hypoxia, previous CO, cyanide or methanol poisoning, drug toxicity and X-irradiation. Several mitochondrial disorders cause white matter lesions. These are characterised by intramyelinic vacuolation or by gliosis and cavitation; calcification of blood vessels may be a prominent feature.

## 5.2 Immunosuppressed Patients

Immunosuppression does not increase the risk of developing herpes encephalitis but does predispose to atypical forms of the disease, most cases of which have been reported in patients with AIDS [33, 35, 41, 55, 67, 123, 127, 145]. The encephalitis may involve a site other than the temporal or frontal lobes, usually the brain stem, and is often more slowly progressive than classical herpes encephalitis, with little or no necrosis and persistence of viral antigen as well as DNA.

Patients with depressed cell-mediated immunity, most often due to AIDS, are at increased risk of CNS infection by two other viruses in the family Herpesviridae: varicella-zoster virus (VZV) and cytomegalovirus (CMV). VZV can cause several patterns of disease in the CNS, with lesions involving the cerebral white matter,

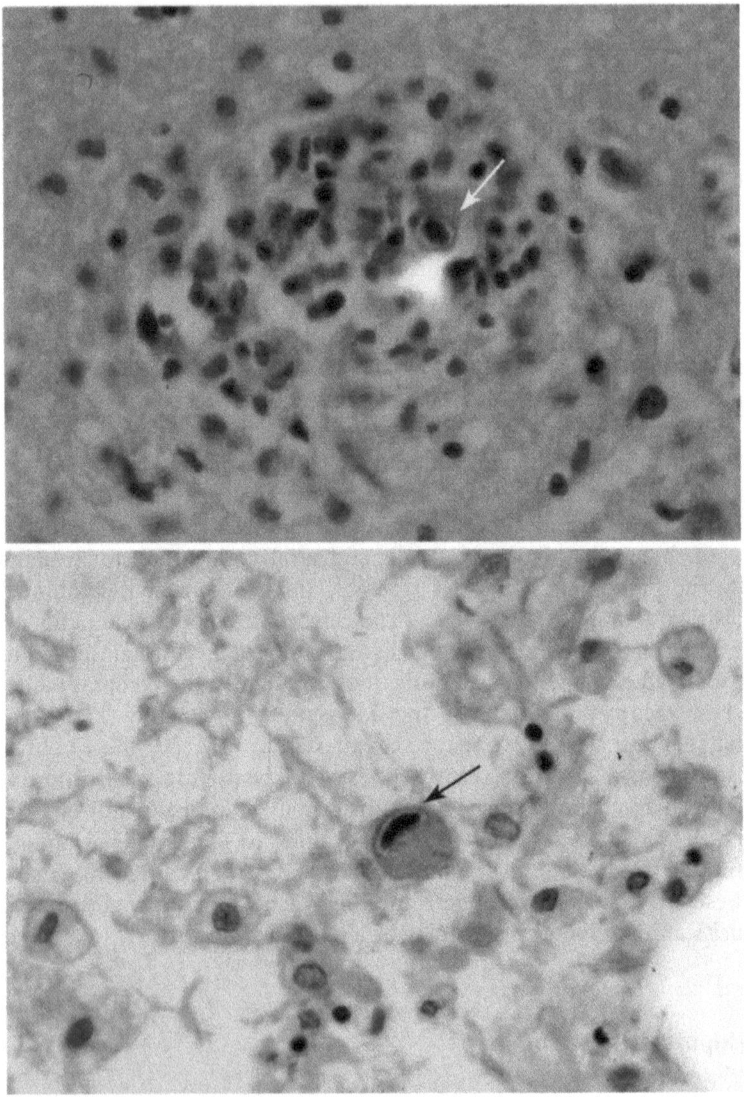

a

b

**Fig. 20 a, b.** Cytomegalovirus infection in patients with AIDS. **a** Microglial nodule encephalitis. Note the central cytomegalic inclusion cell (*arrow*). Courtesy of Prof. C. A. Wiley. **b** Necrotising periventricular infection. The figure includes scattered foamy macrophages and a cytomegalic inclusion cell (*arrow*) optic pathways, periventricular regions, brain stem or spinal cord [34, 36, 64, 120]. In all cases, the lesions are associated with a perivascular and parenchymal infiltrate of lymphocytes and macrophages, and are usually partly necrotic. Blood vessels may show changes of necrotising vasculitis. Well-circumscribed, eosinophilic, intranuclear inclusions are often visible in neurons and glia, and viral antigen can be demonstrated immunohistochemically.

CMV infection of the CNS is a relatively frequent complication of AIDS (Fig. 20) [62, 188]. Most often, this takes the form of a low-grade encephalitis with scattered microglial nodules. Cytomegalic inclusion cells may or may not be present within the nodules and may also occur without adjacent inflammation. Other patterns of involvement include (1) ventriculo-encephalitis, in which there is necrotising periventricular inflammation, (2) large necrotising parenchymal lesions, and (3) myeloradiculitis, which may be associated with microvascular infection and thrombosis within the affected nerve roots [5, 12, 62, 161, 188].

Rarely, adenovirus infection causes an acute necrotising encephalitis [7, 32, 42]. Most reported cases have been in children with immunosuppression (due to bone marrow transplantation or AIDS).

Immunosuppressed patients are susceptible to several other, subacute or chronic forms of viral encephalitis. The most common of these is progressive multifocal leukoencephalopathy (PML). Others include a subacute form of measles encephalitis (measles inclusion body encephalitis) and chronic enteroviral meningoencephalomyelitis. As noted above, immunosuppressed patients may also develop atypical, subacute forms of HSV encephalitis.

PML is caused by a papovavirus, JC virus. This is almost exclusively a disease of patients with depressed cell-mediated immunity, due to AIDS, organ transplantation, leukaemia or lymphoma [66, 81, 151, 157, 196]. The presenting neurological features vary according to the site of the lesions, which are usually asymmetrical and most often involve the cerebral white matter, although the cerebellum, deep grey nuclei, brain stem and even, occasionally, spinal cord can be affected. The disease is usually progressive and fatal within a few months, although remissions have been reported in patients whose underlying cause of immunosuppression has been effectively treated, including AIDS patients receiving combinations of antiretroviral drugs. Macroscopic examination of the fixed, sliced brain reveals multiple small or confluent foci of grey discolouration in affected regions (Fig. 21 a). The abnormal white matter may appear pitted or gelatinous (Fig. 21 b). Microscopy shows loss of myelin and relative preservation of axons within these foci (Fig. 21 c, d). There may be considerable loss of axons or even central cavitation in the larger lesions. Foamy macrophages are usually present in large numbers but lymphocytes very sparse. Intranuclear inclusions tend to be most prominent in oligodendrocytes at the edge of the lesions (Fig. 21 e, f). The affected oligodendrocytes have enlarged nuclei filled with homogeneous amphophilic material. The lesions may include large astrocytes with pleomorphic hyperchromatic nuclei (Fig. 21 d, f). These cells resemble those in glioblastomas, but only rarely contain mitotic figures and are not neoplastic.

Measles inclusion-body encephalitis is an uncommon complication of immunosuppression [4, 75, 144]. Patients present with increasing confusion, seizures and various focal neurological deficits weeks or months after having made a good clinical recovery from the acute exanthem. The disease is usually fatal within a few

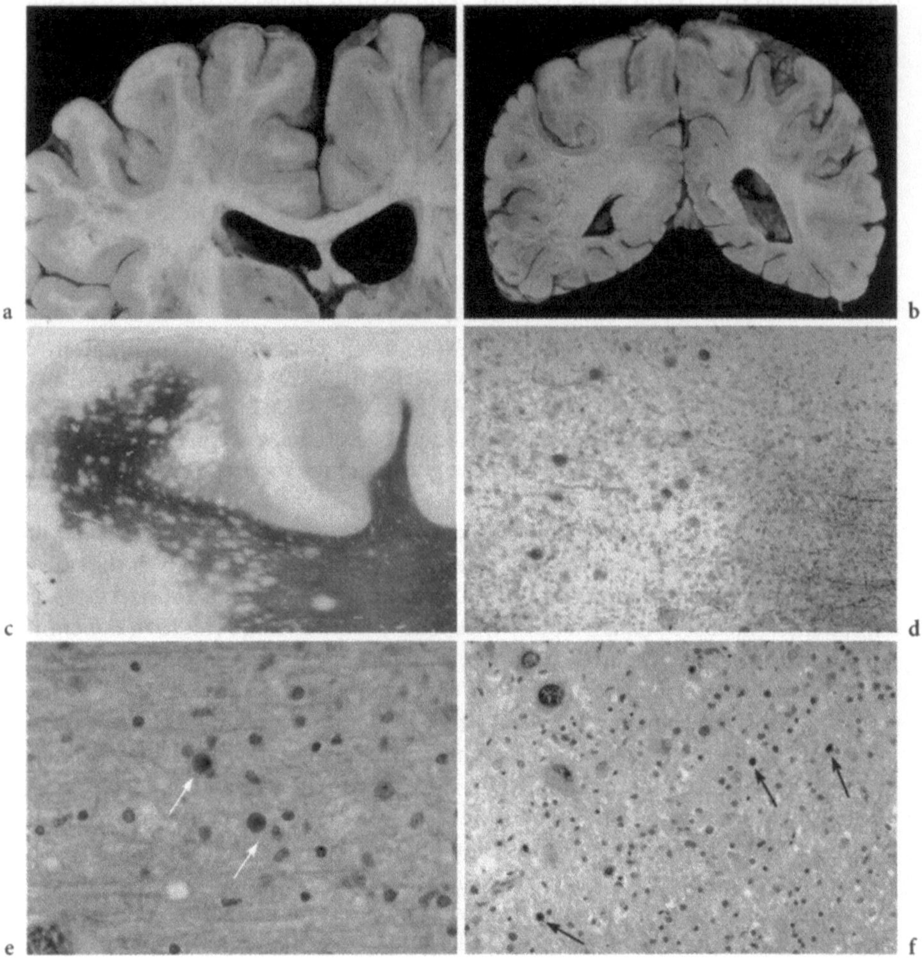


**Fig. 21 a–f.** Progressive multifocal leukoencephalopathy (PML). **a** Multiple small foci of slight grey or brown discolouration are visible in the cortical ribbon and white matter, particularly in the left frontal lobe. **b** Confluent lesions in the left parietal lobe give the white matter a pitted appearance. The loss of myelin is apparent at low magnification in **c** and higher magnification in **d**, in sections stained for myelin with luxol fast blue and cresyl violet. **d** also shows the numerous foamy macrophages and large, pleomorphic astrocytes that are usually present in the lesions of PML. **e** Infected oligodendrocytes (*arrows*) have enlarged nuclei containing homogeneous, amphophilic material. **f** Section through part of a focus of demyelination. The pleomorphic astrocytes are within the zone of demyelination (towards the *left* of the figure) and the inclusion-bearing oligodendrocytes (*arrows*) predominantly at the edge of the lesion

weeks. Neuropathological examination reveals scattered foci of hypercellularity, with reactive astrocytes and microglia, sparse lymphocytes and occasional multinucleated cells. Within these foci, many of the neurons and some of the astrocytes and oligodendrocytes contain large, eosinophilic inclusion bodies (Fig. 22). Abundant measles viral antigen can be demonstrated immunohistochemically.

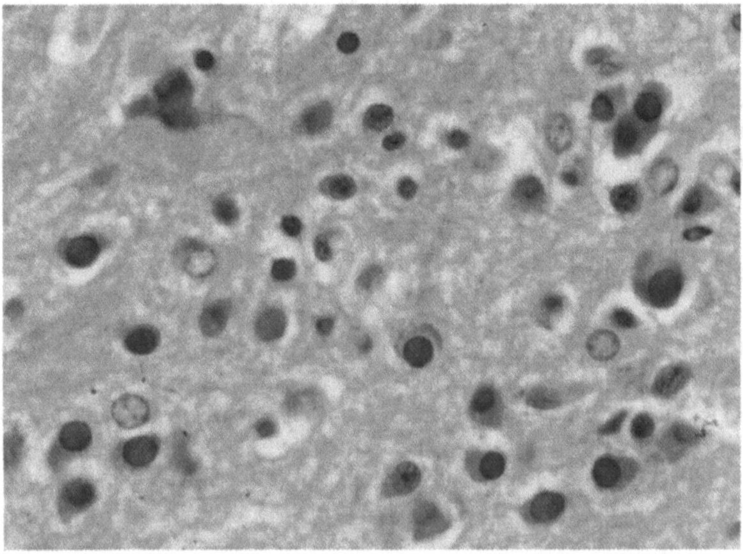

**Fig. 22.** Measles inclusion body encephalitis. Focus of hypercellularity in the cerebral cortex within which several neurons, astrocytes and oligodendrocytes, contain eosinophilic nuclear inclusions. Eosinophilic inclusion material is also present in the cytoplasm of some of the cells

Patients with X-linked agammaglobulinaemia or combined variable immunodeficiency occasionally develop a chronic enteroviral meningoencephalitis, often in association with dermatomyositis or other manifestations of chronic enteroviral infection [104, 110, 116, 150, 197]. Echovirus is most often responsible. The presentation is usually insidious and the progression variable. Encephalopathic or myelopathic features may predominate. Histology reveals a patchy, non-necrotising, chronic meningoencephalitis with infiltration by lymphocytes and macrophages, the formation of microglial nodules, and variable neuronal loss and gliosis.

Immunosuppression predisposes to several fungal infections of the CNS. Most of these cause meningitis, abscesses or granulomas rather than more diffuse parenchymal disease, and are discussed in Sects. 2.2 and 3.2. In some patients with fungal infection, the inflammation is widespread and diffuse, and histology may not reveal typical abscesses or granulomatous inflammation. The possibility of *Candida* infection, in particular, should always be considered in immunosuppressed patients with patchy encephalitis of uncertain aetiology.

Some of the parasitic diseases described in Sect. 3.2 may produce quite diffuse parenchymal CNS disease and should be included in the differential diagnosis of necrotising encephalitis in an immunosuppressed patient. Toxoplasmosis usually causes discrete space-occupying lesions in immunosuppressed patients, as previously noted. However, the lesions may be small and numerous, with scattered microglial nodules, resembling those of viral infections. Two other parasitic encephalitides that occur predominantly in patients who are immunosuppressed and can produce quite extensive parenchymal inflammation and necrosis are granulomatous amoebic encephalitis, and necrotising encephalitis due to *Trypanosoma cruzi*. Granulomatous amoebic encephalitis is due to *Acanthamoeba* species or *Balamuthia mandrillaris* [109]. Microscopy shows necrotising inflammation that is usually granulomatous. The lesions tend to be related to arteries and veins around which are large numbers of *Acanthamoeba* or *Balamuthia* trophozoites and cysts. Reactivation of *T. cruzi* infection in immunosuppressed patients may result in the development of multifocal granulomatous or necrotising cerebral lesions that contain numerous intracellular amastigote parasites [31, 48].

### 5.3 Neonates

Enterovirus infection in neonates can cause severe, multi-organ disease [1, 116]. The CNS lesions consist of clusters of lymphocytes and microglia, predominantly in the grey matter, but white matter may also be involved. Some lesions show focal haemorrhage or necrosis. There are no viral inclusions. The inflammation is usually most marked in the brain stem and spinal cord but lesions may be scattered throughout the cerebellum and cerebrum.

The pattern of HSV infection in neonates differs from that in older age groups. Most cases are due to HSV-2 and are acquired during delivery, as a result of contact of the foetus with infected maternal genital lesions. A small proportion of neonatal infections, mostly with HSV-1, is acquired postnatally. Approximately 45 % of infected neonates develop lesions of the skin, eyes and mouth but not encephalitis. Some of the remaining 55 % or so develop haematogenously disseminated infection, with encephalitis, hepatitis, pneumonitis and other organ involvement. Others develop an isolated encephalitis, initially involving the temporal lobes in a distribution resembling that in older age groups. However, by the time of autopsy, the lesions in all cases of neonatal herpes encephalitis tend to be widespread, with extensive foci of necrotising panencephalitis in the cerebrum, cerebellum and brain stem. Nuclear inclusions, viral antigen and DNA are abundant during the first few days of infection. Long-term survivors may show changes of cystic encephalomalacia.

## 6 Acute Disseminated Encephalomyelitis

Acute disseminated encephalomyelitis (ADEM) is a multifocal inflammatory disorder of the CNS, often preceded by viral, mycoplasma or bacterial infection or, much less commonly, by vaccination [48, 81, 102]. ADEM is believed to be due to a T-cell-mediated hypersensitivity reaction. Measles, mumps and mycoplasma pneumonia are the most commonly identified antecedent infections but the specific cause of the preceding illness is often not determined. The interval between this and the development of encephalitis ranges from a few days to about 3 weeks. Patients present with headache, vomiting and low-grade pyrexia, and may develop a range of neurological abnormalities including ataxia, weakness, sensory loss and visual impairment. Over the subsequent weeks, most patients make a good recovery, but some die during the acute illness or are left with persistent neurological deficits. Neuropathological examination of cases coming to autopsy reveals multifocal, lymphocytic perivenular inflammation and demyelination. In addition to demyelination, there is usually some loss of axons. Most of the lesions are in the white matter. Their distribution within the cerebrum, cerebellum and brain stem is often approximately symmetrical but can be markedly asymmetrical in some cases.

## 7 Taking Specimens for Microbiological Investigation

### 7.1 Cerebrospinal Fluid

The simplest way to obtain an uncontaminated specimen for bacterial or fungal culture is to reflect the dura with the brain in situ, gently part the cerebral hemispheres and insert the needle of a sterile syringe about 30° to the vertical through the corpus callosum and into the lateral ventricle. Slight negative pressure should then be applied to the plunger of the syringe whilst slowly withdrawing the needle. When the tip of the needle enters the lateral ventricle, the fluid will be drawn into the syringe. CSF can also be obtained from the interpeduncular cistern or, after removing the brain, from the cisterna magna, but it is more difficult to obtain reasonably large samples of CSF that are free of contamination from these sites. In addition, swabs should be taken from the subarachnoid space, particularly in the region of any exudates – to do so use fine forceps to elevate the leptomeninges, make a small cut into the meninges with a sterile blade and insert the swab into the subarachnoid space.

If viral infection is suspected, samples of CSF, brain (see below) and serum or clotted blood should be frozen, ideally at –70 °C. The frozen samples can later be used for viral culture, PCR studies and serology, as needed.

In suspected primary amoebic meningoencephalitis, swabs of CSF should be sent together with brain tissue to an appropriate laboratory for culture (see also below).

### 7.2 Abscess or Empyema

In most cases, the nature of the infection will not be in doubt. However, if identification of the responsible micro-organisms is needed, the purulent material should be cultured, in which case it should be aspirated into a sterile syringe, expelled into a sterile universal container and taken to a microbiology laboratory with as little delay as possible. The likelihood of recovering the responsible microorganisms is greater if the contents of the abscess are aspirated than if only swabs are taken.

### 7.3 Brain or Spinal Tissue

Samples of abnormal tissue for bacterial or fungal culture should be removed with a sterile scalpel, placed in a sterile universal container and taken to a microbiology laboratory as soon as possible.

In suspected viral infection, several small blocks of tissue (1–2 g is ample) should be taken from regions showing macroscopic abnormalities and, together with samples of CSF and serum or clotted blood (see above), frozen at –70 °C for later culture or polymerase chain reaction (PCR) studies. The regions sampled in suspected herpes encephalitis should include the anterior part of the temporal lobes and the inferior part of the frontal lobes. Occasionally, it may be appropriate to divide the brain mid-sagittally to sample deep structures for virological studies.

The diagnosis of most parasitic diseases of the CNS can usually be achieved by a combination of serological studies, and morphological and immunohistochemical examination of the parasites or their ova in paraffin sections. The identification of *Naegleria fowleri* may be facilitated by culture of CSF and brain tissue; the swabs and tissue should be transported to an appropriate laboratory as soon as possible, should not be refrigerated prior to transport to and should kept moist by the addition of sterile water, if needed, and not saline, to which the amoebae are highly sensitive. *Acanthamoebae* species and *Balamuthia mandrillaris* are rarely recoverable from CSF but can be cultured from infected brain tissue (although *Balamuthia mandrillaris* does not grow on agar plates but only on cell monolayers).

## References

1. Abzug MJ, Keyserling HL, Lee ML, Levin MJ, Rotbart HA (1995) Neonatal enterovirus infection: virology, serology, and effects of intravenous immune globulin. Clin Infect Dis 20:1201–1206
2. Adams JH, Miller D (1973) Herpes simplex encephalitis: a clinical and pathological analysis of twenty-two cases. Postgrad Med J 49:393–397
3. Adams M, Rhyner PA, Day J, DeArmond S, Smuckler EA (1987) Whipple's disease confined to the central nervous system. Ann Neurol 21:104–108
4. Alcardi J, Goutieres F, Arsenio-Nunes ML, Lebon P (1977) Acute measles encephalitis in children with immunosuppression. Pediatrics 59:232–239
5. Anders HJ, Goebel FD (1999) Neurological manifestations of cytomegalovirus infection in the acquired immunodeficiency syndrome. Int J STD AIDS 10:151–159
6. Anders K, Steinsapir KD, Iverson DJ, Glasgow BJ, Layfield LJ, Brown WJ, Cancilla PA, Verity MA, Vinters HV (1986) Neuropathologic findings in the acquired immunodeficiency syndrome (AIDS). Clin Neuropathol 5:1–20
7. Anders KH, Park CS, Cornford ME, Vinters HV (1990) Adenovirus encephalitis and widespread ependymitis in a child with AIDS. Ped Neurosurg 16:316–320
8. Araujo AdQ, Alfonso CR, Schor D, Leite AC, de Andrada-Serpa MJ (1993) Clinical and demographic features of HTLV-1 associated myelopathy/tropical spastic paraparesis (HAM/TSP) in Rio de Janeiro, Brazil. Acta Neurol Scand 88:59–62
9. Araujo AQ, Leite AC, Dultra SV, Andrada-Serpa MJ (1995) Progression of neurological disability in HTLV-I-associated myelopathy/tropical spastic paraparesis (HAM/TSP). J Neurol Sci 129:147–151
10. Baker AB (1957) Poliomyelitis: a study of pulmonary edema. Neurology 7:743–751
11. Banuelos AF, Williams PL, Johnson RH, Bibi S, Fredricks DN, Gilroy SA, Bhatti SU, Aguet J, Stevens DA (1996) Central nervous system abscesses due to Coccidioides species. Clin Infect Dis 22:240–250
12. Baudrimont M, Moulignier A (1997) Nervous system lesions due to cytomegalovirus in AIDS. Arch Anat Cytol Pathol 45:135–141
13. Bell JE (1998) The neuropathology of adult HIV infection. Rev Neurol 154:816–829
14. Berger JR (1991) Neurosyphilis in human immunodeficiency virus type 1-seropositive individuals. A prospective study. Arch Neurol 48:700–702

15. Bia FJ, Thornton GF, Main AJ, Fong CK, Hsiung GD (1980) Western equine encephalitis mimicking herpes simplex encephalitis. JAMA 244:367–369
16. Boon AP, Adams DH, Buckels J, McMaster P (1990) Cerebral aspergillosis in liver transplantation. J Clin Pathol 43:114–118
17. Bordon J, Martinez-Vazquez C, Alvarez M, Miralles C, Ocampo A, de la Fuente-Aguado J, Sopena-Perez Arguelles B (1995) Neurosyphilis in HIV-infected patients. Eur J Clin Microbiol Infect Dis 14:864–869
18. Bradsher RW (1988) Systemic fungal infections: diagnosis and treatment. I. Blastomycosis. Infect Dis Clin N Am 2:877–898
19. Brook I (1995) Brain abscess in children: microbiology and management. J Child Neurol 10:283–288
20. Budka H, Costanzi G, Cristina S, Lechi A, Parravicini C, Trabattoni R, Vago L (1987) Brain pathology induced by infection with the human immunodeficiency virus (HIV). A histological, immunocytochemical, and electron microscopical study of 100 autopsy cases. Acta Neuropathol 75:185–198
21. Budka H, Wiley CA, Kleihues P, Artigas J, Asbury AK, Cho ES, Cornblath DR, Dal Canto MC, DeGirolami U, Dickson D et al. (1991) HIV-associated disease of the nervous system: review of nomenclature and proposal for neuropathology-based terminology. Brain Pathol 1:143–152
22. Burman LA, Norrby R, Trollfors B (1985) Invasive pneumococcal infections: incidence, predisposing factors, and prognosis. Rev Infect Dis 7:133–142
23. Burrow JN, Whelan PI, Kilburn CJ, Fisher DA, Currie BJ, Smith DW (1998) Australian encephalitis in the Northern Territory: clinical and epidemiological features, 1987–1996. Austr N Z J Med 28:590–596
24. Centers for Disease Control (1982) Subacute sclerosing panencephalitis surveillance – United States. MMWR 31:585–588
25. Centers for Disease Control (1987) Epidemiologic notes and reports B-virus infection in humans – Pensacola, Florida. MMWR 36:289–290, 295–296
26. Centers for Disease Control (1989) Epidemiologic notes and reports B virus infections in humans – Michigan. MMWR 38:453–454
27. Centers for Disease Control (1998) Fatal Cercopithecine herpesvirus 1 (B virus) infection following a mucocutaneous exposure and interim recommendations for worker protection. MMWR 47:1073–1076
28. Cernescu C, Ruta SM, Tardei G, Grancea C, Moldoveanu L, Spulbar E, Tsai T (1997) A high number of severe neurologic clinical forms during an epidemic of West Nile virus infection. Rom J Virol 48:13–25
29. Chapelon C, Ziza JM, Piette JC, Levy Y, Raguin G, Wechsler B, Bitker MO, Bletry O, Laplane D, Bousser MG et al. (1990) Neurosarcoidosis: signs, course and treatment in 35 confirmed cases. Medicine 69:261–276
30. Chimelli L, Mahler-Araujo MB (1997) Fungal infections. Brain Pathol 7:613–627
31. Chimelli L, Scaravilli F (1997) Trypanosomiasis. Brain Pathol 7:599–611
32. Chou SM, Roos R, Burrell R, Gutmann L, Harley JB (1973) Subacute focal adenovirus encephalitis. J Neuropathol Exp Neurol 32:34–50
33. Chretien F, Belec L, Hilton DA, Flament-Saillour M, Guillon F, Wingertsmann L, Baudrimont M, de Truchis P, Keohane C, Vital C, Love S, Gray F (1996) Herpes simplex virus type 1 encephalitis in acquired immunodeficiency syndrome. Neuropathol Appl Neurobiol 22:394–404
34. Chretien F, Belec L, Lescs MC, Authier FJ, De Truchis P, Scaravilli F, Gray F (1997) Central nervous system infection due to varicella and zoster virus in AIDS. Arch Anat Cytol Pathol 45:142–152
35. Chretien F, Belec L, Wingerstmann L, de Truchis P, Baudrimont M, Perronne C, Gray F (1997) Central nervous system infection due to Herpes simplex virus in AIDS. Arch Anat Cytol Pathol 45:153–158
36. Chretien F, Gray F, Lescs MC, Geny C, Dubreuil-Lemaire ML, Ricolfi F, Baudrimont M, Levy Y, Sobel A, Vinters HV (1993) Acute varicella-zoster virus ventriculitis and meningo-myelo-radiculitis in acquired immunodeficiency syndrome. Acta Neuropathol 86:659–665

37. Chua KB, Goh KJ, Wong KT, Kamarulzaman A, Tan PSK, Ksiazek TG, Zaki SR, Paul G, Lam SK, Tan CT (1999) Fatal encephalitis due to Nipah virus among pig -farmers in Malaysia. Lancet 354:1257–1259
38. Chun RW (1983) Clinical aspects of La Crosse encephalitis: neurological and psychological sequelae. Prog Clin Biol Res 123:193–201
39. Connolly KJ, Hammer SM (1990) The acute aseptic meningitis syndrome. Infect Dis Clin N Am 4:599–622
40. Conti DJ, Rubin RH (1988) Infection of the central nervous system in organ transplant recipients. Neurol Clin 6:241–260
41. Cornford ME, McCormick GF (1997) Adult-onset temporal lobe epilepsy associated with smoldering herpes simplex 2 infection. Neurology 48:425–430
42. Davis D, Henslee PJ, Markesbery WR (1988) Fatal adenovirus meningoencephalitis in a bone marrow transplant patient. Ann Neurol 23:385–389
43. De Coene B, Gilliard C, Indekeu P, Duprez T, Trigaux JP (1996) Whipple's disease confined to the central nervous system. Neuroradiology 38:325–327
44. Deayton J, French P (1997) Incidence of early syphilis acquired in former Soviet Union is increasing. BMJ 315:1018–1019
45. Dill SR, Cobbs CG, McDonald CK (1995) Subdural empyema: analysis of 32 cases and review. Clin Infect Dis 20:372–386
46. Domingo Z, Peter JC (1994) Brain abscess in childhood. A 25-year experience. S Afr Med J 84:13–15
47. Elifson KW, Boles J, Darrow WW, Sterk CE (1999) HIV seroprevalence and risk factors among clients of female and male prostitutes. J Acq Imm Def Syndr Hum Retrovirol 20:195–200
48. Ellison DE, Love S (1998) Neuropathology. A reference text of CNS pathology. Mosby, London
49. Embil JA, Camfield P, Artsob H, Chase DP (1983) Powassan virus encephalitis resembling herpes simplex encephalitis. Arch Int Med 143:341–343
50. Esiri MM (1982) Herpes simplex encephalitis. An immunohistological study of the distribution of viral antigen within the brain. J Neurol Sci 54:209–226
51. Esiri MM, Kennedy PGE (1997) Viral diseases. In: Graham DI, Lantos PL (eds) Greenfield's neuropathology, vol. 2: 6th edition. Arnold, London, pp 3–63
52. Falangola MF, Reichler BS, Petito CK (1994) Histopathology of cerebral toxoplasmosis in human immunodeficiency virus infection: a comparison between patients with early-onset and late-onset acquired immunodeficiency syndrome. Hum Pathol 25:1091–1097
53. Farrington CP (1991) Subacute sclerosing panencephalitis in England and Wales: transient effects and risk estimates. Statist Med 10:1733–1744
54. Flood JM, Weinstock HS, Guroy ME, Bayne L, Simon RP, Bolan G (1998) Neurosyphilis during the AIDS epidemic, San Francisco, 1985–1992. J Infect Dis 177:931–940
55. Fodor PA, Levin MJ, Weinberg A, Sandberg E, Sylman J, Tyler KL (1998) Atypical herpes simplex virus encephalitis diagnosed by PCR amplification of viral DNA from CSF. Neurology 51:554–559
56. Francis BM, Gilbert GL (1992) Survey of neonatal meningitis in Australia: 1987–1989. Med J Austr 156:240–243
57. Gadoth N, Weitzman S, Lehmann EE (1979) Acute anterior myelitis complicating West Nile fever. Arch Neurol 36:172–173
58. Gellin BG, Weingarten K, Gamache FWJ, Hartman BJ (1991) Epidural abscess. In: Scheld WM, Whitley RJ, Durack DT (eds) Infections of the central nervous system. Raven Press, New York, pp 499–514
59. Gerbase AC, Rowley JT, Mertens TE (1998) Global epidemiology of sexually transmitted diseases. Lancet 351 (Suppl 3): 2–4
60. Germain M, Gourdeau M, Hebert J (1994) Case report: familial chronic mucocutaneous candidiasis complicated by deep candida infection. Am J Med Sci 307:282–283
61. Graham E, James DG (1988) Neurosarcoidosis. Sarcoidosis 5:125–131
62. Gray F (1993) Atlas of the Neuropathology of HIV Infection. Oxford University Press, Oxford
63. Gray F (1997) Bacterial infections. Brain Pathol 7:629–647

64. Gray F, Mohr M, Rozenberg F, Belec L, Lescs MC, Dournon E, Sinclair E, Scaravilli F (1992) Varicella-zoster virus encephalitis in acquired immunodeficiency syndrome: report of four cases. Neuropathol Appl Neurobiol 18:502-514
65. Gray F, Nordmann P (1997) Bacterial infections. In: Graham DI, Lantos PL (eds) Greenfield's neuropathology, vol 2: 6th edition. Arnold, London, pp 113-233
66. Greenlee JE (1989) Progressive multifocal leukoencephalopathy. Curr Clin Topics Infect Dis 10:140-156
67. Hamilton RL, Achim C, Grafe MR, Fremont JC, Miners D, Wiley CA (1995) Herpes simplex virus brainstem encephalitis in an AIDS patient. Clin Neuropathol 14:45-50
68. Hammer SM, Connolly KJ (1992) Viral aseptic meningitis in the United States: clinical features, viral etiologies, and differential diagnosis. Curr Clin Topics Infect Dis 12:1-25
69. Heck AW, Phillips LHd (1989) Sarcoidosis and the nervous system. Neurol Clin 7:641-654
70. Hemachudha T, Phuapradit P (1997) Rabies. Curr Opin Neurol 10:260-267
71. Hofman P, Michiels JF, Saint-Paul MC, Galibert A, Marty P, Durant J, Fuzibet JG, Mouroux J, Le Fichoux Y, Loubiere R (1993) Toxoplasmosis in AIDS patients. Pathoclinical study of 78 cases. Annales Pathol 13:233-240
72. Holtom PD, Larsen RA, Leal ME, Leedom JM (1992) Prevalence of neurosyphilis in human immunodeficiency virus-infected patients with latent syphilis. Am J Med 93:9-12
73. Hristeva L, Booy R, Bowler I, Wilkinson AR (1993) Prospective surveillance of neonatal meningitis [see comments]. Arch Dis Child 69:14-18
74. Huang C-C, Liu C-C, Chang Y-C, Chen C-Y, Wang S-T, Yeh T-F (1999) Neurologic complications in children with enterovirus 71 infection. N Eng J Med 341:936-942
75. Hughes I, Jenney ME, Newton RW, Morris DJ, Klapper PE (1993) Measles encephalitis during immunosuppressive treatment for acute lymphoblastic leukaemia. Arch Dis Child 68:775-778
76. Ishii T, Matsushita M, Hamada S (1977) Characteristic residual neuropathological features of Japanese B encephalitis. Acta Neuropathol 38:181-186
77. Izumo S, Ijichi T, Higuchi I, Tashiro A, Takahashi K, Osame M (1992) Neuropathology of HTLV-I-associated myelopathy–a report of two autopsy cases. Acta Paed Japon 34:358-364
78. Izumo S, Umehara F, Kashio N, Kubota R, Sato E, Osame M (1997) Neuropathology of HTLV-1-associated myelopathy (HAM/TSP). Leukemia 11:82-84
79. Jabbour JT, Garcia JH, Lemmi H, Ragland J, Duenas DA, Sever JL (1969) Subacute sclerosing panencephalitis. A multidisciplinary study of eight cases. JAMA 207:2248-2254
80. Joesoef MR, Linnan M, Barakbah Y, Idajadi A, Kambodji A, Schulz K (1997) Patterns of sexually transmitted diseases in female sex workers in Surabaya, Indonesia. Int J STD AIDS 8:576-580
81. Johnson RT (1998) Viral Infections of the Nervous System:2nd Edition. Philadelphia: Lippincott-Raven
82. Jones A, Bradley L, Alterman L, Tarlow M, Thompson R, Kinnon C, Morgan G (1996) X linked agammaglobulinaemia with a 'leaky' phenotype. Arch Dis Child 74:548-549
83. Kaplan AM, Koveleski JT (1978) St Louis encephalitis with particular involvement of the brain stem. Arch Neurol 35:45-46
84. Kaplan JE, Osame M, Kubota H, Igata A, Nishitani H, Maeda Y, Khabbaz RF, Janssen RS (1990) The risk of development of HTLV-I-associated myelopathy/tropical spastic paraparesis among persons infected with HTLV-I. J Acq Imm Def Synd 3:1096-1101
85. Katz DA, Berger JR, Duncan RC (1993) Neurosyphilis. A comparative study of the effects of infection with human immunodeficiency virus. Arch Neurol 50:243-249
86. Kennedy PG, Adams JH, Graham DI, Clements GB (1988) A clinico-pathological study of herpes simplex encephalitis. Neuropathol Appl Neurobiol 14:395-415
87. Kevy SV, Tefft M, Vawier GF, Rosen FS (1968) Hereditary splenic hypoplasia. Pediatrics 42:752-757
88. Kira R, Ihara K, Watanabe K, Kanemitsu S, Ahmed SU, Gondo K, Takeshita K, Hara T (1999) Molecular epidemiology of C9 deficiency heterozygotes with an Arg95Stop mutation of the C9 gene in Japan. J Hum Genet 44:109-111

89. Kleihues P, Lang W, Burger PC, Budka H, Vogt M, Maurer R, Luthy R, Siegenthaler W (1985) Progressive diffuse leukoencephalopathy in patients with acquired immune deficiency syndrome (AIDS). Acta Neuropathol 68:333–339
90. Kleinschmidt-DeMasters BK, Amlie-Lefond C, Gilden DH (1996) The patterns of varicella zoster virus encephalitis. Hum Pathol 27:927–938
91. Knoper SR, Galgiani JN (1988) Systemic fungal infections: diagnosis and treatment. I. Coccidioidomycosis. Infect Dis Clin N Am 2:861–875
92. Kornyey S (1978) Contribution to the histology of tick-borne encephalitis. Acta Neuropathol 43:179–183
93. Krauss WE, McCormick PC (1992) Infections of the dural spaces. Neurosurg Clin N Am 3:421–433
94. Kumar R, Mathur A, Kumar A, Sharma S, Saksena PN, Chaturvedi UC (1988) Japanese encephalitis–an important cause of acute childhood encephalopathy in Lucknow, India. Postgrad Med J 64:18–22
95. Lankoande S, Meda N, Sangare L, Compaore IP, Catraye J, Sanou PT, van Dyck E, Cartoux M, Sankara O, Curtis V, Soudre RB (1998) Prevalence and risk of HIV infection among female sex workers in Burkina Faso. Int J STD AIDS 9:146–150
96. Le DH (1986) Clinical aspects of Japanese B encephalitis in North Vietnam. Clin Neurol Neurosurg 88:189–192
97. Lehmann NI, Gust ID, Doherty R (1976) Isolation of Murray Valley encephalitis virus from the brains of three patients with encephalitis. Med J Austr 2:450–454
98. Lehrer RI, Cline MJ (1969) Leukocyte myeloperoxidase deficiency and disseminated candidiasis: the role of myeloperoxidase in resistance to Candida infection. J Clin Invest 48:1478–1488
99. Levy RM, Bredesen DE, Rosenblum ML, Davis RL (1989) Central nervous system disorders in AIDS. Immunology Series 44:371–401
100. Linglof T (1995) Rapid increase of syphilis and gonorrhea in parts of the former USSR. Sex Trans Dis 22:160–161
101. Lipton SA, Hickey WF, Morris JH, Loscalzo J (1984) Candidal infection in the central nervous system. Am J Med 76:101–108
102. Love S, Wiley CA (in press) Viral infections. In: Graham DI, Lantos PL (eds) Greenfield's neuropathology, vol. 2: 7th edition. Arnold, London
103. Lum LCS, Wong KT, Lam SK, Chua KB, Goh AYT, Lim WL, Ong BB, Paul G, AbuBakar S, Lambert M (1998) Fatal enterovirus 71 encephalomyelitis. J Pediatr 133:795–798
104. Lyon G, Griscelli C, Fernandez-Alvarez E, Prats-Vinas J, Lebon P (1980) Chronic progressive encephalitis in children with x-linked hypogammaglobulinemia. Neuropadiatrie 11:57–71
105. Mallouh AA, Abu-Osba YK (1987) Bacterial infections in children with glucose-6-phosphate dehydrogenase deficiency. J Pediatr 111:850–852
106. Mandybur TI (1990) The distribution of Alzheimer's neurofibrillary tangles and gliosis in chronic subacute sclerosing panencephalitis. Acta Neuropathol 80:307–310
107. Mandybur TI, Nagpaul AS, Pappas Z, Niklowitz WJ (1977) Alzheimer neurofibrillary change in subacute sclerosing panencephalitis. Ann Neurol 1:103–107
108. Mangano MF, Plotkin SA (1991) Viral vaccines that protect the central nervous system. In: Scheld WM, Whitley RJ, Durack DT (eds) Infections of the central nervous system. Raven Press, New York, pp 233–258
109. Martinez AJ, Visvesvara GS (1997) Free-living, amphizoic and opportunistic amebas. Brain Pathol 7:583–598
110. McKinney REJ, Katz SL, Wilfert CM (1987) Chronic enteroviral meningoencephalitis in agammaglobulinemic patients. Rev Infect Dis 9:334–356
111. Mendel E, Khoo LT, Go JL, Hinton D, Zee CS, Apuzzo ML (1999) Intracerebral Whipple's disease diagnosed by stereotactic biopsy: a case report and review of the literature. Neurosurgery 44:203–209
112. Minamoto G, Armstrong D (1988) Fungal infections in AIDS. Histoplasmosis and coccidioidomycosis. Infect Dis Clin North Am 2:447–456
113. Misra UK, Kalita J (1997) Anterior horn cells are also involved in Japanese encephalitis. Acta Neurol Scand 96:114–117

114. Misra UK, Kalita J (1997) Movement disorders in Japanese encephalitis. J Neurol 244:299–303
115. Misra UK, Kalita J, Jain SK, Mathur A (1994) Radiological and neurophysiological changes in Japanese encephalitis. J Neurol Neurosurg Psychiat 57:1484–1487
116. Modlin JF (1997) Update on enterovirus infections in infants and children. Adv Ped Infect Dis 12:155–181
117. Modlin JF, Jabbour JT, Witte JJ, Halsey NA (1977) Epidemiologic studies of measles, measles vaccine, and subacute sclerosing panencephalitis. Pediatrics 59: 505–512
118. Montgomery RD (1989) HTLV-1 and tropical spastic paraparesis. 1. Clinical features, pathology and epidemiology. Trans Roy Soc Trop Med Hyg 83:724–728
119. Moreno MT, Vargas S, Poveda R, Saez-Llorens X (1994) Neonatal sepsis and meningitis in a developing Latin American country. Ped Infect Dis J 13:516–520
120. Moulignier A, Pialoux G, Dega H, Dupont B, Huerre M, Baudrimont M (1995) Brain stem encephalitis due to varicella-zoster virus in a patient with AIDS. Clin Infect Dis 20:1378–1380
121. Mrak RE, Young L (1994) Rabies encephalitis in humans: pathology, pathogenesis and pathophysiology. J Neuropathol Exp Neurol 53:1–10
122. Muir P, van Loon AM (1997) Enterovirus infections of the central nervous system. Intervirology 40:153–166
123. Nakajima H, Furutama D, Kimura F, Shinoda K, Nakagawa T, Shimizu A, Ohsawa N (1995) Herpes simplex virus type 2 infections presenting as brainstem encephalitis and recurrent myelitis. Int Med 34:839–842
124. Ndinya-Achola JO, Ghee AE, Kihara AN, Krone MR, Plummer FA, Fisher LD, Holmes KK (1997) High HIV prevalence, low condom use and gender differences in sexual behaviour among patients with STD-related complaints at a Nairobi primary health care clinic. Int J STD AIDS 8:506–514
125. Netto EM, Dye C, Raviglione M (1999) Global Tuberculosis Control. Geneva, Switzerland: World Health Organization. Global Tuberculosis Programme
126. Netto EM, Dye C, Schmidt S, Raviglione M (1998) Global Tuberculosis Control. Geneva, Switzerland: World Health Organization. Global Tuberculosis Programme
127. Nicoll JA, Kinrade E, Love S (1992) PCR-mediated search for herpes simplex virus DNA in sections of brain from patients with multiple sclerosis and other neurological disorders. J Neurol Sci 113:144–151
128. Nicoll JA, Maitland NJ, Love S (1991) Autopsy neuropathological findings in 'burnt out' herpes simplex encephalitis and use of the polymerase chain reaction to detect viral DNA. Neuropathol Appl Neurobiol 17:375–382
129. Nilsson UR, Nilsson B, Storm KE, Sjolin-Forsberg G, Hallgren R (1992) Hereditary dysfunction of the third component of complement associated with a systemic lupus erythematosus-like syndrome and meningococcal meningitis. Arthritis Rheum 35:580–586
130. Parker JC, Jr., McCloskey JJ, Lee RS (1981) Human cerebral candidosis – a postmortem evaluation of 19 patients. Hum Pathol 12:23–28
131. Pendlebury WW, Perl DP, Munoz DG (1989) Multiple microabscesses in the central nervous system: a clinicopathologic study. J Neuropathol Exp Neurol 48:290–300
132. Peters M, Gottschalk D, Boit R, Pohle HD, Ruf B (1993) Meningovascular neurosyphilis in human immunodeficiency virus infection as a differential diagnosis of focal CNS lesions: a clinicopathological study. J Infect 27:57–62
133. Pittella JEH (1997) Neurocysticercosis. Brain Pathol 7:681–693
134. Pittella JEH (1997) Neuroschistosomiasis. Brain Pathol 7:649–662
135. Poneprasert B (1989) Japanese encephalitis in children in northern Thailand. SE Asian J Trop Med Pub Health 20:599–603
136. Purevdawa E, Moon TD, Baigalmaa C, Davaajav K, Smith ML, Vermund SH (1997) Rise in sexually transmitted diseases during democratization and economic crisis in Mongolia. Int J STD AIDS 8:398–401
137. Ramaiah C, Boynton RF (1998) Whipple's disease. Gastroenterol Clin N Am 27:683–695, vii
138. Ramjee G, Karim SS, Sturm AW (1998) Sexually transmitted infections among sex workers in KwaZulu-Natal, South Africa. Sex Trans Dis 25:346–349

139. Relman DA, Schmidt TM, MacDermott RP, Falkow S (1992) Identification of the uncultured bacillus of Whipple's disease. N Engl J Med 327:293–301
140. Reyes MG, Gardner JJ, Poland JD, Monath TP (1981) St Louis encephalitis. Quantitative histologic and immunofluorescent studies. Arch Neurol 38:329–334
141. Robson DK, Faraj BB, Hamal PB, Ironside JW (1990) Whipple's disease with cerebral involvement. Postgrad Med J 66:724–726
142. Roman GC, Roman LN (1988) Tropical spastic paraparesis. A clinical study of 50 patients from Tumaco (Colombia) and review of the worldwide features of the syndrome. J Neurol Sci 87:121–138
143. Roos KL, Tunkel AR, Scheld WM (1991) Acute bacterial meningitis in children and adults. In: Scheld WM, Whitley RJ, Durack DT (eds) Infections of the central nervous system. Raven Press, New York, pp 335–410
144. Roos RP, Graves MC, Wollmann RL, Chilcote RR, Nixon J (1981) Immunologic and virologic studies of measles inclusion body encephalitis in an immunosuppressed host: the relationship to subacute sclerosing panencephalitis. Neurology 31:1263–1270
145. Rose JW, Stroop WG, Matsuo F, Henkel J (1992) Atypical herpes simplex encephalitis: clinical, virologic, and neuropathologic evaluation. Neurology 42:1809–1812
146. Rosemberg S (1980) Neuropathology of S. Paulo south coast epidemic encephalitis (Rocio flavivurus). J Neurol Sci 45:1–12
147. Rosenfeld EA, Rowley AH (1994) Infectious intracranial complications of sinusitis, other than meningitis, in children: 12-year review. Clin Infect Dis 18:750–754
148. Ross SC, Densen P (1984) Complement deficiency states and infection: epidemiology, pathogenesis and consequences of neisserial and other infections in an immune deficiency. Medicine 63:243–273
149. Rotbart HA (1995) Enteroviral infections of the central nervous system. Clin Infect Dis 20:971–981
150. Rudge P, Webster AD, Revesz T, Warner T, Espanol T, Cunningham-Rundles C, Hyman N (1996) Encephalomyelitis in primary hypogammaglobulinaemia. Brain 119:1–15
151. Sadler M, Nelson MR (1997) Progressive multifocal leukoencephalopathy in HIV. Int J STD AIDS 8:351–357
152. Sarkar S, Islam N, Durandin F, Siddiqui N, Panda S, Jana S, Corbitt G, Klapper P, Mandal D (1998) Low HIV and high STD among commercial sex workers in a brothel in Bangladesh: scope for prevention of larger epidemic. Int J STD AIDS 9:45–47
153. Scaravilli F, Cook GC (1997) Parasitic and fungal infections. In: Graham DI, Lantos PL (eds) Greenfield's neuropathology, vol. 2: 6th edition. Arnold, London, pp 65–111
154. Scheld WM, Whitley RJ, Durack DT (1991) Infections of the Central Nervous System. New York: Raven Press
155. Schlesinger M, Nave Z, Levy Y, Slater PE, Fishelson Z (1990) Prevalence of hereditary properdin, C7 and C8 deficiencies in patients with meningococcal infections. Clin Exp Immunol 81:423–427
156. Schmidbauer M, Budka H, Okeda R, Cristina S, Lechi A, Trabattoni GR (1990) Multifocal vacuolar leucoencephalopathy: a distinct HIV-associated lesion of the brain. Neuropathol Appl Neurobiol 16:437–443
157. Schmidbauer M, Budka H, Shah KV (1990) Progressive multifocal leukoencephalopathy (PML) in AIDS and in the pre-AIDS era. A neuropathological comparison using immunocytochemistry and in situ DNA hybridization for virus detection. Acta Neuropathol 80:375–380
158. Schmidbauer M, Huemer M, Cristina S, Trabattoni GR, Budka H (1992) Morphological spectrum, distribution and clinical correlation of white matter lesions in AIDS brains. Neuropathol Appl Neurobiol 18:489–501
159. Schoedon G, Goldenberger D, Forrer R, Gunz A, Dutly F, Hochli M, Altwegg M, Schaffner A (1997) Deactivation of macrophages with interleukin-4 is the key to the isolation of Tropheryma whippelii. J Infect Dis 176:672–677
160. Schofer H, Imhof M, Thoma-Greber E, Brockmeyer NH, Hartmann M, Gerken G, Pees HW, Rasokat H, Hartmann H, Sadri I, Emminger C, Stellbrink HJ, Baumgarten R, Plettenberg A (1996) Active syphilis in HIV infection: a multicentre retrospective survey. The German AIDS Study Group (GASG). Genitour Med 72:176–181

161. Setinek U, Wondrusch E, Jellinger K, Steuer A, Drlicek M, Grisold W, Lintner F (1995) Cytomegalovirus infection of the brain in AIDS: a clinicopathological study. Acta Neuropathol 90:511–515
162. Seydoux C, Francioli P (1992) Bacterial brain abscesses: factors influencing mortality and sequelae. Clin Infect Dis 15:394–401
163. Sharer LR (1992) Pathology of HIV-1 infection of the central nervous system. A review. J Neuropathol Exp Neurol 51:3–11
164. Skoldenberg B (1996) Herpes simplex encephalitis. Scand J Infect Dis – Suppl 100:8–13
165. Smacchia C, Parolin A, Di Perri G, Vento S, Concia E (1998) Syphilis in prostitutes from Eastern Europe. Lancet 351:572
166. Smith AL, Haas J (1991) Neonatal bacterial meningitis. In: Scheld WM, Whitley RJ, Durack DT (eds) Infections of the central nervous system. Raven Press, New York, pp 313–333
167. Solomon T, Kneen R, Dung NM, Khanh VC, Thuy TT, Ha DQ, Day NP, Nisalak A, Vaughn DW, White NJ (1998) Poliomyelitis-like illness due to Japanese encephalitis virus. Lancet 351:1094–1097
168. Stein DK, Sugar AM (1989) Fungal infections in the immunocompromised host. Diag Microbiol Infect Dis 12:221S–228 S
169. Stern BJ, Krumholz A, Johns C, Scott P, Nissim J (1985) Sarcoidosis and its neurological manifestations. Arch Neurol 42:909–917
170. Strittmatter C, Lang W, Wiestler OD, Kleihues P (1992) The changing pattern of human immunodeficiency virus-associated cerebral toxoplasmosis: a study of 46 postmortem cases. Acta Neuropathol 83:475–481
171. Synnott MB, Morse DL, Hall SM (1994) Neonatal meningitis in England and Wales: a review of routine national data. Arch Dis Child 71: F75–80
172. Takashima I (1998) Epidemiology of tick-borne encephalitis in Japan. Comp Immunol Microbiol Infect Dis 21:81–90
173. Taratuto AL, Venturiello SM (1997) Echinococcosis. Brain Pathol 7:673–679
174. Tenenbaum MJ, Greenspan J, Kerkering TM (1982) Blastomycosis. Crit Rev Microbiol 9:139–163
175. Thomas PK, Landon DN, King RHM (1997) Diseases of the peripheral nerves. In: Graham DI, Lantos PL (eds) Greenfield's neuropathology, vol. 2: 6th edition. Arnold, London, pp 367–487
176. Thong YH, Simpson DA, Muller-Eberhard HJ (1980) Homozygous deficiency of the second component of complement presenting with recurrent bacterial meningitis. Arch Dis Child 55:471–473
177. Tichonova L, Borisenko K, Ward H, Meheus A, Gromyko A, Renton A (1997) Epidemics of syphilis in the Russian Federation: trends, origins, and priorities for control. Lancet 350:210–213
178. Townsend JJ, Baringer JR, Wolinsky JS, Malamud N, Mednick JP, Panitch HS, Scott RA, Oshiro L, Cremer NE (1975) Progressive rubella panencephalitis. Late onset after congenital rubella. N Engl J Med 292:990–993
179. Townsend JJ, Stroop WG, Baringer JR, Wolinsky JS, McKerrow JH, Berg BO (1982) Neuropathology of progressive rubella panencephalitis after childhood rubella. Neurology 32:185–190
180. Townsend JJ, Wolinsky JS, Baringer JR (1976) The neuropathology of progressive rubella panencephalitis of late onset. Brain 99:81–90
181. Tsai TF, Popovici F, Cernescu C, Campbell GL, Nedelcu NI (1998) West Nile encephalitis epidemic in southeastern Romania. Lancet 352:767–771
182. Tsiang H (1993) Pathophysiology of rabies virus infection of the nervous system. Adv Vir Res 42:375–412
183. Tunkel AR, Wispelwey B, Scheld WM (1990) Pathogenesis and pathophysiology of meningitis. Infect Dis Clin N Am 4:555–581
184. Turner G (1997) Cerebral malaria. Brain Pathol 7:569–582
185. Uchiyama T (1997) Human T cell leukemia virus type I (HTLV-I) and human diseases. Ann Rev Immunol 15:15–37
186. Unhanand M, Mustafa MM, McCracken GH Jr, Nelson JD (1993) Gram-negative enteric bacillary meningitis: a twenty-one-year experience. J Ped 122:15–21

187. Verhagen WI, Huygen PL, Dalman JE, Schuurmans MM (1996) Whipple's disease and the central nervous system. A case report and a review of the literature. Clin Neurol Neurosurg 98:299–304
188. Vinters HV, Anders KH (1990) Neuropathology of AIDS. Florida: CRC Press
189. Walsh TJ, Hier DB, Caplan LR (1985) Aspergillosis of the central nervous system: clinicopathological analysis of 17 patients. Ann Neurol 18:574–582
190. Watanabe T (1997) HTLV-1-associated diseases. Int J Hematol 66:257–278
191. Wheat LJ (1988) Systemic fungal infections: diagnosis and treatment. I. Histoplasmosis. Infect Dis Clin N Am 2:841–859
192. Wheat LJ, Batteiger BE, Sathapatayavongs B (1990) Histoplasma capsulatum infections of the central nervous system. A clinical review. Medicine 69:244–260
193. Whitley RJ (1991) Arthropod-borne encephalitides. In: Scheld WM, Whitley RJ, Durack DT (eds) Infections of the central nervous system. Raven Press, New York, pp 87–111
194. Whitley RJ, Lakeman F (1995) Herpes simplex virus infections of the central nervous system: therapeutic and diagnostic considerations. Clin Infect Dis 20:414–420
195. Whitley RJ, Soong SJ, Linneman C, Jr, Liu C, Pazin G, Alford CA (1982) Herpes simplex encephalitis. Clinical assessment. JAMA 247:317–320
196. Wiley CA, Grafe M, Kennedy C, Nelson JA (1988) Human immunodeficiency virus (HIV) and JC virus in acquired immune deficiency syndrome (AIDS) patients with progressive multifocal leukoencephalopathy. Acta Neuropathol 76:338–346
197. Wilfert CM, Buckley RH, Mohanakumar T, Griffith JF, Katz SL, Whisnant JK, Eggleston PA, Moore M, Treadwell E, Oxman MN, Rosen FS (1977) Persistent and fatal central-nervous-system ECHOvirus infections in patients with agammaglobulinemia. N Engl J Med 296:1485–1489
198. Wilson KH, Blitchington R, Frothingham R, Wilson JA (1991) Phylogeny of the Whipple's-disease-associated bacterium. Lancet 338:474–475
199. Wispelwey B, Dacey RGJ, Scheld WM (1991) Brain abscess. In: Scheld WM, Whitley RJ, Durack DT (eds) Infections of the central nervous system. Raven Press, New York, pp 457–486
200. Woods GL, Goldsmith JC (1990) Aspergillus infection of the central nervous system in patients with acquired immunodeficiency syndrome. Arch Neurol 47:181–184
201. World Health Organization http://www.who.int/emc-documents/rabies/docs/wsr94/wsr94_1.html (1994) World Survey of Rabies N° 30 for the Year 1994
202. World Health Organization. Emerging and other Communicable Diseases SaC (1996) Report of the 3rd International Symposium on Rabies in Asia. Wuhan, China, 11–15 September 1996
203. Wroe SJ, Pires M, Harding B, Youl BD, Shorvon S (1991) Whipple's disease confined to the CNS presenting with multiple intracerebral mass lesions. J Neurol Neurosurg Psychiat 54:989–992
204. Zimran A, Rudensky B, Kramer MR, Tedesco F, Ehrenfeld M, Raz R, Greif Z, Gelber M, Lishner M, Golan E et al. (1987) Hereditary complement deficiency in survivors of meningococcal disease: high prevalence of C7/C8 deficiency in Sephardic (Moroccan) Jews. Q J Med 63:349–358

# Cerebrovascular Disease – Practical Issues in Surgical and Autopsy Pathology

H. V. VINTERS



## 1 Introduction

This chapter will deal with practical approaches to the pathologic diagnosis of cerebrovascular diseases. Many forms of 'stroke' and cerebrovascular disease pay little respect to arbitrary boundaries defined by age, whereas others [e.g., cerebral amyloid angiopathy, (CAA)] are clearly most prevalent in the elderly, and a few are primarily disorders of the young. In this chapter, these will all be considered in the appropriate clinical context. Many principles important in understanding anoxic-ischemic brain injury are relevant to the developed brain, regardless of age, but are different when applied to the infant/developing central nervous system (CNS) [128]. This chapter is divided into consideration of (1) practical approaches to the autopsy or biopsy examination in suspected stroke, (2) anoxic-ischemic encephalopathy, (3) cerebral infarcts and ischemic lesions, and (4) encephalic hemorrhage. It should, however, be noted that many of the disease processes discussed in this chapter may have both ischemic and hemorrhagic components. Any extensive review of human cerebrovascular disease and 'stroke' owes a massive debt to the monograph of W.E. STEHBENS [139], which remains an authoritative classic in the field almost 30 years after its publication. More recent volumes and reviews on clinicopathologic aspects of cerebrovascular disease are also recommended to the interested reader [3, 7, 8, 22, 53, 68], as are sections devoted to 'stroke' and cerebrovascular disease in standard textbooks of neuropathology [47, 81, 156].

Current Topics in Pathology, Vol. 95
S. Love (Ed.): Neuropathology

The magnitude of the 'stroke' problem is immense. In the USA there are approximately 0.5 million new 'strokes' diagnosed annually, and 3 million survivors of a previous 'stroke'. As a recent review has stated, stroke is the third most frequent cause of death, the second most common cause of dementia found in a memory clinic, and a major reason for severe (acquired) disability and long-term dependency in developed nations; hence it is a major public health issue [90]. Stroke has an incidence of 250–400 per 100,000 and a mortality of 25%–30%, and is the third leading cause of death in industrialized countries [42]. The incidence of cerebrovascular disease increases with age, being about 100/100,000 for individuals of age 45–54 years, but 1,800/100,000 for those over 85 years of age [47]. Among North Americans, brain infarcts are about ten times as common as hemorrhages, whereas in the Orient spontaneous encephalic hemorrhage is almost as common as ischemic infarct. Epidemiologic surveys have found that African-American men (ages 35–74 years) were 2.5-fold, and women 2.4-fold, as likely as whites to die of stroke [63].

## 2 Practical Approaches to the Pathological Assessment of 'Stroke' at Autopsy or in Surgical Specimens

Anatomical pathologists are frequently asked to evaluate at necropsy a patient who may have had a 'stroke' during life. Asked to perform such an autopsy, the pathologist should ask several questions of the clinician requesting the examination:

1. Since 'stroke' is a clinical term that simply describes a syndrome of rapidly evolving neurologic deficit, what is the evidence that the deceased in fact had a stroke rather than, for example, a brain abscess or rapidly growing CNS tumor, either of which may present as a stroke?
2. If cerebrovascular disease was indeed suspected or proven during life, was the stroke thought to be the result of an ischemic infarct or an intraparenchymal hemorrhage? (Detailed information about neuroimaging studies is usually helpful.)
3. If stroke were the result of an ischemic infarct, was it felt to be embolic or the consequence of thrombosis of a major cervical or intracranial artery? If the latter, how well was this documented? (Knowledge of the cerebral angiograms is invaluable.)

In a young patient with spontaneous fatal intracerebral hemorrhage, occult structural lesions are possible causes (small vascular malformation, berry aneurysm), but the possibility of a bleed related to recreational drug use (e.g., amphetamines, cocaine) should be kept in mind. Therefore, in such a patient gastric contents, blood, and other body fluids should be retained in the event that they may be required for toxicologic analysis. Increasingly recognized are familial stroke syndromes – e.g., rare familial forms of cerebral microvasculopathy causing cerebral hemorrhage (see below) – and familial syndromes of vascular dementia, such as CADASIL (cerebral autosomal dominant arteriopathy with subcortical infarcts and leukoencephalopathy). The family history of the stroke patient may therefore be crucial in interpreting the neuropathologic findings and providing important feedback to the patient's family [153].

At autopsy, the pathologist must establish both the topography and extent of brain injury, and its likely cause(s). This involves not only examination of the brain, but also removal of the cervical carotid arteries including, when relevant, the intraosseous and intracavernous segments or, failing this, establishing a likely locus of arterial occlusion by a more limited dissection. Full exposure and removal of the vertebral arteries, which run through the cervical spine, are only occasionally necessary but can be accomplished in situ, within about 15 min through an anterior approach. This involves sawing parasagitally through the cervical pedicles at their junction with the vertebral bodies, levering the bodies away from the column and then using a bone nibbler to trace the intraosseous part of the vertebral arteries from their origin, upwards to their entry into the cranial cavity.

Careful review of the heart for evidence of valvular abnormalities, septal defects, or other congenital anomalies is mandatory, especially in young patients, in whom cardioembolic infarcts are much more common as a cause of stroke than is atherosclerosis. In young patients with stroke the possibility of a hematologic abnormality must also be considered, as should the possible existence of antiphospholipid antibodies – almost half of patients with systemic lupus, for instance, have high levels of these antibodies which carry a high risk of thrombotic disease including recurrent strokes [47]. Inherited disorders of coagulation (protein C

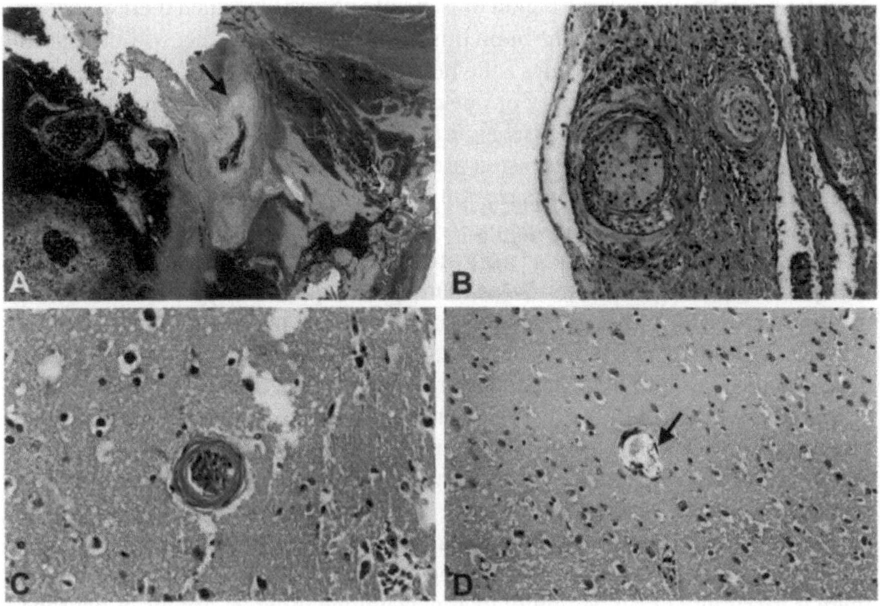


**Fig. 1 A – D.** Intraparenchymal blood clot resected from an elderly patient with many medical problems. In addition to blood, several fragments of brain were removed. Several changes were found. **A** Note abundant acute hemorrhage, and a prominently thickened, arteriosclerotic artery (*arrow*), one of many found among the clot fragments (H&E). **B** Section stained with elastica van Gieson shows smaller thickened arterioles, with intimal thickening (probably including macrophages) between the elastica and vessel lumen. **C, D** Brain fragments showed thickened arterioles which, when stained with Congo red (**C**) demonstrated apple/yellow green birefringence (*arrow*, **D**) typical of amyloid angiopathy. **A** ×35, **B** and **D** ×180, **C** ×355

deficiency, Factor V Leiden mutation, protein S deficiency) increase the risk of brain infarcts, especially in the young.

In neuropathology practice, surgical specimens from patients with stroke are relatively frequent. Carotid endarterectomy specimens usually show features of severe, complicated atherosclerosis [129, 130]. Arteriovenous malformations and other types of angioma are often resected (see below). Rarely, surgically evacuated blood clot may contain evidence of a vascular malformation, even when this was not suspected clinically. Stains for elastica and collagen are useful in confirming this diagnosis. In general, clot removed surgically from brain parenchyma needs to be examined carefully for other disease that may have caused the bleed, e.g., primary or metastatic neoplasm, vasculitis, etc. [74]. Microangiopathies associated with spontaneous intracerebral hemorrhage can be diagnosed in such seemingly trivial surgical material, and may influence subsequent clinical management of the affected patient (Fig. 1) [1]. Patients with HIV infection and hemorrhagic brain lesions are likely to have an opportunistic infectious or a neoplastic cause for them (e.g., fungal infection, hemorrhagic component of a primary CNS lymphoma), though a rare form of HIV-associated vasculopathy is described [154].

## 3 Anoxic-Ischemic Encephalopathy

An infarct can be defined as a region of ischemic necrosis in which there is irreversible injury to all cell types. In the brain this is usually situated either within a specific arterial territory or in the border zone between two arterial territories, and results from occlusion of a major artery or one of its branches by a thrombus or embolus (see below). By contrast, anoxic-ischemic encephalopathy (AIE) usually results from a sustained drop in cerebral perfusion pressure below the threshold for autoregulation (global brain ischemia) or perfusion of the brain by poorly oxygenated blood. Relative hypoxia may occur in the brain as a function of hypoxemic hypoxia (low oxygen content in the blood, e.g., near drowning, respiratory arrest, carbon monoxide poisoning), stagnant hypoxia (an inadequate supply of oxygenated blood, e.g., cardiac arrest with prolonged asystole, intraoperative hypotension), or histotoxic hypoxia (inability of cerebral tissues to utilize oxygen, e.g., inhibition of mitochondrial enzymes involved in oxidative respiration as a result of cyanide intoxication).

Within the brain, there is a distinctive hierarchy of susceptibility to anoxia of different cell types (e.g., neurons are more vulnerable than oligodendroglia, astrocytes, or microvascular endothelium) and different cells within a given set – especially neurons. Among neurons, the 'hierarchy' of anatomic regions showing greatest to least vulnerability to anoxia (in adults) is hippocampus, neocortex, cerebellum, deep central gray matter, and brain stem. Even within these regions, there is variability of susceptibility to anoxia among different groups of neurons – e.g., the CA1 field of pyramidal cells in the hippocampus is vulnerable, the CA2 zone relatively resistant, and within cerebellum the Purkinje cells show a susceptibility to anoxic injury not shared by the more resistant granule cells. Determinants of selective vulnerability are complex, but include (1) variable oxygen and energy requirements among different neurons, (2) glutamate receptor densities – glutamate acts as an excitotoxic neurotransmitter, and (3) activation of immediate early genes (e.g., heat shock proteins) by ischemia-induced free radicals [42, 47, 171].

An increase in the level of intracellular calcium in ischemic cells acts as a second messenger and may initiate a series of cellular events that contributes to tissue injury after either generalized or focal ischemia. These include the activation of proteolytic enzymes that act to degrade both structural (cytoskeletal) and extracellular matrix (e.g., laminin) proteins. Lipid peroxidation and membrane damage may result from activation of phospholipase $A_2$ and cyclooxygenase, which generates superoxide and other potentially harmful free radicals. Nitric oxide (NO) generated by nitric oxide synthase (NOS) may react with superoxide to form peroxynitrite, a highly reactive species that promotes tissue damage [42]. In focal cerebral ischemia, this cascade of events may result in extensive tissue damage and neuronal loss surrounding the central region of complete necrosis. Peri-infarct depolarizations, inflammation, and apoptosis may all aggravate the neurologic deficit associated with even a comparatively small focal infarct. Many strategies for treating ischemic brain infarcts are aimed at minimizing tissue injury in the marginally perfused, potentially salvageable peri-infarct penumbra [42]. There is growing interest in the inflammatory response to ischemic brain lesions, in particular because modifying this may be one rational approach to ameliorating the devastating sequelae of stroke [38].

The diagnosis of acute anoxic-ischemic encephalopathy is made when neurons showing characteristic eosinophilic cytoplasmic change with nuclear pyknosis, are seen multifocally or throughout the brain – especially in anoxia-sensitive regions (see above). Eventually, these neurons disappear, leaving glial scars. In particularly severe hypoxia or with profound hypotension (e.g., after prolonged cardiac arrest followed by resuscitation) regions of the brain may show laminar necrosis, characterized by patchy regions of necrosis of the deep cortical layers along segments of the cortical ribbon (Fig. 2) [47]. In severe cases, there may be essentially pancortical neuronal necrosis.

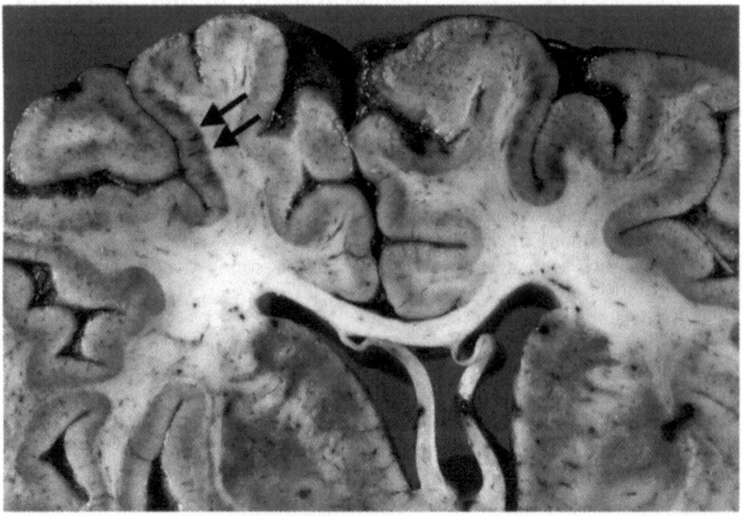

**Fig. 2.** Cortical laminar necrosis (LN) and anoxic-ischemic encephalopathy. Coronal section of brain shows patchy, focally prominent gray/black discoloration (e.g., *arrows*) within deep cortex throughout the specimen. Basal ganglia (bottom of the photograph) also show mottling and discoloration, indicative of severe anoxic-ischemic encephalopathy

# 4 Ischemic Brain Infarcts

## 4.1 Vascular Disease Causing Stroke

Table 1 presents a classification of the major types of cerebral vascular disease that may cause stroke and/or dementia. Subdividing vascular disease affecting the CNS into 'macro-' and 'micro-' vascular components represents an oversimplification of the 'real world' situation [153]. The major forms of vasculopathy – atherosclerosis, arteriosclerosis, and/or cerebral amyloid angiopathy (CAA) – often coexist in the elderly and probably share major risk factors, an important one being aging.

**Table 1.** Major categories of arterial disease that affect the human nervous system[a]

1. Arteriopathies affecting (primarily) large arteries
   a. Atherosclerosis ('simple'/complicated)
   b. Fibromuscular dysplasia (FMD)
   c. Moyamoya disease
   d. Arterial dissection (cystic medial necrosis?)
   e. HIV-associated vasculopathy
   f. Vasculitis/angiitis/arteritis
      Giant cell (temporal) arteritis
      Takayasu arteritis
2. Arteriopathies affecting small arteries
   a. Arteriosclerosis/arteriolosclerosis/lipohyalinosis
   b. Cerebral amyloid (congophilic) angiopathy
      Sporadic (associated with aging, AD/SDAT)
      Familial CAA syndromes (HCHWA-D, HCCAA-HCHWA-I, British CAA, Transthyretin)
   c. Vasculitis/angiitis/arteritis
      Primary (including granulomatous) angiitis of the CNS [often associated with CAA in the elderly]
      Polyarteritis nodosa
      Wegener's granulomatosis
      Systemic lupus (SLE)
      Behçet disease
      Hypersensitivity vasculitis
      Lymphomatoid granulomatosis (LG)[b]
      Vasculitis secondary to systemic infection, connective tissue disease, malignancy, sarcoidosis, etc.
   d. Associated with dementia
      Binswanger's subcortical (arteriosclerotic) leukoencephalopathy (BSLE)
      CADASIL
      Cerebral amyloid angiopathy (see above)
   e. Thrombotic thrombocytopenic purpura (TTP)
   f. ?MELAS (mitochondrial cytopathies with stroke-like episodes)
   g. Cerebroretinal vasculopathy/HERNS (Hereditary endotheliopathy, retinopathy, nephropathy, and stroke)

[a] Neuropathologic entities that are an 'incidental' finding at autopsy (siderocalcinosis of arteries in the basal ganglia) are not included in this table.
[b] LG is a controversial entity with features of both a vasculitis and a lymphoproliferative disorder.

**Macroangiopathy.** Atherosclerosis remains a leading factor contributing to the importance of cardiovascular and cerebrovascular disease as major causes of morbidity and mortality in most developed countries, especially among the elderly. The pathogenesis of atherosclerosis is now understood in considerable detail, thanks to advances in the development of animal models, cell and molecular biological tools that can be utilized to study its initiating factors and progression [116, 129, 130].

Early events that precede the formation of atherosclerotic 'plaques' include endothelial dysfunction (with abnormally increased permeability to lipoproteins and other plasma components) – possibly mediated by NO and platelet-derived

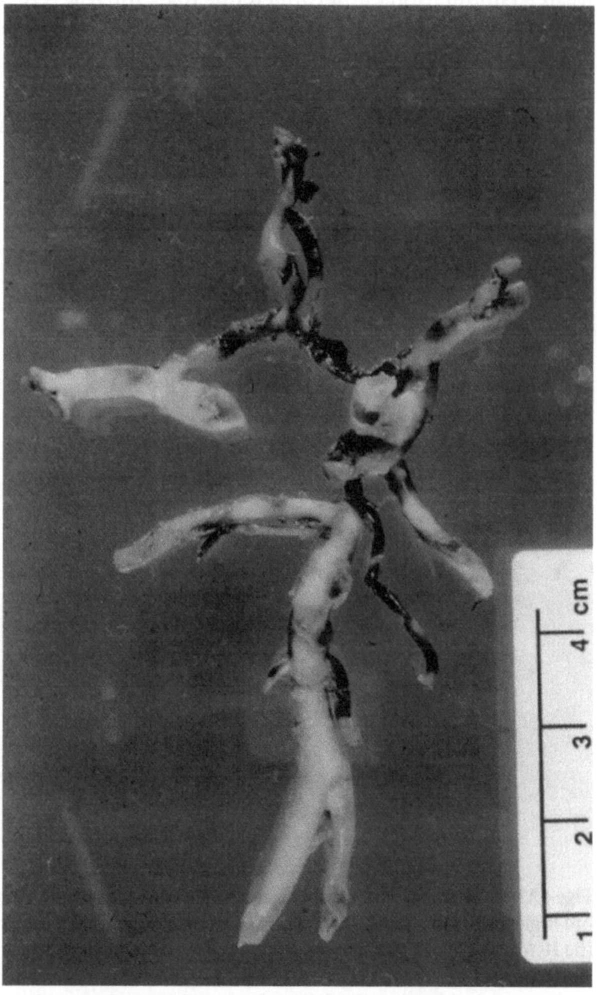


**Fig. 3.** Atherosclerosis on the circle of Willis. Note patchy, focally accentuated atheroma on branches of the circle of Willis, e.g., in the mid-portion of the basilar artery and the MCAs. The right posterior communicating artery was thin and fragmented during removal of the circle of Willis from base of the brain

growth factor, upregulation of leukocyte adhesion molecules such as integrins and L-selectin, and endothelial adhesion molecules, and migration of white blood cells (WBCs) into the arterial wall. Lesions of 'complicated' atherosclerosis develop after a fibrous cap forms over a fatty streak; this cap eventually overlies a necrotic core that includes a mixture of WBCs, lipids, and amorphous debris, and itself results from lipid accumulation, necrosis, and proteolytic activity [129, 130]. Unstable plaques, often resulting in symptomatic plaque rupture, probably result from thinning of the protective fibrous cap associated with continued influx and activation of macrophages. Bleeding into this unstable plaque (with or without its rupture into the arterial lumen) may occur from vasa vasorum or fragile microvessels within plaque itself, and may lead to mural or occlusive thrombus in an affected artery.

Atherosclerosis often involves major branches of the circle of Willis (Fig. 3). In western populations, atheroma tends to be most severe in basal arteries, whereas in Japanese individuals, atherosclerosis is more severe in peripheral arterial branches [125]. An arterial segment in or near the circle of Willis may undergo thrombosis with resultant brain infarction. Commonly, however, the brain is injured because of severely stenotic or occlusive atherosclerosis in the intracervical, extracranial carotid, and vertebral arterial systems [25, 52, 143, 144]. The extent of atheroma in

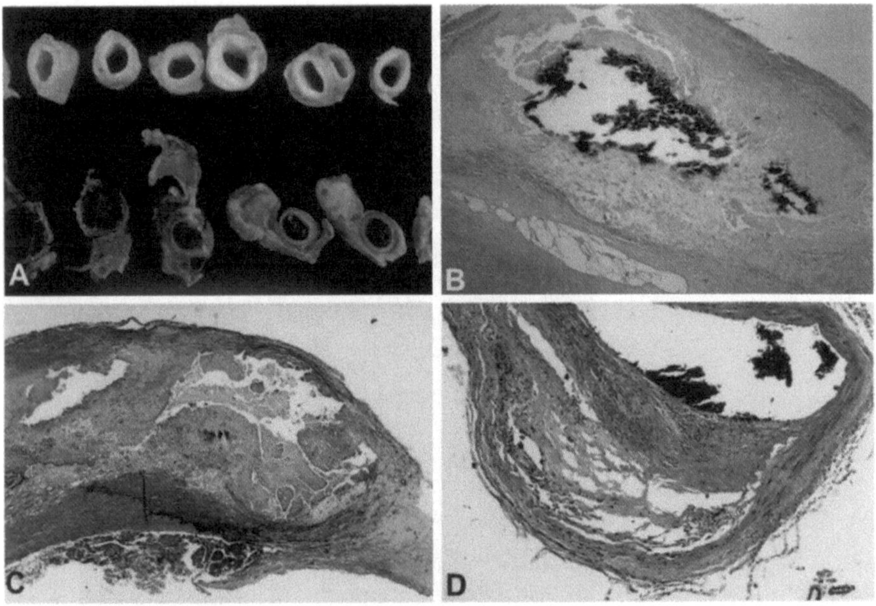


**Fig. 4 A–D.** Atherosclerosis of the cervical carotid artery. **A** Autopsy specimen from a 62-year-old male who had complete thrombosis of the left common carotid artery. Sections at top are of the ICA, showing moderate eccentric atheroma, including a semilunar area of intimal thickening, but relatively mild stenosis of the arterial lumen. Sections at bottom show thrombosed common carotid artery. **B, C** Histologic sections of carotid endarterectomy specimens from various patients. **B** shows a prominently calcified portion of plaque, while **C** shows cholesterol clefts in a region of intimal fibromuscular hyperplasia. **D** Severe atherosclerosis of intracranial (meningeal) artery in a patient with dementia. **B, C,** and **D** stained with H&E; **B** and **C** ×35, **D** ×90

neck arteries can be predicted with considerable success using ultrasonic and angiographic imaging techniques [44, 96, 123]. Carotid endarterectomy (CEA) is now routinely carried out as prophylaxis against stroke in patients with severe stenosis at the carotid bifurcation; not surprisingly, the surgical specimens that result show typical features of complicated atheroma (Fig. 4) [113]. Fragile, often ulcerated, atheroma, strategically located within cervical arteries, may lead to artery-to-artery emboli of either platelet-fibrin or atheromatous material (Fig. 5), causing ischemic stroke [24, 98].

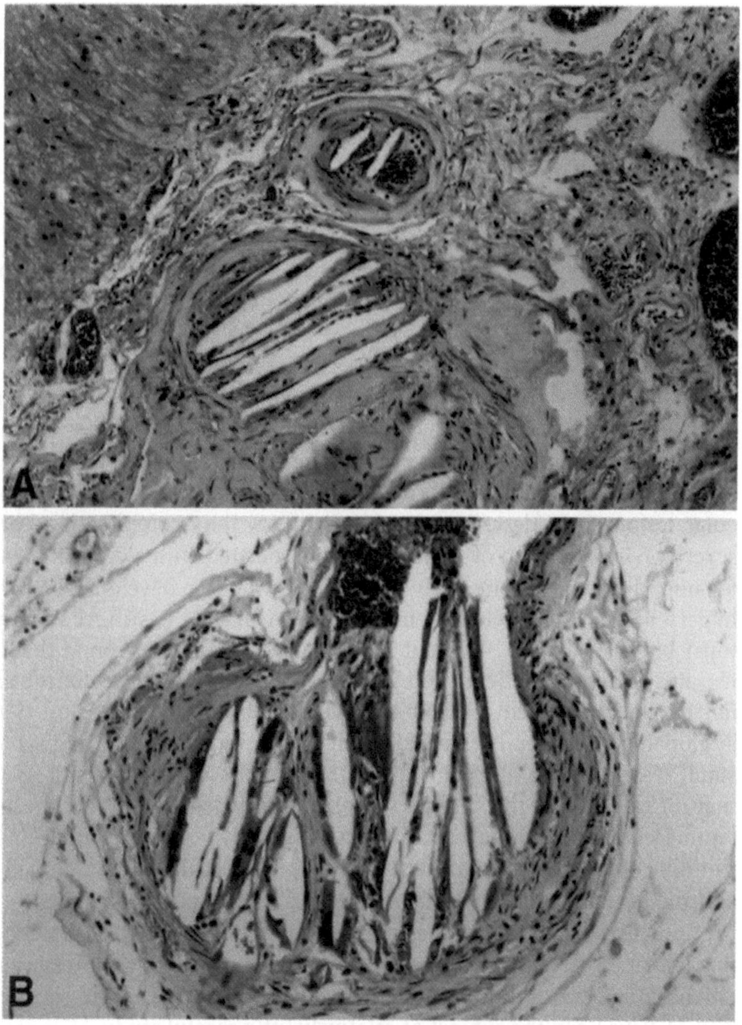


**Fig. 5 A, B.** Atheroemboli. Brain sections from patient who had experienced multiple stroke-like episodes over months prior to death. Small vessels occluded by atheromatous material were scattered throughout the brain. Note cholesterol clefts, surrounded by multinucleated giant cells, characteristic components of atheromatous plaque in situ. H&E; **A** ×110, **B** ×220

Patterns of ischemic brain infarcts resulting from thrombotic and embolic occlusions of the carotid arteries have been examined in a meticulous necropsy study of almost 1,000 patients [79, 80]. The close association between cardiovascular disease and severe carotid atherosclerosis was emphasized. Cerebral infarcts were found in 78% of patients with thromboembolic carotid occlusions. While the middle cerebral artery (MCA) territory of the cerebral hemisphere was most commonly infarcted in association with carotid occlusion, anterior and middle cerebral artery territories had also sometimes undergone necrosis [144]. In a companion investigation, the same investigators analyzed the extent and clinicopathologic correlates of ischemic cerebrovascular disease within brain – this was found in almost $^1/_3$ of the 994 patients examined [79, 80].

Rarely, severe atheroma in the circle of Willis – especially involving the basilar artery – may cause ectasia or fusiform enlargement of the artery. This aneurysmal dilatation may result in symptoms caused by compression of nearby structures, e.g., brain stem in the case of a basilar aneurysm [136, 150]. Cross sections of these aneurysms show severe complicated atheroma, frequently with superimposed mural hemorrhage, rupture, and infiltration by chronic inflammatory cells. They may become occluded to produce brain stem and/or cerebellar infarcts.

Other rare arteriopathies affecting large arteries (e.g., fibromuscular dysplasia/FMD, moyamoya disease, HIV-associated vasculopathy) are a major diagnostic consideration when ischemic stroke occurs children and young or middle-aged adults [47, 150, 153].

**Microangiopathy.** By comparison with atherosclerosis, the molecular pathogenesis of arteriosclerosis/arteriolosclerosis (AS), one of the two most common forms of cerebral microangiopathy (the other being cerebral amyloid angiopathy; see below) is poorly understood. There is a lack of uniform agreement on the brain microvascular lesions best described by the term AS, thus complicating comparisons of severity. The evolution of AS is strongly associated with a clinical history of hypertension. However, despite fairly effective treatment in developed countries of severe hypertension, arteriosclerotic microvascular disease is still frequently seen in autopsy brain specimens. A recent autopsy investigation has found that of 70 patients in whose brains significant cerebral small vessel disease was found, almost a third failed to meet stringent clinicopathologic criteria for hypertension. Cerebral microangiopathy was hypothesized to result from conditions that might have enhanced small vessel permeability during life [87]. Microscopic features of AS, when severe, may include hyaline thickening (sometimes with degeneration of the internal elastic lamina), intimal fibromuscular hyperplasia, variable degrees of luminal narrowing, thinning of the media, concentric 'onion-skin' type smooth muscle cell proliferation and the presence of foamy macrophages in the arterial wall (Fig. 6) [139, 153]. Fibrinoid necrosis usually occurs only with malignant hypertension. Microatheroma may also be seen in medium-sized meningeal – and sometimes even intraparenchymal – arteries. Pathophysiologic mechanisms important in the genesis of cerebral AS have been the subject of relatively little careful study. AS is sometimes used interchangeably with the term 'lipohyalinosis' (LH), the latter deriving from an assumption of events likely to have been important in the pathogenesis of the microangiopathy, i.e., lipid deposition and hyalinization. Consequences of AS/LH, including lacunar infarcts and parenchymal brain hemorrhage, are discussed below.

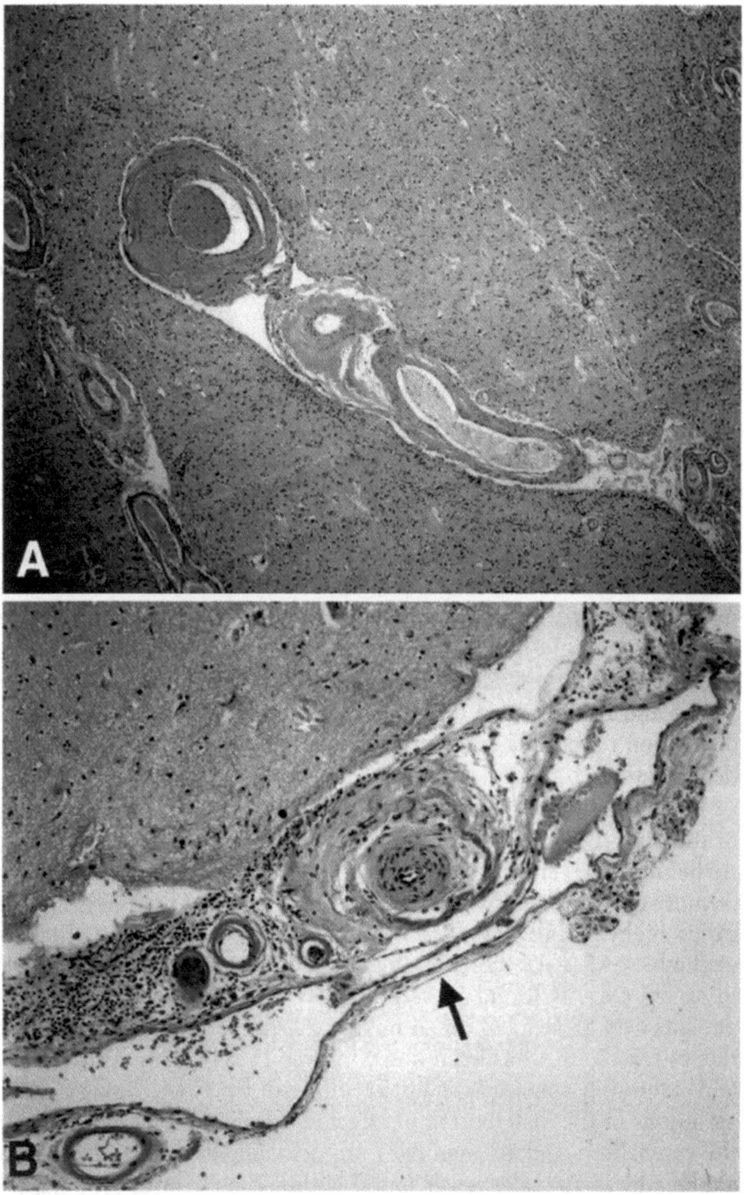


**Fig. 6 A, B.** Severe arteriosclerotic change in an elderly patient with ischemic-vascular dementia. Both panels show extensive onion-skin type and hyaline thickening of a severe degree. AS/LH involves both parenchymal (**A**) and meningeal (*arrow*, **B**) arterioles. H&E; **A** ×45, **B** ×110

Cerebral amyloid (congophilic) angiopathy (CAA) – a vascular lesion more commonly associated with brain hemorrhage than ischemia – describes a microvascular lesion that involves both parenchymal and leptomeningeal arterioles, whereby their medial and/or adventitial components are replaced by an eosinophilic hyaline material with distinctive biochemical properties [148, 162, 163]. CAA is associated with both stroke and dementia. This microvascular lesion is one of the key microscopic lesions which, when found 'in excess' in the CNS, provide morphologic support for the clinical diagnosis of Alzheimer disease (AD) [152]. The most common form of CAA is that associated with deposition, within arterial walls, of A$\beta$ protein, a small, unique, approximately 4.2 kDa peptide cleaved from the amyloid precursor protein (APP), encoded by a gene on chromosome 21 [152, 163]. AD is associated with excessive deposition of A$\beta$ in both the brain parenchyma (as senile plaques, SPs) and as CAA.

Relatively rare familial forms of CAA are also found in various geographic locations. In a circumscribed coastal region of the Netherlands, a familial type of severe CAA (hereditary cerebral hemorrhage with amyloidosis, Dutch type/HCHWA-D) is attributed to a unique APP gene mutation (at codon 693). Massive A$\beta$ deposition occurs within the media of cerebral arterioles, and fatal cerebral parenchymal hemorrhages frequently result [16, 92, 115, 160]. An Icelandic form of CAA leading to hemorrhagic stroke, hereditary cerebral hemorrhage with amyloidosis, Icelandic type (HCHWA-I), results from mutation in the gene encoding cystatin C/gamma-trace – hence this condition is also sometimes described as hereditary cystatin C amyloid angiopathy (HCCAA). It causes cerebral bleeds in young and middle-aged adults. Brains from HCHWA-I patients show extensive deposition of gamma-trace protein within arteriolar walls, associated with their degeneration [120, 165].

Setting aside the relatively rare examples of familial CAA, over 80% of brains originating from patients with autopsy-confirmed AD/SDAT (senile dementia of Alzheimer type) show some degree of (A$\beta$) CAA, involving cerebral vessels in one or more cortical regions [46]. Brains with moderate to severe CAA have a significantly higher frequency of ischemic or hemorrhagic lesions than do those with negligible CAA. CAA increases in extent and severity with advancing age. Moderate to severe CAA is found in as many as 12%–13% of brains from (unselected) patients over 85 years of age. Among consecutive autopsies on AD patients, moderate to severe CAA has been noted in over 25% [65, 66]. All regions of neocortex and overlying meninges may be affected by CAA, though there are minor variations in the distribution of affected arteries among lobes [99, 157]. Whereas the cerebellum and its meninges are occasionally involved by CAA, the microangiopathy is virtually never found within deep central gray matter, subcortical white matter, or brain stem. Selected light microscopic and immunohistochemical features of CAA are highlighted in Figs. 1 and 7.

The severity of CAA within a region of brain, or even a single affected arteriolar segment, can be graded, depending upon the degree of smooth muscle cell (SMC) replacement by amyloid within the media. Grade 1 CAA defines deposition of amyloid protein among SMC in an otherwise intact arteriolar segment, whereas grade 3 CAA describes arteriolar media entirely replaced by amyloid, with associated disruption of the vessel wall [164]. The extent of amyloid deposition within vessel walls correlates with an increasing risk of cerebral hemorrhage. A variety of CAA-

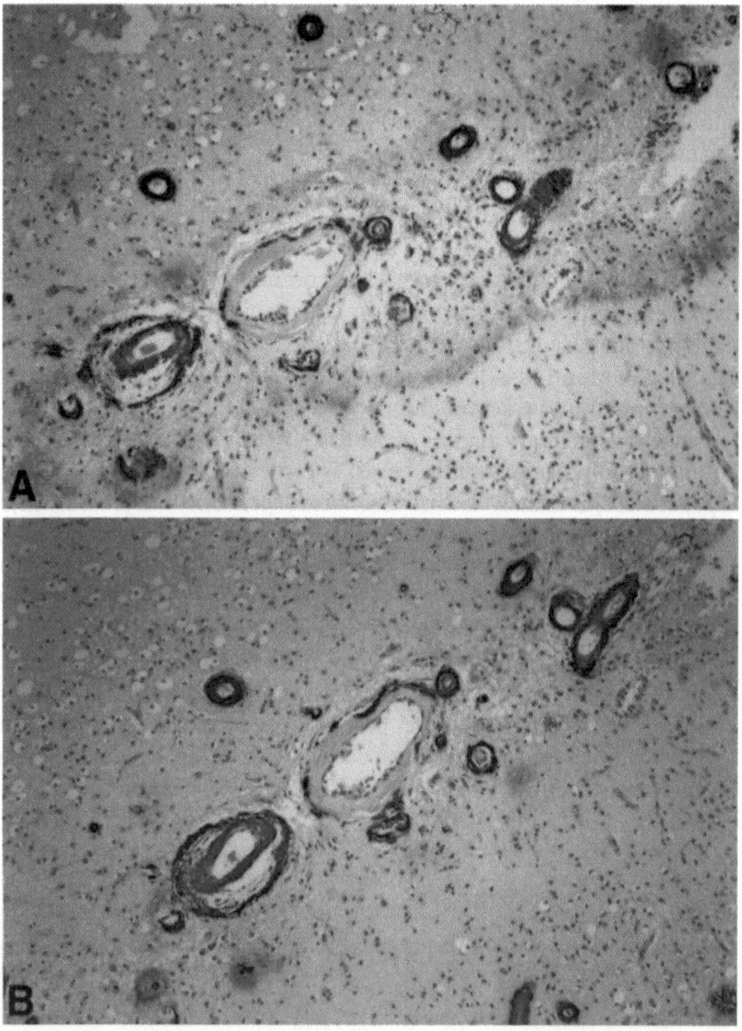


**Fig. 7 A, B.** CAA. **A** Biopsy specimen from a patient with brain hemorrhage caused by CAA. Sections stained with primary antibodies to A$\beta$ 1–42 (**A**) and A$\beta$ 1–40 (**B**) show abundant immunoreactive amyloid material in the media of parenchymal arterioles and both media and adventitia of meningeal arteries. Negligible parenchymal amyloid is seen, apart from subpial A$\beta$ immunoreactivity in **A** and scattered, rare senile plaques. Large artery at the center shows non-A$\beta$-immunoreactive thickening and fibrosis, a manifestation of CAA-associated microangiopathy. **A, B** ×110

associated microangiopathies (CAA-AM) have been described, including fibrosis, microaneurysm formation, chronic (including granulomatous) inflammation, 'double-barreling', fibrinoid necrosis and (very rarely) vessel wall calcification [94, 151, 162]. The pathogenesis of CAA is incompletely understood. SMCs appear to be able to synthesize APP mRNA and A$\beta$ protein [84, 114, 135]. Various types of A$\beta$ peptide, including ones that carry the amino acid substitution encoded by the

HCHWA-D codon 693 APP mutation, show pronounced cytotoxicity when added to SMC cultures [36, 166].

**Vasculitis.** As a cause of stroke, vasculitis (angiitis) is much less common than either atherosclerosis or arteriosclerosis. However, because vasculitis is potentially treatable, recognizing its manifestations is crucial for optimal patient management. The CNS may be affected by systemic vasculitides, or primary angiitis involving only the brain. Key reviews have summarized the pathogenesis of these comparatively rare conditions [21, 31, 126]. Whereas entities such as polyarteritis nodosa and Wegener granulomatosis commonly involve both the CNS and PNS, hypersensitivity vasculitis rarely (in less than 10% of cases) results in neurologic dysfunction. Vasculitic lesions are usually classified by (1) the size, type and distribution of blood vessels affected, and (2) the nature of the inflammatory infiltrate that accompanies vessel wall injury or destruction (fibrinoid necrosis).

Reviews of primary angiitis of the CNS (PACNS) report a preponderance of males among pathologically verified cases. The age at diagnosis (in both biopsy and autopsy studies) is usually in the fifth or sixth decades of life [21, 31, 126]. Patients with PACNS experience a range of neurologic symptoms, varying from headaches or diffuse neurologic dysfunction to ischemic or hemorrhagic stroke. Histopathologic features of PACNS may vary from a dense lymphocytic infiltrate with or without fibrinoid necrosis, to granulomatous inflammation with prominent multinucleated giant cells (Fig. 8). In recent years it has been recognized that severe CAA in elderly patients may be associated with a severe granulomatous angiitis; thus in geriatric patients who show vasculitis on brain biopsy or in a fragment of brain evacuated together with clot material (from a patient with intraparenchymal hemorrhage), A$\beta$ immunohistochemistry on the surgical material is clearly indicated [4, 162].

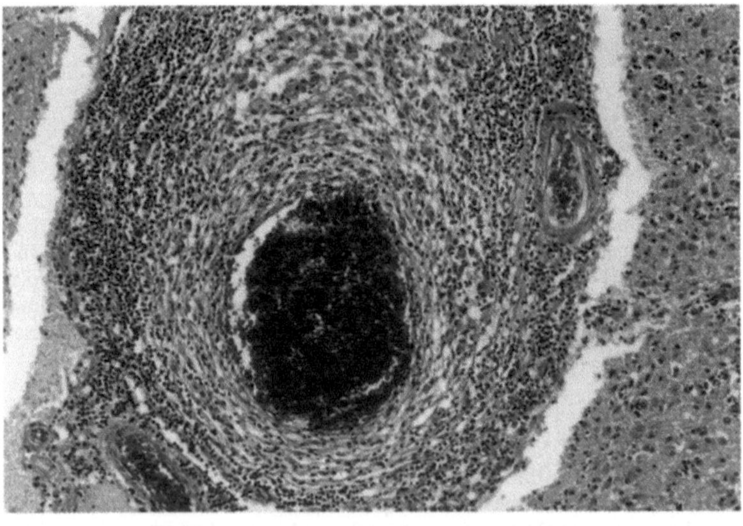

**Fig. 8.** Primary angiitis of the CNS. Note vessel wall is totally replaced, thickened, and effaced by chronic inflammatory cells. In this case, multinucleated giant cells were not present. H&E, ×110

Arguably the most common form of vasculitis among the elderly is giant cell arteritis/angiitis (GCA). Its annual incidence has been estimated to be as high as 17–18 per 100,000, over the age of 50 years [76]. This form of angiitis is eminently responsive to steroid therapy. The multifocal nature of the angiitis is reflected in its various patterns of presentation, which may include headache, visual complaints, and the syndrome of polymyalgia rheumatica [58, 133]. Vessels commonly involved (at autopsy) include the aorta, coronary and cerebral arteries (including the central retinal artery), and arteries of the head and neck [58, 133, 172]. Devastating ischemic infarcts have been documented in patients with GCA who develop occlusion of the MCA and anterior cerebral artery (ACA) [77]. Frequently, patients undergo temporal artery biopsy to confirm the diagnosis. An affected vessel shows a transmural lymphohistiocytic infiltrate, among which multinucleated giant cells may be prominent. 'Skip' areas may occur in a biopsy, so special care must be utilized in its assessment, including the examination of the specimen at multiple levels and in step-serial sections. Typical histopathologic features of GCA may persist in affected arteries even after successful steroid therapy [48].

The etiology of GCA is not well understood. An etiologic association between GCA and varicella zoster infection of the arterial wall has been suggested but seems unlikely [117]. Humoral immunity may be involved in its pathogenesis, given the finding of intracellular and extracellular immunoglobulin and complement deposition within the inflamed arterial wall. The polyclonal lymphocytic infiltrate in GCA is mainly of T-cell type, with CD4 (T-helper) cells exceeding CD8 (T-suppressor) cells, and cellular immunity is likely to be important in disease causation. Interleukin (IL)-1 and IL-2 are present within GCA lesions, and serum IL-6 and thrombomodulin levels are elevated. The inflammatory infiltrate noted within affected arterial walls may represent a reaction to an as-yet-unidentified microbial pathogen [59, 64].

## 4.2 Brain Embolism

Embolic brain infarcts may result whenever a mass of solid or undissolved material, usually (though not always) consisting of platelet-fibrin aggregates or thrombus, is carried in the blood-stream and lodges in blood vessels supplying the brain. In general, the solid material forms within, or is introduced into, the systemic arterial circulation, or forms in the venous circulation but has unrestricted passage to the arterial circulation, e.g., via a right-to-left cardiac shunt [47]. Most emboli that cause brain infarcts originate within either (1) an atheromatous plaque (atheroemboli) [12, 85] or (2) the heart. Other sources of emboli to the brain include fat (following bone fractures) and particulate material that enters the circulation during cardiothoracic surgical procedures, cerebral angiography or interventional embolotherapy procedures.

Table 2 summarizes the most common sources of cardiogenic emboli that cause cerebral infarct [12, 73, 149]. In most large series, embolic infarcts are less common than infarcts resulting from thrombi in the major cranial or cervical arteries, and probably account for 5%–25% of ischemic brain infarcts. Patients at risk for thrombotic occlusion of a cervical or intracranial artery are also the ones likely to develop a cardiac lesion – e.g., a hypokinetic myocardial wall segment with mural thrombus following a myocardial infarct – that predisposes to an embolic event. As many as

Table 2. Potential sources of cardiogenic emboli (adapted and modified from [12])

1. Isolated arrhythmias (40%–45%)
   Most commonly atrial fibrillation and sick sinus syndrome
2. Isolated myocardial abnormalities (25%–30%)
   Post-myocardial infarct:
   Global or focal left ventricular akinesia, with/without thrombus
   Ventricular aneurysm
   Patent foramen ovale
   Left atrial myxoma or thrombus
3. Isolated valvular abnormalities (20%–25%)
   Mitral valve prolapse or stenosis, prosthetic valve(s)
   Infectious and non-bacterial thrombotic (marantic) endocarditis
   Mitral annulus calcification
   Mitral valve prolapse/myxomatous degeneration
4. Arrhythmias and myocardial abnormalities (3%–5%)
5. Arrhythmias and valvular abnormalities (3%–5%)

2.5% of patients with an acute myocardial infarct develop a stroke within 2–4 weeks of the heart attack [26]. Neurologic features suggestive of embolic (rather than thrombotic) brain infarct include abrupt onset of maximal neurologic deficit, headache and loss of consciousness at stroke onset, and clinical or imaging evidence for at least two distinct sites of embolization – either within the brain, or involving the brain and a non-CNS site. However, the use of purely clinical criteria to distinguish thrombotic from embolic stroke often leads to an inaccurate diagnosis. Non-rheumatic atrial fibrillation is clearly associated with an age-dependent stroke incidence that rises from 2.8% in the sixth decade of life, to 7.1% in the ninth [26].

Cardiogenic emboli usually migrate to the MCA bifurcation in the Sylvian fissure or to distal MCA branches, less commonly to the vertebrobasilar system; in the latter, they often lodge at the 'tip' (upper end) of the basilar artery, producing neurologic symptoms referable to the visual cortex. In deciding whether an occluded artery has undergone embolic occlusion or in situ thrombosis, a pathologist must consider the degree of complicated atherosclerosis in the affected vessel. Thrombus superimposed on a large, focally calcified and ulcerated plaque – and attached to intima – is likely to have developed in situ. A platelet-fibrin plug, clearly detached from the intima or focally adherent to it, in a relatively normal artery is more likely to be embolic (Fig. 9).

Valvular abnormalities are of several types:

- Endocarditis. Infective endocarditis (IE) may affect a native or prosthetic heart valve, usually the mitral, aortic, or both. Neurologic abnormalities may be the presenting feature of IE. Native valves most likely to develop IE are those which show either congenital or acquired abnormalities, e.g., secondary to rheumatic valvular disease. Normal valves may become colonized by microorganisms as a consequence of intravenous drug use or hyperalimentation, immunosuppression or nosocomial infection. An estimated 15%–25% of patients with IE develop embolic infarcts. While most brain infarcts associated with IE are comparatively small, those seen with *Staphylococcus aureus* infection may be very large. Other neurologic complications of IE include abscesses, 'mycotic' (infective) aneurysms, meningitis, encephalopathy, and intraparenchymal hemorrhage.

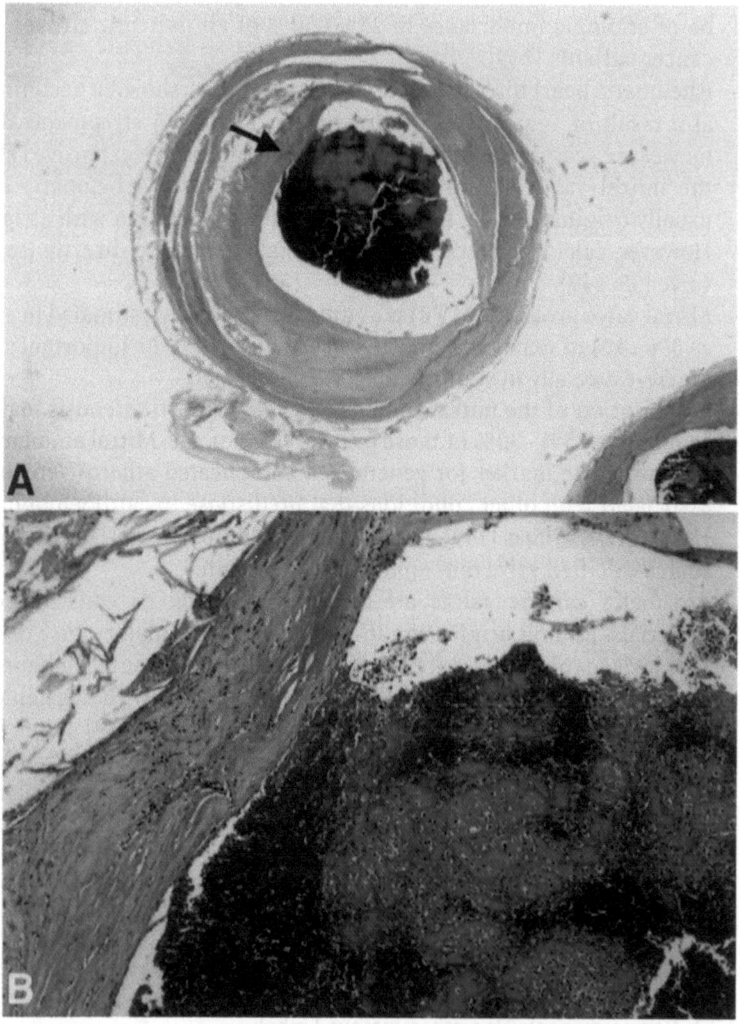


**Fig. 9 A, B.** Embolus. An artery showing only moderate atheroma, although the lumen contains occlusive platelet-fibrin material. The relatively minimal atherosclerotic change in this artery and absence of intimal ulceration suggest that this is an embolus rather than in situ thrombosis. *Arrow* (**A**) indicates region that is shown enlarged in **B**, indicating site of attachment of the embolus to arterial wall. H&E; **A** ×20, **B** ×110

- Non-bacterial thrombotic endocarditis (NBTE), also described as marantic endocarditis, an entity of uncertain pathogenesis, may complicate a wasting disease such as AIDS or widespread malignancy [10, 26, 149]. It is also seen with various non-neoplastic diseases of the heart, gastrointestinal tract, and lungs. Aortic and mitral valves are the ones most commonly affected. Brain embolism is documented in approximately $^1/_3$ of patients. Patients who come to autopsy following acute stroke in conjunction with any condition that has placed them at risk for developing NBTE should be suspected to have this entity until proven otherwise by a thorough examination of the heart. NBTE has been suggested to be of etiologic importance in 25%–30% of all ischemic strokes countered in cancer patients [149].

- Rheumatic heart disease has, over recent decades, shown a declining prevalence as a result of aggressive early treatment of group A streptococcal infection. It may cause scarring and deformation, sometimes with extensive calcification, of the mitral valve. Cerebral emboli in patients with rheumatic heart disease usually originate in the left atrium, often in association with atrial fibrillation. However, calcified debris or thrombus may embolize directly from the mitral valve [55, 149].
- Mitral valve prolapse (MVP) is a controversial entity estimated to affect as many as 3%–4% of males and over 5% of females [149]. Its importance as a cause of stroke, especially in young people, is still debated.
- Calcification of the mitral annulus and calcific aortic stenosis may be found in as many as 25%–30% of those over 90 years of age. Mitral annular calcification is a surrogate marker for generalized complicated atherosclerosis, and is also associated with other conditions that predispose to cardioembolic stroke, e.g., IE and arrhythmias [149]. Rarely, calcified embolic material that originates from such a calcified valve may embolize to the brain.
- Prosthetic cardiac valves are either mechanical or constructed from biomaterials. Emboli originating in both types are a major cause of brain infarct [147]. Mechanical valves are associated with a significantly higher risk of thromboembolism than are bioprostheses; hence, patients with mechanical valves are usually maintained on long-term anticoagulation [26, 149]. When such patients develop an acute neurologic deficit, anticoagulant-related intraparenchymal cerebral hemorrhage is an important diagnostic consideration. Late prosthetic valve IE develops with roughly equal frequency on mechanical and bioprosthetic valves; however, major neurologic complications (with a higher mortality) are more common with mechanical valves, especially those replacing the native mitral valve.

### 4.2.1 Non-cardiogenic/Non-atheromatous Emboli

Fat emboli are usually associated with fractures of long bones or the pelvis (often after a motor-vehicle accident), but may complicate soft tissue trauma and cardiothoracic surgical procedures [40, 47, 82]. Encephalopathic signs may predominate, with restlessness confusion, stupor, or coma, but respiratory insufficiency often dominates the clinical picture, and some of the neurologic signs and symptoms are probably attributable to hypoxia. Cerebral findings at autopsy include widespread petechial hemorrhages in the white matter. Fat emboli within small arteries may be demonstrable by fat stains carried out on frozen sections of involved brain regions.

Other types of emboli include fragments of neoplasm, which may embolize to the brain in patients with widespread malignancy. Parasites or parasitic ova may do likewise. Air embolism occurs with decompression sickness and can complicate cardiac bypass surgery. Cardiac surgery may also result in unintentional embolization to the CNS of material or debris that is either released from a lesion or introduced during the procedure itself. Emboli of intervertebral disc material have been demonstrated in the spinal cord [47]. Surgical and autopsy pathologists should keep in mind that intentional iatrogenic embolization is now an accepted way of treating many cerebral vascular malformations (especially arteriovenous malformations) and even certain extra-axial brain tumors. These procedures have been in widespread use for at least 15–20 years, and materials injected into CNS lesions or ones that go 'astray' upon injection may be encountered years later, because many of them are not effectively resorbed after lodging within the brain. A large variety of embolotherapy materials are used, and many elicit a brisk granulomatous inflammatory reaction that can persist for months or years – in some cases perhaps indefinitely [134, 159].

## 4.3 Brain Infarcts – Gross and Microscopic Features

Cerebral infarcts can be classified as either hemorrhagic or non-hemorrhagic, though in reality many have both components. Bland infarcts have historically been attributed to complete obstruction of blood flow to a region of brain, whereas hemorrhagic infarcts have been thought to result from reperfusion of an infarcted brain region. Hemorrhagic infarcts more commonly result from emboli than from in situ thrombosis [3, 22, 47, 81, 156]. Post-anoxic-ischemic tissue edema may lead to venous compression and elevated intravascular pressures, exacerbating the likelihood of hemorrhage into necrotic tissue.

Early changes of coagulative necrosis occur 8–48 h after a region of brain is rendered ischemic [47, 81, 156]. The cortex-white matter junction becomes effaced, and affected cortex becomes dusky, secondary to hyperemia due to vascular dilatation. Cerebral edema reaches a maximum at 48–96 h after an infarct has occurred – during this time, the risk of fatal brain herniation is maximal. Infarcted tissue becomes clearly delineated from intact CNS and a separation of necrotic from relatively normal brain may appear as a 'cracking artefact'. Between 7 days and 3–4 weeks after infarction, liquefactive necrosis develops. After approximately 3 weeks, cavitation of brain substance begins, and abundant macrophages may be seen within the necrotic tissue cavity by light microscopy. The infarct is eventually replaced by an irregular fluid-filled cyst traversed by fine blood vessels and irregular glial fibers. Overlying meninges may become thickened and somewhat opaque. Usually, there is preservation of an intensely gliotic molecular layer of cortex overlying the infarct. If resolution of the infarct occurs, collapse and contraction of surrounding tissues may be prominent, while an adjacent ventricle may enlarge. The lining of a large cystic cavity resulting from an infarct (e.g., in the MCA territory) will often collapse as the brain is removed from the calvarium at autopsy (Fig. 10).

Microscopic features of evolving infarct follow a characteristic sequence, though with variation among patients (Fig. 11) [47, 81, 139, 156]. Between 6 and 24 h after irreversible ischemia, neurons become shrunken and angulated and the cytoplasm takes on an intense eosinophilia (in hematoxylin and eosin-stained sections). Within white matter, axons become swollen and fragmented, myelin pale and eventually myelin sheaths disintegrate. Astrocytes and endothelial cells also swell. Microvacuolation becomes visible, even by light microscopy. Polymorphonuclear leuko-

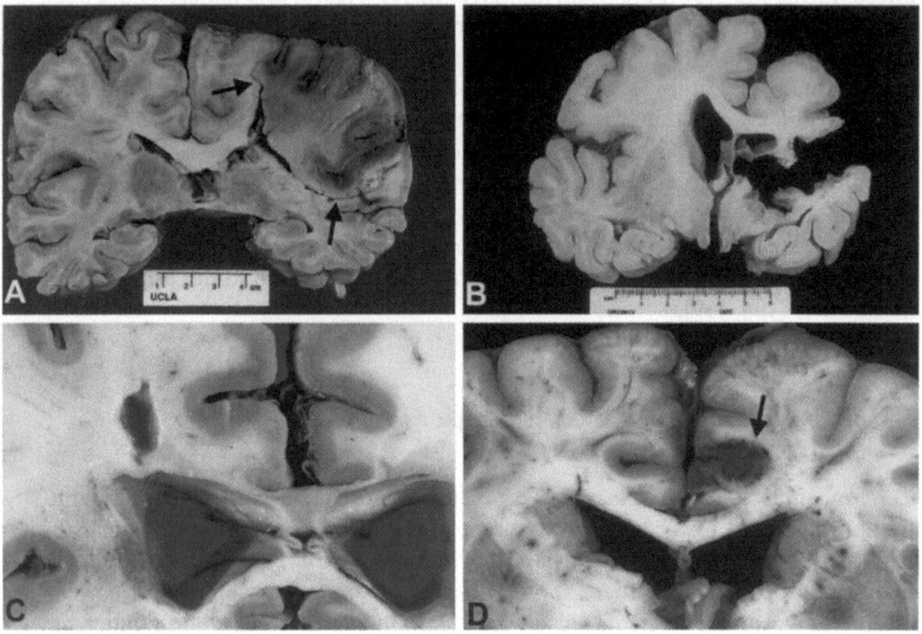


**Fig. 10 A–D.** Appearances of cerebral infarcts in coronal sections of fixed brain. Each panel represents image from a different patient. **A** Relatively recent infarct (exact time of occurrence prior to death unknown, but appearance suggests less than a week). *Arrows* indicate area of gray discoloration and softening in the right MCA territory. Note 'cracking' separation of infarcted brain from intact brain tissue. **B** Old (years) right MCA territory infarct shows a large cyst in right cerebral hemisphere, with collapse of surrounding tissue around the cavity. **C** Old left ACA territory infarct, showing region of cystic cavitation at base of the left cingulate gyrus and involving the corpus callosum. **D** Small hemorrhagic infarct (*arrow*) in right mesial frontal region, also in the ACA territory

cytes (PMNs) may migrate into the region of the infarct within 1–3 days after its occurrence, though this occurs much less consistently than after infarcts in other organs, e.g., the heart. Approximately 48 h after infarction, macrophages appear in increasing numbers at the edge of an infarct, phagocytose breakdown products of neurons, axons, and myelin, and take on a foamy/granular appearance. Most of the macrophages that infiltrate brain infarcts are bone marrow-derived cells, but some may have lived inconspicuously as resident microglia within the brain [141]. Macrophage density tends to be highest 2–3 weeks following an infarct. Thereafter, they decrease in number, though many may persist at the edges or center of an infarct that was clearly documented to have occurred years prior to a patient's death.

**Fig. 11 A–C.** Microscopic features of cerebral infarct. **A, B** Regions of white matter (**A**) and cortex (**B**) from a patient with 2- to 3-day history suggestive of large cerebral infarct. White matter (**A**) shows geographic, well-delineated regions of vacuolization separated by islands of intact tissue. Cortex (**B**) shows confluent areas of necrosis and microvacuolization within which prominent neuronal eosinophilia was noted. **C** Old infarct. Center of micrograph shows many histiocytes, while surrounding tissue is packed with gemistocytic (reactive) astrocytes. H&E; A and B ×35, C ×90

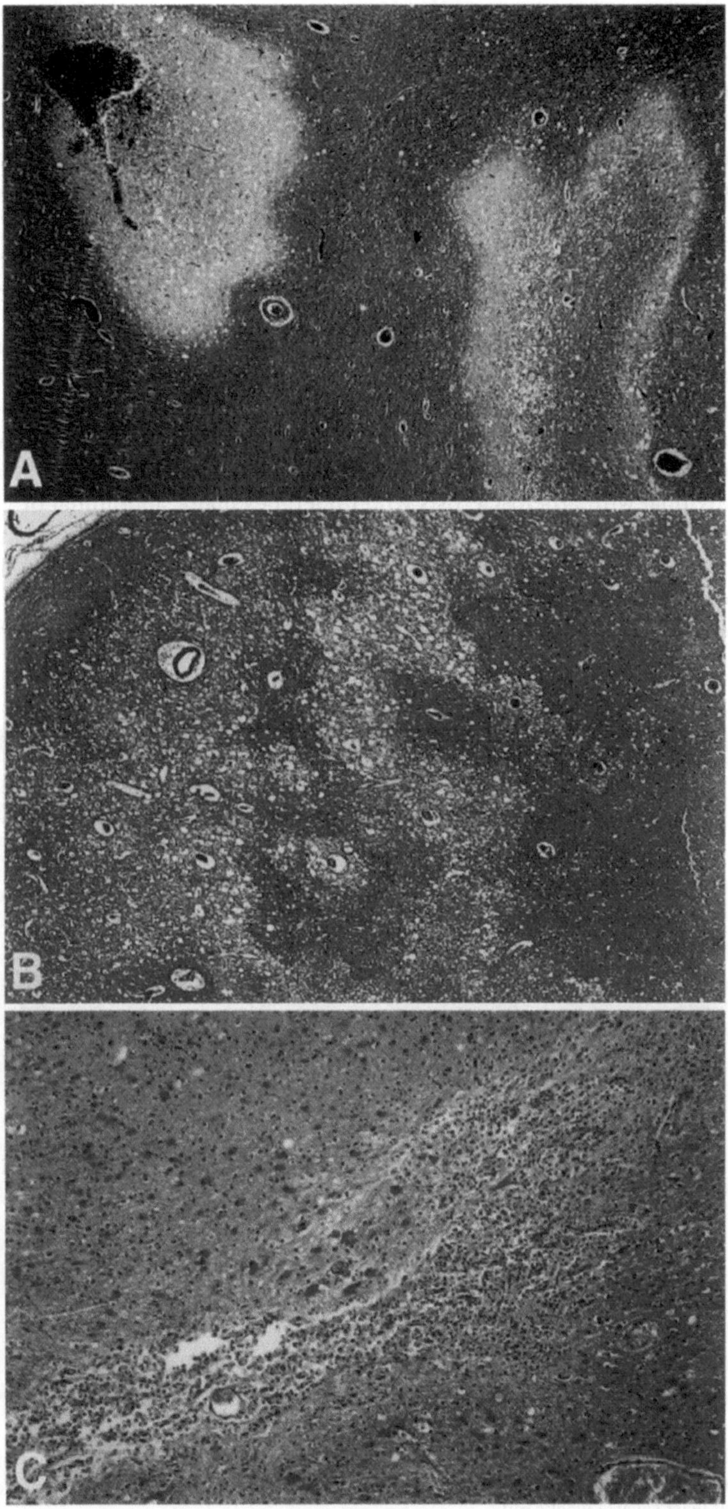
A
B
C

Between 2 and 4 weeks after infarction, endothelial proliferation with neovascularization occurs. Reactive astrocytes proliferate at the margins of the infarct and become hypertrophic, often taking on the appearance of gemistocytes. Eventually, 4–5 weeks after infarction, capillaries become less prominent, necrotic debris and macrophages are less conspicuous or may disappear altogether, and a dense glial scar forms around the infarct cavity.

**Watershed or Border-Zone Infarcts.** These occur along the boundaries between two arterial territories, generally of major vessels such as the ACA and MCA. However, watershed infarcts may affect the brain stem, basal ganglia, and cerebellum (Fig. 12) [142]. When present in the cerebral hemispheres, borderzone infarcts are often symmetrical bilaterally in both size and location. Several hypotheses as to their pathogenesis have been proposed, including profound hypotension and microemboli [2, 19]. Borderzone infarcts are most commonly associated with a sharp, often sustained, drop in systemic blood pressure – e.g., in an elderly individual with atherosclerosis who undergoes major abdominal or cardiovascular surgery. Decrease in blood flow under such circumstances appears to be most severe in the arterial 'end-fields'. The regional reduction in blood flow may itself cause neuronal death or frank infarction, but may also promote the deposition of emboli composed of cholesterol crystals or atheromatous debris from a plaque.

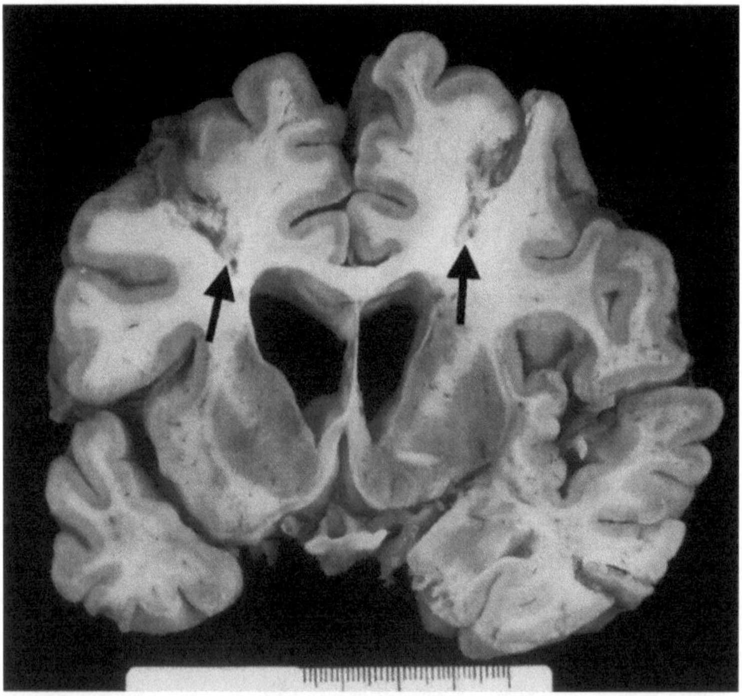

**Fig. 12.** Watershed/borderzone infarcts. *Arrows* indicate symmetrical regions of wedge-shaped encephalomalacia in the border zones between ACA and MCA territories. Infarcts appear to be at least several weeks old

**Lacunar Infarcts.** As mentioned above, arteriosclerosis (AS) or lipohyalinosis (LH) have been associated with lacunar infarcts and parenchymal brain hemorrhage. Lacunar infarcts are small (less than 15 mm maximal size) regions of cystic cavitation, most often seen within basal ganglia, thalamus, pons, internal capsule, and deep subcortical white matter (Fig. 13) [104–106]. When found in abundance within the subcortical white matter, they may be associated with the clinical syndrome of Binswanger's subcortical leukoencephalopathy (BSLE), a variant of vascular dementia. Lacunar infarcts are to be distinguished from prominently enlarged perivascular spaces, which they may almost perfectly mimic on gross – and sometimes even microscopic – examination of the brain at necropsy [27]. Despite the historical association between lacunas, AS/LH and high blood pressure, a history of hypertension is not found in as many as 35%–40% of individuals with these small, deep brain infarcts [107]. It has even been suggested that lacunes result from carotid atherosclerosis (and are due to hemodynamic changes and/or atheroemboli) or even non-atheromatous emboli [167]. Lacunar infarcts have been associated with several stroke syndromes. One large study found that, while lacunar stroke syndromes are highly predictive of finding lacunas on appropriate imaging studies, in approximately 25% of patients such syndromes are associated with nonlacunar types of infarction [57]. Small areas of cystic cavitation resembling lacunar infarcts may rarely result from non-hypertensive vascular disease, e.g., meningovascular syphilis.

Occluded arteries of varying caliber may be found in close proximity to lacunar infarcts. When the abnormal artery is of diameter 40–200 µm, it may show typical features of AS/LH, whereas larger arteries (of up to 500 µm diameter) may contain microatheroma within their lumens and walls [6, 168]. Defining the clinicopatho-

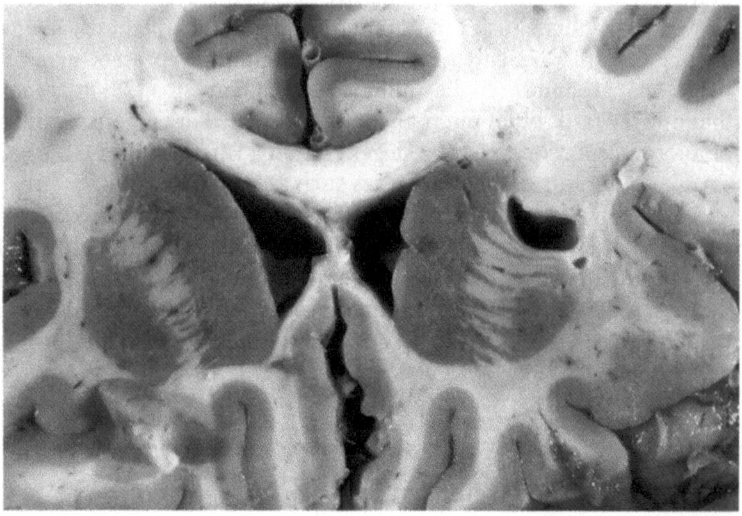

**Fig. 13.** Lacunar infarct. Small cystic infarct, with a smooth cavity lining, is noted in right internal capsule and adjacent basal ganglia. These infarcts are classically associated with longstanding hypertension and AS/LH (see text), though they may occasionally be the result of large artery atherosclerosis

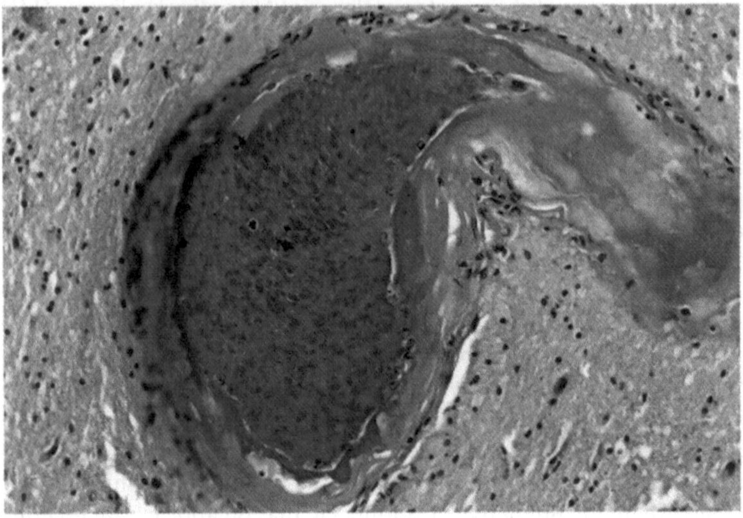

**Fig. 14.** Charcot-Bouchard microaneurysm, a characteristic complication of cerebral arteriolar degeneration, regardless of cause. In this patient, it was seen in the context of longstanding arteriosclerosis/lipohyalinosis. Upper right shows 'parent artery', from which a balloon-like outpouching (center of micrograph) has developed. H & E, ×220

logic substrates of lacunes is especially difficult, given that the lesions are frequently asymptomatic [145].

Miliary microaneurysms of Charcot-Bouchard (C-B) type have been reported to be present in many hypertensive patients with parenchymal hemorrhage [30]. More recent study of cerebral microvessels in the brains of hypertensive patients, by use of cytochemistry and microradiographic methods, suggests that C-B aneurysms are rare and may sometimes simply represent arteriolar 'coils and twists' that are interpreted as miliary microaneurysms [28]. It is the author's view that miliary (C-B type) microaneurysms (Fig. 14) are a nonspecific manifestation of microvascular or arteriolar degeneration – whether this be the result of AS/LH, CAA, or other less-common entities such as CADASIL.

Infarcts in specific vascular territories, the result of atherosclerotic or embolic occlusion of major branches of the circle of Willis, or more proximal segments of the carotid or vertebrobasilar systems, produce characteristic neurologic syndromes. A detailed discussion of these is beyond the scope of this chapter, but the reader is referred to detailed descriptions of their clinicopathologic features [7, 11, 37, 39, 56, 72, 86, 139].

## 4.4 Venous Thrombosis

Thrombosis of dural venous sinuses occurs as an infrequent complication of various infectious and noninfectious processes, including polycythemia, sickle cell anemia (or trait), paroxysmal nocturnal hemoglobinuria, trauma, vasculitis, pregnancy, use of oral contraceptives, congenital heart disease, presence of circulating lupus anticoagulants, dehydration, marasmus, and compression by mass lesions such as neoplasms or aneurysms [17, 41, 50, 88, 137, 170]. Recent reviews have emphasized that cerebral venous thrombosis (CVT) is more common than previously thought, has a wide variety of clinical presentations, may have a favorable outcome, and is treatable with heparin or selective catheterization and urokinase infusion [45, 75].

The cavernous sinuses, located at the skull base superior and lateral to the sphenoid sinuses, are the ones most commonly involved by septic thrombosis. The most common primary site of infection associated with cavernous sinus thrombosis is the medial part of the face. Common causal pathogens include gram-positive bacteria, especially *Staph. aureus* [41]. Infection of the ethmoid and sphenoid air sinuses and dental infections are also conditions that predispose to septic cavernous sinus thrombosis.

Thrombosis in the cavernous sinus can extend to involve other dural sinuses, e.g., the petrosal, sigmoid, lateral and inferior sinuses [137]. Spread of infection to the pituitary gland, and its resultant necrosis, have been described, as have complications such as meningitis, brain abscess formation, and cortical vein thrombosis with brain infarction. Septic lateral sinus thrombosis is nearly always associated with spread of infection from the mastoid air cells after otitis media [41, 137]. Pathogens usually associated with otitis media or mastoiditis include *Proteus* species, *Staph. aureus*, anaerobes or *E. coli*. Lateral sinus thrombosis may extend to involve the superior sagittal sinus. Primary septic thrombosis of the superior sagittal sinus occurs less commonly than thrombosis of the cavernous or lateral sinuses. The most common predisposing condition is bacterial meningitis, especially in children.

## 5 Intracranial Hemorrhage

Hemorrhage into the various intracranial compartments will be considered separately, beginning with the most superficial. This is an arbitrary separation, since some etiologic mechanisms operative in (as one example) subarachnoid hemorrhage are also important in the pathogenesis of parenchymal bleeding. Furthermore, hematomas in one 'compartment' can easily extend into another – primary intraparenchymal bleeds may extend into the ventricular cavities, thence into the subarachnoid space.

### 5.1 Extradural/Epidural Hemorrhage

Extradural/epidural hemorrhage (EDH) is usually considered in relation to craniocerebral trauma, with which it is almost invariably linked. Spontaneous EDH is an extraordinarily rare event [47]. In a large series of fatal head injuries from an Irish neurosurgical unit, neuropathologic findings included EDH in 18% of patients, acute intracerebral hematoma in 27%, subdural hematoma (SDH) in

45%, and skull fracture in 69% [9]. Other studies suggest that over 90% of EDH patients are likely to have a skull fracture [35]. After a closed head injury, EDH can present with a rapidly evolving neurologic deficit, because hemorrhage is usually from a high-pressure arterial source (typically, the middle meningeal artery) adjacent to a skull fracture. However, because the dura is often firmly adherent to the inner surface of the skull, the accumulation of blood in the extradural space and the resulting development of neurologic symptoms and signs may be delayed by several hours (the lucid interval). Rarely, EDH results from the tearing of a venous sinus. EDH may occur together with SDH. EDH is found in 5%–15% of non-missile head injuries. The blood clot most commonly occupies the temporal fossa in adults, the posterior fossa in children. Mortality from this condition is highest in the geriatric population. However, if treated early by drainage of the clotted blood, patients may make a satisfactory recovery, provided substantial damage to underlying brain tissue has not occurred.

Documentation of a fatal EDH must be made at the time of necropsy; if this is not done immediately after removal of the calvarium, another opportunity will not arise. On removing the calvarium, the hematoma is readily seen between the fractured skull and the dura. After removal of the brain, further accumulation of blood is usually visible through the dura covering one middle fossa or part of the posterior fossa. As patients who have succumbed to EDH are often the subject of a forensic or medicolegal investigation, the size and site of any (causal) skull fracture and the volume of the hematoma needs to be assessed – bleeds of 75–100 ml are usually fatal. The dura should be stripped for detailed examination of the skull. The pathologist should also document effects of the hematoma on the brain (e.g., distortion, herniations) and any associated scalp lesions, brain contusions and lacerations, and other effects of trauma.

## 5.2 Subdural Hemorrhage

Subdural hemorrhages (SDHs) may be either acute or chronic, and are a major problem in the elderly. They have protean clinical manifestations, and frequently insidious evolution and presentation. Unlike EDH, they are not consistently associated with clinically perceived, documented, or reported trauma. Their clinical evolution may occur with a more indolent tempo, since bleeding is usually from a venous source, i.e., bridging veins between the dura and the leptomeninges. In a small number of patients, SDH may represent dissection of blood from the subarachnoid space – where it has originated from an arterial source such as a ruptured berry aneurysm or arteriovenous malformation (see below) [47, 139, 156].

The pathogenesis of acute SDH is usually traumatic, involving the head being subjected to rapid acceleration or deceleration. Under these circumstances, movement of the brain, having inertia of some 1,250–1,400 g, lags in relation to that of the skull. This causes stretching, and possible tearing, of the aforementioned bridging veins between the brain surface and dura mater, the latter being tightly adherent to the inner table of the skull. Chronic SDH begins with rupture of the same bridging veins, but acute hemorrhage is followed by cycles of organization and rebleeding due to the formation of richly vascular granulation tissue (pseudomembrane) around the hematoma [47, 54, 156]. Patients with impaired hemostasis (disease-associated or iatrogenic coagulopathy, platelet abnormalities) may develop spontaneous acute or chronic SDH, as may patients with dural tumors (metastases, meningiomas) or vascular malformations. In patients with hematologic malignancies or abnormal coagulation, 'smear' subdural hematomas, of no clinical importance, are commonly found at autopsy (Fig. 15).

SDH, which may be bilateral, should be suspected and looked for in any patient who has experienced head trauma. The clinical diagnosis of chronic SDH in the elderly is often difficult and a history of trauma is often lacking [43, 138]. Progression of clinical signs and symptoms may be 'stuttering' or slow; in some patients, dementia may be the presenting feature. Chronic SDH is especially common in people with cerebral atrophy due to aging or Alzheimer's disease, in whom dementia secondary to the SDH may be difficult to differentiate from that due to underlying brain parenchymal disease. The increased risk of SDH in these patients is presumably because the bridging veins in these patients have a longer course and the atrophic brain is more mobile in relation to the skull. In patients who come to autopsy with SDH the precise size and location of the clot, and its impact on brain substance, need to be carefully documented.

In children, the demonstration of SDH should prompt consideration of possible non-accidental injury. Careful review of the clinical history is particularly important in this age group. If non-accidental injury is a possibility, the autopsy investigation should include detailed postmortem radiology, and documentation and histologic assessment of all other cutaneous, skeletal, and visceral injuries. The eyes and attached intraorbital segments of optic nerve should be preserved for careful examination. Detailed review of the findings in non-accidental injury is beyond the scope of this chapter.

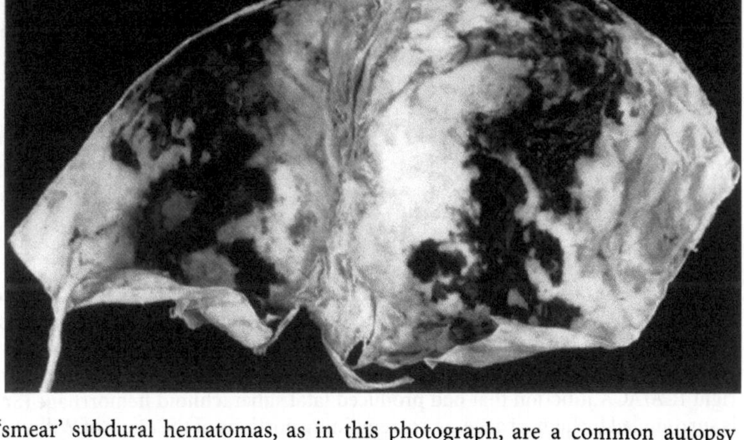

**Fig. 15.** Thin, 'smear' subdural hematomas, as in this photograph, are a common autopsy finding in patients who have coagulopathy or thrombocytopenia. They are almost always asymptomatic

## 5.3 Subarachnoid Hemorrhage

Hemorrhage into the subarachnoid space is a major cause of morbidity and mortality in people of all age groups beyond childhood. Subarachnoid hemorrhage (SAH) may be secondary to intraparenchymal brain hemorrhage (IPH), i. e., when there is extension of parenchymal hemorrhage into the subarachnoid space, or it may represent the result of rupture of an aneurysm on the circle of Willis, one of its branches or a distal arterial segment, a vascular malformation (hemangioma) within brain parenchyma or (rarely) involving the circle of Willis, a neoplasm, or systemic causes such as hematologic malignancy.

**Berry/Saccular Aneurysms.** An aneurysm may be defined as a localized and persistent pathologic dilatation of the heart or a blood vessel that results from the yielding of its wall components [139]. Berry aneurysms, also referred to as saccular or (incorrectly) congenital intracranial aneurysms, usually occur at major bifurcation points of the circle of Willis (Fig. 16). Over half involve anterior portions of the

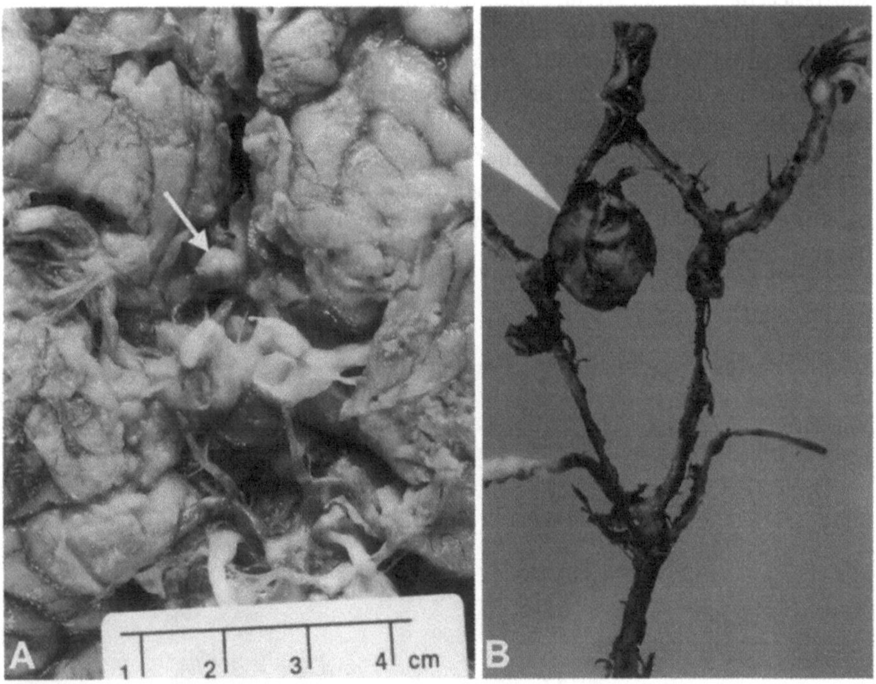


**Fig. 16. A** Berry (saccular) aneurysm (*arrow*) found at the right ACA/anterior communicating artery junction, in an elderly patient who underwent autopsy to determine cause of dementia. The aneurysm had been asymptomatic throughout her life, and there was no histologic evidence of prior subarachnoid hemorrhage. **B** Large berry aneurysm (indicated by *arrow*) at right ICA/ACA junction that had produced fatal subarachnoid hemorrhage (SAH). Aneurysm is surrounded by hemorrhage, as are remaining portions of the circle of Willis (abundant blood filled the basal cisterns at autopsy). Rupture site is visible in the aneurysm, immediately distal to tip of the *arrow*

circle of Willis, usually at the internal carotid (ICA)-posterior communicating artery or anterior choroidal artery junction, MCA bi/trifurcation in the Sylvian fissure, or anterior cerebral artery (ACA)-anterior communicating artery junction. Berry aneurysms may present with SAH at any age but usually do so between the ages of 40 and 70 years. In the Framingham Study, mean age at presentation with a SAH was essentially identical for men and women (62–63 years), whereas other studies suggest a mean age of aneurysmal rupture at around 55–60 years [110, 131]. Berry aneurysms are approximately 1.5- to 2 times more common in women than men. From 10% to 30% of patients have multiple aneurysms [169]. A typical aneurysm, since it expands gradually into the subarachnoid space, rarely produces symptoms prior to rupture. However, cranial nerves may be compressed as they exit the brain stem, leading to isolated palsies. Giant aneurysms (larger than 2.5 cm in diameter) may present as space-occupying lesions within the brain, in some cases producing longstanding neurobehavioral abnormalities [14]. Warning signs of an impending SAH (usually a small hemorrhage or 'sentinel bleed') are described in as many as 20% of patients who progress to having a larger bleed [169].

Though referred to as congenital, berry/saccular aneurysms are only rarely encountered in children or infants. The fact that the aneurysms themselves are not truly congenital does not rule out the possibility that an aneurysm found in later life represents expansion of a focus of congenital vascular weakening. This theory has, however, been disputed [139]. Alternatively, berry aneurysms may develop as a result of degenerative changes within cerebral blood vessels, possibly secondary to loss of tensile strength due to weakening of connective tissues and/or elastica within their walls. Theories on the pathogenesis of berry aneurysms abound [110, 131, 139]. An increased incidence of intracerebral aneurysm is seen in many systemic diseases, including polycystic kidney disease, Marfan and Ehlers-Danlos syndromes, pseudoxanthoma elasticum, fibromuscular dysplasia, sickle cell disease, and coarctation of the aorta. African-Americans have approximately twice the risk of SAH seen in the Caucasian population.

Rupture of a berry aneurysm usually produces life-threatening SAH (Fig. 17), though bleeding may occur directly into brain parenchyma, especially if the rupture site on the dome of the aneurysm is embedded within brain substance. Intraventricular hemorrhage may also occur, though usually this is secondary to extensive bleeding within the subarachnoid space. When an intraparenchymal hematoma is encountered in any patient, but especially a young person, berry aneurysm should be considered high in the etiologic differential diagnosis. The mortality from SAH secondary to a ruptured berry aneurysm is, unfortunately, as high as 35%–50% [15, 119]. Post-hemorrhage vasospasm, leading to multiple infarcts within the CNS, is a feared complication of a large SAH [83, 169]. Other causes of major post-bleed morbidity include the development of hydrocephalus (secondary to scarring of the meninges) or rebleeding. Successful clipping of an aneurysm by a skilled neurosurgeon with minimal postoperative complications may, however, be associated with an essentially normal life expectancy. Fig. 16 illustrates an example of an aneurysm found incidentally at autopsy, and another that had produced fatal subarachnoid hemorrhage.

Berry aneurysms are encountered as an incidental finding at autopsy, with an estimated frequency that varies tremendously – figures from 4%–17% are quoted [110, 169]. This variability probably reflects the 'size threshold' accepted by a given

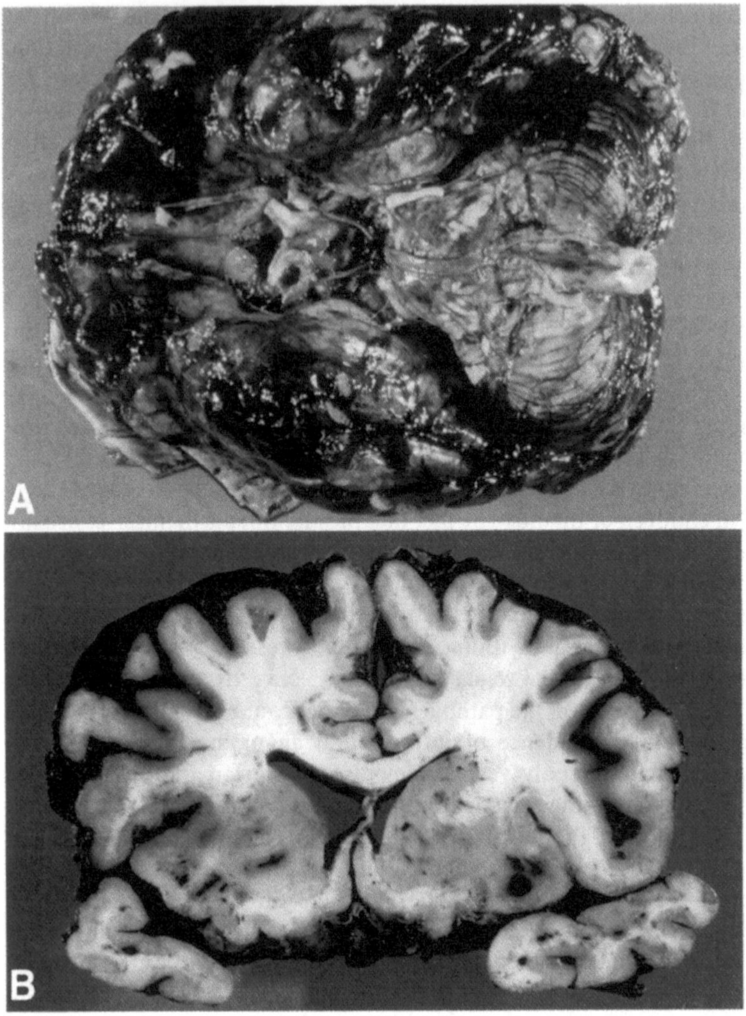


**Fig. 17.** **A** Acute, fatal SAH – note extensive blood at base of the brain. **B** Coronal section of fixed brain (same patient) shows a thick 'coating' of blood in the subarachnoid space, especially overlying the left cerebral hemisphere

**Fig. 18 A–C.** Berry (saccular) aneurysm, microscopic features. **A** Normal artery, stained with elastica van Gieson, to show internal elastic membrane. **B** Wall of a berry aneurysm (also stained for elastica) shows its complete absence in a somewhat thickened aneurysm wall. **C** Parallel section to that shown in **B**, stained with Masson trichrome, to show segmental fibrosis of the aneurysm wall. **A** ×180, **B** and **C** ×90

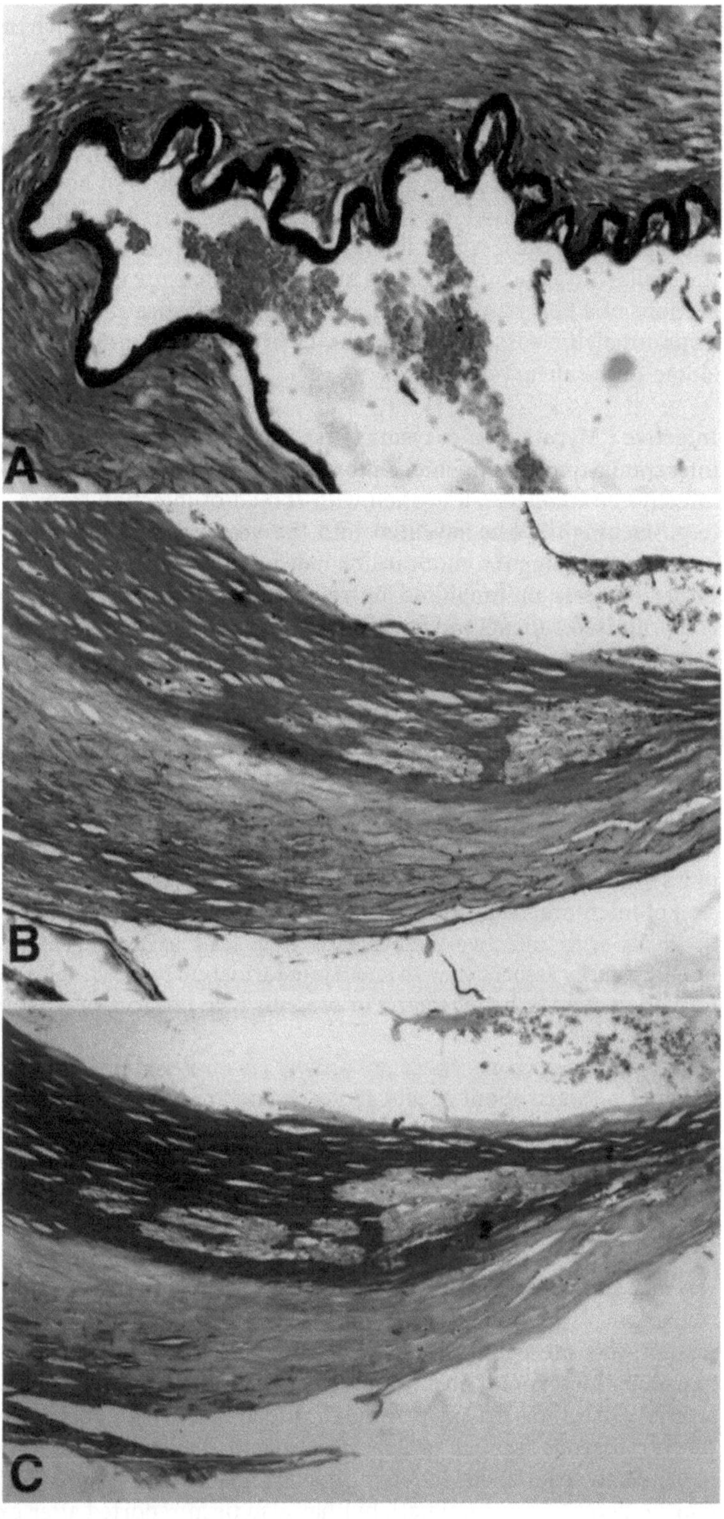

pathologist for calling a lesion aneurysmal, or the care with which these tiny lesions are sought by the prosector. When seen in the elderly, 'incidental' (unruptured) berry aneurysms often show significant superimposed atherosclerotic change. There is controversy as to the factors (and especially the critical size of aneurysm) that precipitate SAH. Aneurysms smaller than 10 mm in diameter have a low rate of rupture. The location of an aneurysm also appears to be important in determining the likelihood of its bleeding: ICA-posterior communicating artery aneurysms and those within the vertebrobasilar system (especially those located at the basilar 'tip') are more likely to hemorrhage than are others [23, 140]. Histologic sections of a berry aneurysm show loss of the elastica associated with fibrosis or thinning of the vascular media, the latter especially around the rupture site or 'dome' of the aneurysm (Fig. 18).

**Infective ('Mycotic') Aneurysms (IAs).** These lesions, accounting for 3%–6% of intracranial aneurysms, are almost always associated with subacute or acute infective endocarditis, less often with spread of infection from a contiguous site (e.g., meningitis, osteomyelitis) into the vessel wall [47, 110, 127, 132]. Microorganisms causing the endocarditis may be varied and are often of low virulence. Either bacteria or fungi can be responsible, the latter especially in immunocompromised patients and intravenous drug abusers. IAs, unlike berry aneurysms, usually affect peripheral branches of the arterial circulation. Rupture of an IA may result in SAH or IPH. An aneurysm, friable and weakened because of polymorphonuclear leukocytes in the vessel wall, may be resected in the course of removal of an intracerebral clot and should be sought in any such specimen from an 'at-risk' patient. Stainable microorganisms may be seen among inflammatory cells in sections through an IA [47].

The pathogenesis of an IA due to endocarditis is thought to involve the lodging of a septic embolus within a branch of a cerebral artery and the subsequent extension of microorganisms from the embolus into the vessel wall. Septic emboli in individuals with infective endocarditis may lead to a pyogenic arteritis that is not necessarily associated with aneurysm formation but leads to hemorrhagic transformation of an ischemic infarct or presents with intracerebral hemorrhage [100].

**Dissecting Aneurysms.** These are usually encountered in young and middle-aged patients, between about 25 and 45 years, and are rare in those over 65 [49, 69, 70, 112, 121]. Dissection may occur in extracranial or intracranial branches of the carotid or vertebrobasilar system. FARRELL et al. [49] meticulously described the autopsy findings in seven affected individuals with the syndrome of intracranial arterial dissection. When dissection had occurred in the anterior circulation, its site was between the internal elastic lamina and the media, with resultant intravascular thrombosis. When dissection had occurred in the posterior circulation, transmural dissection had often resulted in SAH. Variable degrees of acute inflammation were present at sites of dissection. Specific degenerative or inflammatory vasculopathies could not, however, be identified with certainty. Extracranial arterial dissections may involve the carotid artery, usually above the bifurcation, or the intraosseous segment of a vertebral artery.

Clinically, arterial dissection is often associated with trauma to the neck (which may be perceived as minimal), but has also been reported after exercise or neck manipulation, after administration of heparin, or in the context of fibromuscular dysplasia, though none of these antecedent events or conditions is necessarily present in a given patient. In cases of more severe head injury, the dissection usually occurs in the extracranial part of the carotid artery close to the base of the skull, or within the base of the skull (in which case the dissection is invariably associated with basal skull fractures), or at the point of dural entry of one of the vertebral arteries into the cranial cavity. Intracerebral hemorrhage has been described following transmural dissection of the anterior cerebral artery [67].

**Fusiform Aneurysms.** These lesions present (to the pathologist) as ectatic, often very tortuous or serpentine, basal arteries. They are rarely symptomatic and frequently associated with complicated atherosclerosis [47, 136]. In young patients they may be associated with deficiencies of the arterial muscularis and internal elastic lamina [91]. In a clinicopathologic review of the entity, seven autopsy cases were found to have presented over an age range of 56–65 years [136]. As their name implies, fusiform aneurysms result from enlargement and widening of an arterial segment along its length. Most often, they are found on the basilar artery, though fusiform aneurysms may also occur on the anterior circulation [91]. In the older literature, they have been described as „arteriosclerotic aneurysms“ [34, 71]. They may reach giant proportions (arbitrarily defined as larger than 2.5 cm) and when examined in cross section often contain laminated thrombus overlying severe complicated atheroma. Acute and chronic inflammatory change has been found within the walls of fusiform atherosclerotic aneurysms; this may be a response to severe atheromatous change or related thrombosis or rupture of the aneurysm, and possibly contributes to its becoming symptomatic [136].

Fusiform aneurysms of the basilar artery can enlarge to the point where they cause brain stem displacement and compression, and cranial nerve deficits. Because laminated thrombus is often present within their lumina, platelet-fibrin or atheromatous embolic material may migrate distally in the circulation to produce transient ischemic attacks or infarcts in branches of the vertebrobasilar circulation. These aneurysms may also, rarely, rupture to produce SAH.

## 5.4 Intraparenchymal Brain Hemorrhage

Intraparenchymal brain hemorrhage (IPH) may also be termed encephalic hemorrhage, and describes primary bleeding into the brain substance rather than an adjacent compartment. Obviously, IPH may extend into the ventricular cavities and the subarachnoid space. As a cause of stroke, IPHs are comparatively much less common in western populations than are infarcts resulting from atherothrombotic disease or cerebral emboli [7, 47]. The most common causes of IPH are hypertension, CAA, anticoagulant administration, primary or secondary brain neoplasms, prescription or 'recreational' drug use, AVMs and aneurysms, and miscellaneous other causes [53]. There is some evidence that spontaneous hematomas often occur within cerebral infarcts, and that primary IPH may thus be overdiagnosed [13].

Given the increasing recognition and effective treatment of hypertension, a reasonable prediction would be that high blood pressure (HBP) should be in decline as a major cause of IPH. There is some evidence that this has occurred over recent decades [53]. A population-based study in Japan showed a diminution in the annual incidence of intracerebral hemorrhage between 1961 and 1983 [146]. Among males over age 40 years, this figure decreased from 3.1/1,000 (1961–1970) to 1.2/1,000 (1974–1983). In autopsy series, the incidence of IPH varies markedly from center to center, as do apparent etiologies, often reflecting the unique clinical interests of a given center, the demographics of the population from which individuals are referred, etc. In a setting where hematologic malignancies are treated aggressively in large numbers, for instance, IPH related to leukemia or thrombocytopenia would likely be disproportionately increased by comparison to other etiologies. Clinical and neuroimaging features of IPH are well described in recent and older reviews [7, 8, 53, 124].

**Hypertension.** The assignment of the cause of primary IPH to HBP is usually made on the basis of (1) the presence within brain of a patient who has experienced hemorrhage, of microvascular changes of arteriosclerosis/lipohyalinosis (AS/LH), with or without Charcot-Bouchard (C-B) microaneurysms, and/or (2) a clinical history of documented HBP, and/or (3) autopsy evidence of longstanding HBP, e.g., nephrosclerosis, cardiomegaly with left ventricular hypertrophy. Typical locations for hypertensive IPH include the lateral or medial basal ganglia, thalamus, pons, and cerebellum, though HBP-related hematomas may also be seen in the deep subcortical white matter (Fig. 19). The term 'hypertensive hemorrhage' is sometimes applied to a given IPH with minimal support for the putative etiology [20]. The significance of increased heart weight (cardiomegaly) or left ventricular hypertrophy (LVH) found at autopsy is often not clear. Systemic hypertension is the most common cause of severe LVH, though other causes (e.g., aortic stenosis, ventricular septal defect) must always be considered and ruled out by careful examination of the heart. Using a rigorous autopsy definition of apparent HBP, i.e., heart weight greater than the mean cardiac weight of necropsy controls plus 1.5 standard deviations, one investigator found that less than half of patients with primary intracerebral hemorrhage had cardiac enlargement by this criterion [5, 18].

Microscopic features of AS/LH associated with hypertensive IPH are discussed and illustrated above. Hypertensive IPH results from extravasation of blood from brain parenchymal arterioles that are assumed to have become noncompliant and weakened by replacement of medial smooth muscle cells (SMC) by collagenous fibrous tissue, with fragmentation of their elastica. C-B type microaneurysms may be found on affected arterioles, though they may be absent even when brain parenchyma around a putative hypertensive hemorrhage is sampled extensively [51].

A typical hypertensive hematoma is shown in Fig. 19. The appearance of the hematoma will vary according to its age. Hematomas that are months to years old will show (on gross inspection) a cystic cavity rimmed by yellowish/orange, scarred brain tissue; the appearances may be quite similar to those of an old cystic infarct, except that IPHs are not generally confined to the territory of supply of a major artery, whereas infarcts commonly are. Microscopic sections around the margins of a hematoma will show changes that also reflect the duration of the bleed: subacute hemorrhage (2–4 days) is associated with edematous surrounding tissue containing macrophages, reactive microglia and gemistocytic astrocytes, while the tissue around older bleeds contains hemosiderin-laden macrophages and abundant fibrous astrocytes.

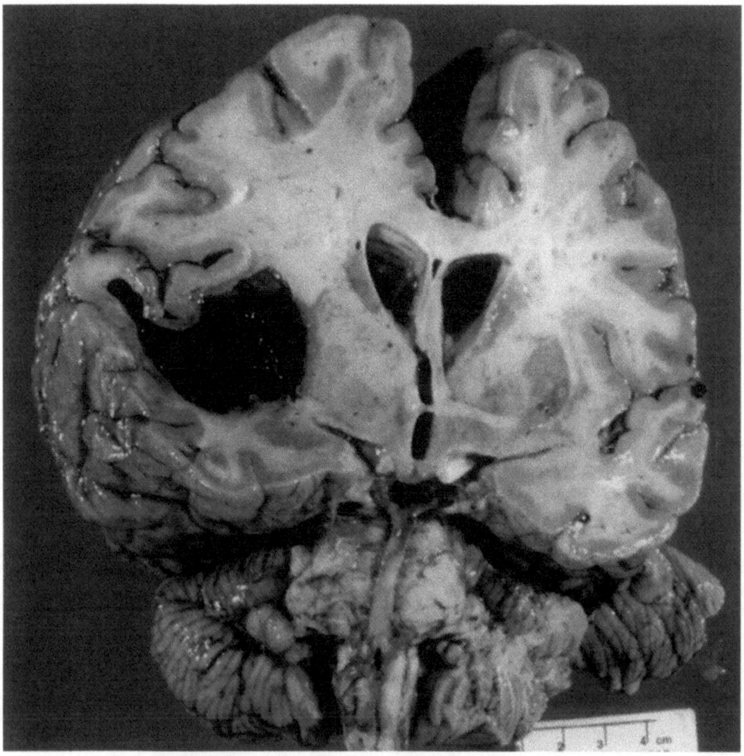

**Fig. 19.** Hypertensive intracerebral hemorrhage. Freshly cut brain shows subacute clotted blood in the right basal ganglia, extending into the right temporal lobe. Hemorrhage probably originated in the right putamen

**Cerebral Amyloid Angiopathy (CAA).** The pathogenesis and microscopic features of this entity are discussed and illustrated above. It is worth re-emphasizing the patchy nature of CAA within brain cortex and leptomeninges, its segmental nature in a given arteriole, and its strong association with aging and Alzheimer's disease [148]. The extent of amyloid deposition within vessel walls correlates with increasing risk of IPH. CAA may have a variety of clinical and neuroradiographic manifestations - including no specific abnormality - but IPH is its most common stroke-related manifestation [32, 61, 62, 78, 118, 155]. Other presentations of CAA include SAH without IPH, leukoencephalopathy, angiitis, and recurrent transient neurologic symptoms (possibly due to microhemorrhages/microinfarcts within the CNS); all of these are relatively rare [151, 162, 163]. An association between CAA and brain ischemic infarcts is less clearly established than that between CAA and IPH.

CAA causes IPHs with distinctive clinicopathologic features (Fig. 20). Hematomas are typically found in patients within the 8th and 9th decades of life, many of whom have overt features of AD/SDAT. The hematomas occur within the cortex and subcortical white matter ('lobar' hemorrhages), and often dissect into the subarachnoid space, less frequently the ventricles. This anatomic predilection

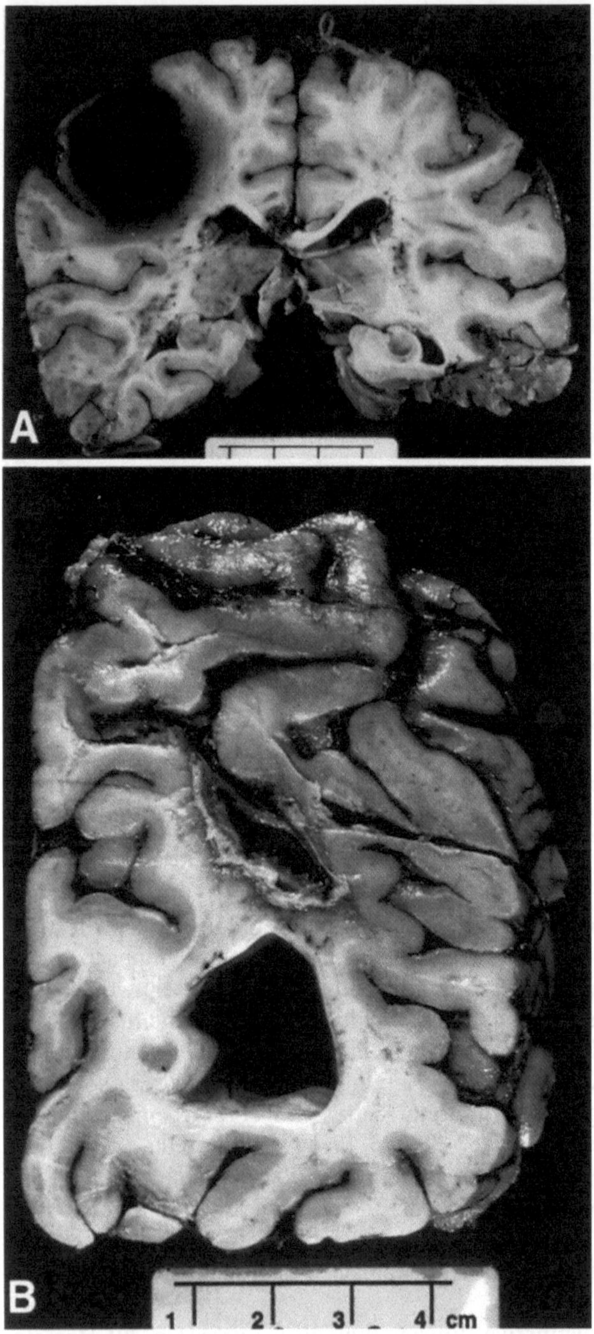


**Fig. 20. A** Recent left frontal (lobar) hematoma in the brain of a patient with severe CAA. Though CAA is a meningocortical microangiopathy, associated hemorrhages often extend into the subcortical white matter and frequently rupture into the subarachnoid space, as in this case. **B** Old (lobar) resorbed hematoma in a patient with longstanding AD and severe CAA. The cavity resembles an old ischemic infarct, though overlying neocortex is somewhat spared

reflects the topography of CAA, a cortical and meningeal vasculopathy [157]. Heightened awareness of CAA as a likely etiology for lobar IPHs is also important for the surgical pathologist; CAA is readily detected in fragments of brain parenchyma evacuated together with a hematoma, particularly if sections are immunostained for A$\beta$ protein [173]. Bleeds may occur, over months or years, into different lobes of the cerebral hemispheres. The cerebellum and pons, commonly involved by hypertensive bleeds, are almost never sites of CAA-related hemorrhage [151, 162]. As many as $^{1}/_{3}$ of patients with CAA-related IPH also have clinical evidence of HBP – mixed microangiopathies, with features of both AS/LH and CAA, may be found within brain of such individuals [118, 148].

Amyloid deposition in the arterial wall causes atrophy of the medial smooth muscle cell (SMC) layer in both leptomeningeal and parenchymal arteries, as the SMC are replaced by fibrillar amyloid [94, 95, 161]. These changes probably impair function of involved vessels by reducing their flexibility and compliance in response to fluctuations in arterial pressure. Fibrillar amyloid disrupts vascular architecture and weakens the affected arterial walls, causing cracks, focal fragmentation, and microaneurysm formation, with or without fibrinoid necrosis [161, 164]. Amyloid deposits within CNS arteriolar walls appear to be comparatively well tolerated up to a certain threshold, e.g., CAA of grades 1 and 2 (see above). However, when grade 3 changes occur, the risk of IPH increases dramatically – in this situation, extrinsic, apparently trivial factors such as minor head trauma may trigger cerebral bleeding.

**Vascular Malformations.** These may involve the CNS parenchyma, overlying dura, or (rarely) both [29, 97, 101, 102, 108, 111, 139]. The most clinically important of these lesions, arteriovenous malformations (AVMs), rarely present beyond the age of 60 years. AVMs (also sometimes described as arteriovenous aneurysms) may cause IPH and/or SAH. They are more frequently encountered as surgical specimens than at autopsy. They most often occur in the MCA territory, classically involving a wedge-shaped area of brain parenchyma and overlying leptomeninges, but may be seen anywhere in the CNS, including posterior fossa structures, and rarely involve the circle of Willis. By definition, an AVM represents an abnormal direct communication between one or more arteries in the brain parenchyma and one or more draining veins, without an intervening capillary bed [29]. Its morphologic features, both grossly and microscopically, are characteristic (Fig. 21). An AVM consists of a collection of vascular channels of varying wall thickness and diameter, embedded within abnormal, gliotic, and occasionally malformed brain parenchyma [29, 47, 97, 101, 102, 156]. The CNS parenchyma may or may not show morphologic evidence of old hemorrhage, but an absence of blood breakdown products (hemosiderin, hematoidin) does not rule out the possibility that the AVM has bled prior to resection. Commonly, thrombosed and recanalized vascular channels are present within an AVM. Other intriguing abnormalities noted within AVMs are hyalinized, sometimes calcified (rarely, ossified), arterial walls, and others that show foci of intimal fibromuscular hyperplasia. Infrequently, 'foreign' particles, covered by endothelium and surrounded by foreign body type giant cells, are seen embedded within vessel walls; these are thought to represent material introduced into the circulation during cerebral angiographic instrumentation [158].

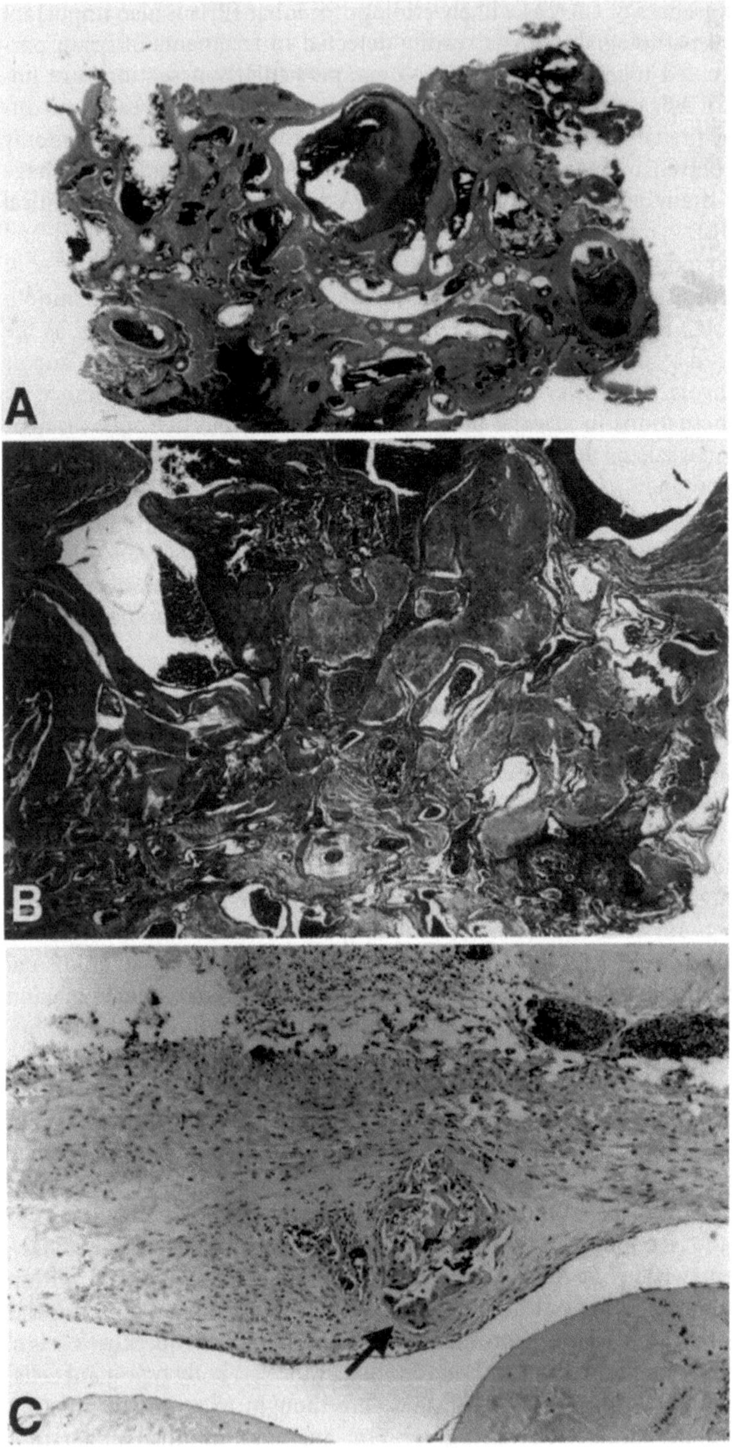
A
B
C

AVMs usually produce symptoms by bleeding (with reactive changes in surrounding brain parenchyma or leptomeninges), direct pressure on surrounding brain substance, or a 'steal' of blood from normal anatomic structures because of significant arteriovenous shunting of blood through the AVM [33]. AVMs are usually treated by excision or iatrogenic embolization (performed with the intention of occluding and obliterating the AVM nidus), the latter resulting in a variety of tissue reactions to embolotherapy agents used [134, 159].

Venous angiomas (VAs) consist of one or more dilated, often grossly apparent, veins and their smaller tributaries, but without an obvious arterial component. A single tortuous vein (e.g., in the spinal subarachnoid space) may be described as a varix. Their component vessels are more dilated and have thicker walls than normal veins, and brain parenchyma between the vessels shows negligible reactive change or (old) hemorrhage [47, 139, 156]. VAs are usually an incidental finding at autopsy, as are capillary telangiectases, composed of multiple dilated capillaries without alterations of the surrounding brain substance. Both VAs and capillary telangiectases appear (at brain cutting) as small, fairly well-defined punctate vascular lesions that resemble a localized region of bleeding or petechial hemorrhages (Fig. 22).

Cavernous hemangiomas (CAs) are less common than AVMs and appear as closely packed blood vessels (of varying wall thickness) without intervening CNS parenchyma, except towards the periphery of the lesion (Fig. 23) [29, 47, 156]. They have a predilection for the pons, subcortical white matter, and the external capsule. In these regions, they may mimic primary CNS neoplasms and behave as space-occupying lesions, producing mass effect and 'irritation' of surrounding brain that causes, for example, seizures. Though they do not usually cause massive IPH, they are almost always surrounded by massive deposits of hemosiderin, suggesting slow or recurrent leaks of blood from the component vessels. A familial syndrome of cavernous angiomas has recently been linked to a gene on chromosome 7q [60, 122]. In the described kindreds, patients became symptomatic at an early age, usually the second or third decade of life.

**Systemic and Miscellaneous Factors.** IPH may result from systemic factors and diseases such as thrombocytopenia, coagulopathy (either iatrogenic or secondary to hepatic failure), hemophilia, disseminated intravascular coagulation, leukemia, and abuse of recreational drugs such as cocaine [7, 8, 22, 47, 89, 103, 109, 156]. Of these, anticoagulant-related bleeds and those associated with hematologic malignancies are relatively common in the geriatric population. The bleeds may mimic, in terms of topography and extent, hematomas associated with HBP and CAA; they may also occur on a background of these common microangiopathies.

**Fig. 21 A–C.** Arteriovenous malformation (AVM) of the brain. **A** Whole mount of a large, recently embolized, AVM. **B** Low-magnification view of a surgically resected AVM. In both panels (**A, B**) note the marked variation in vessel lumen caliber and wall thickness – the vessels include arteries, veins, and arterialized veins showing fragmented, reduplicated, or absent internal elastic lamina. **C** Microscopic detail of wall of an AVM embolized with cyanoacrylate several weeks prior to resection. Intimal fibromuscular 'cushions', such as this one, are common in AVMs. This one also contains fragments of embolotherapy material (*arrow*) surrounded by foreign body giant cells. **A–C**, H&E

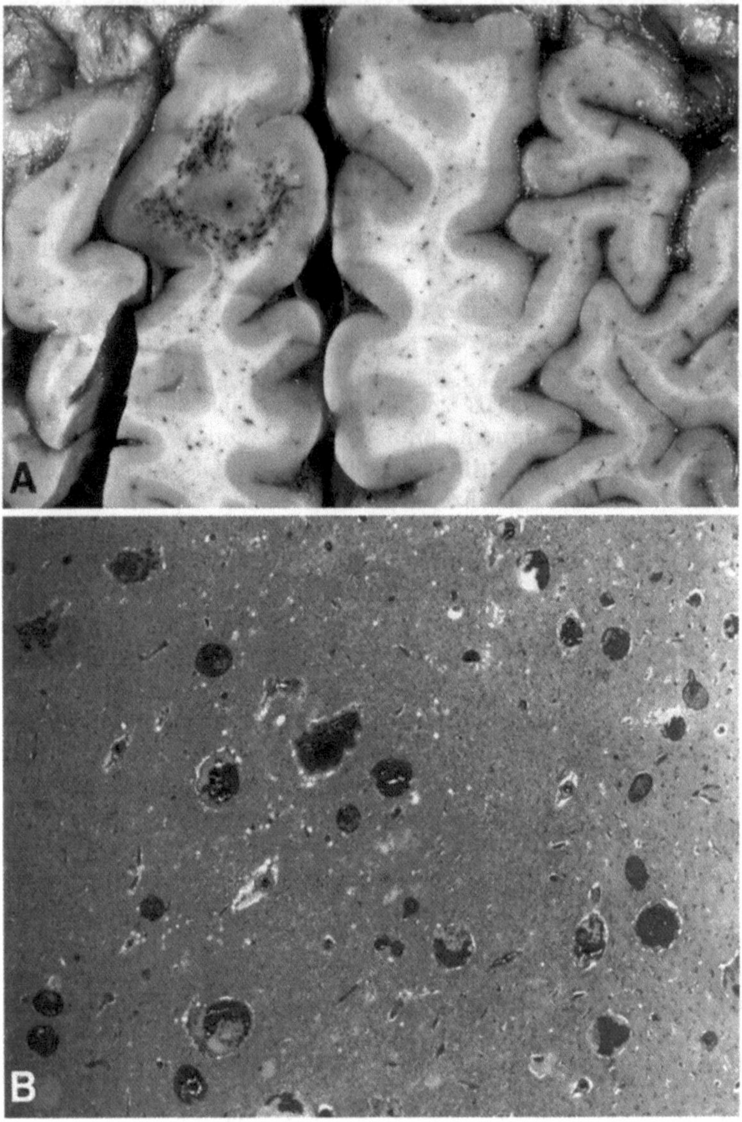

**Fig. 22 A, B.** Venous angioma. **A** This was an incidental finding at autopsy. Note a fairly well circumscribed collection of (what appear to be) petechial hemorrhages in subcortical white matter. **B** Histologic section shows venous channels separated by normal appearing neuroglial tissue, and no evidence of reactive change or remote hemorrhage. **B** H&E, ×55

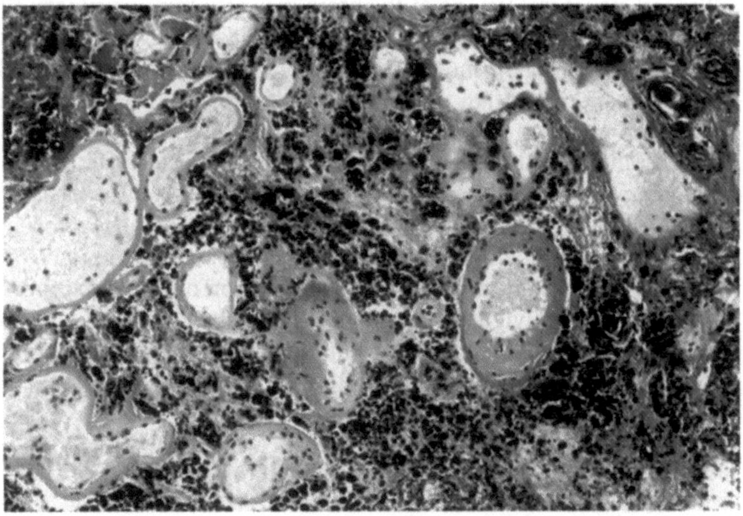

**Fig. 23.** Cavernous hemangioma. Note the prominently hyalinized vessels packed closely together, separated only by abundant hemosiderin, indicative of previous hemorrhage. H&E, ×175

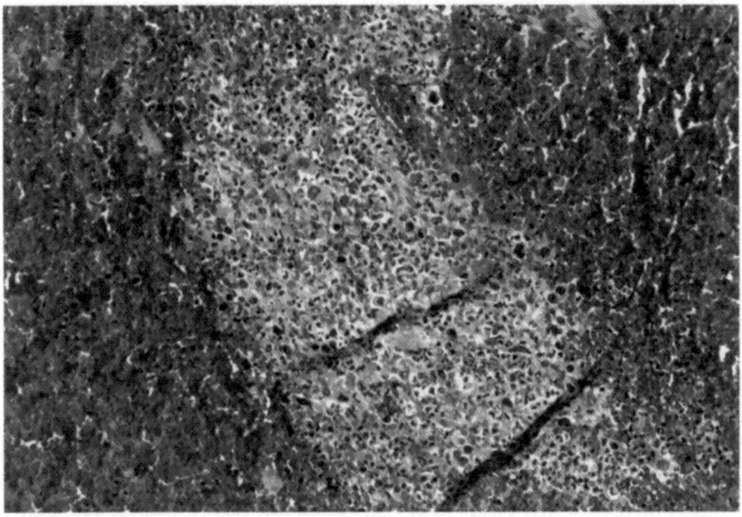

**Fig. 24.** Acute cerebral hemorrhage into a metastatic tumor deposit. This surgical specimen was resected from a 77-year-old male with history of lung carcinoma, who developed an IPH. Abundant acute hemorrhage is noted. Highly atypical, somewhat cohesive, neoplastic cells are seen together with the blood. Hemorrhage into metastatic brain tumor deposits is well documented; occasionally, this is the presenting manifestation of the primary malignancy. ×220

Several structural lesions of the brain may also mimic primary IPH. The most common of these are primary or secondary neoplasms, and infections – in particular by microorganisms that have a propensity to invade vessel walls (e.g., *Aspergillus* species). High-grade glial neoplasms (and both low- or high-grade oligodendrogliomas) probably bleed because of their content of thin-walled, fragile capillaries. Whereas infection-related bleeds usually occur on a background of sepsis and thus can be fairly readily differentiated, on the basis of clinical presentation and neuroimaging, from primary IPH, hemorrhage into a neoplasm may be its initial presentation – even in the case of metastases (Fig. 24) [93]. The neoplasm may become apparent upon evacuation of the clot and careful scrutiny of its contents by a vigilant pathologist. If clot evacuation is not undertaken the tumor will eventually 'declare itself,' although there may be an initial improvement in signs and symptoms associated with resorption of the hematoma.

**Acknowledgement.** Work in the author's laboratory supported by U.S. PHS Grant P01 AG 12435 and P50 AG 16570. Carol Appleton prepared the figures, Annetta Pierro assisted with manuscript preparation, and Justine Garakian and Alexander Brooks cut and stained many of the sections from which micrographs were made.

## References

1. Abrahams NA, Prayson, RA (2000) The role of histopathological examination of intracranial blood clots removed for hemorrhage of unknown etiology. A review of 31 cases. J Neuropathol Exp Neurol 59:430 [abstract]
2. Adams JH, Brierley JB, Connor RCR, Treip CS (1966) The effects of systemic hypotension upon the human brain. Clinical and neuropathological observations in 11 cases. Brain 89:235–268
3. Adams JH, Graham DI (1989) Cerebrovascular disease. In: Anthony PP, Macsween RNM (eds) Recent advances in histopathology. No. 14, Churchill Livingstone, Edinburgh, pp 205–222
4. Anders KH, Wang ZZ, Kornfeld M, Gray F, Soontornniyomkij V, Reed LA et al. (1997) Giant cell arteritis in association with cerebral amyloid angiopathy: immunohistochemical and molecular studies. Hum Pathol 28:1237–1246
5. Bahemuka M (1987) Primary intracerebral hemorrhage and heart weight: a clinicopathologic case-control review of 218 patients. Stroke 18:531–536
6. Bamford JM, Warlow CP (1988) Evolution and testing of the lacunar hypothesis. Stroke 19:1074–1082
7. Barnett HJM, Mohr JP, Stein BM, Yatsu FM (eds) (1998) Stroke. Pathophysiology, Diagnosis, and Management. Third edition. Churchill Livingstone, New York
8. Batjer HH (ed) (1997) Cerebrovascular Disease. Lippincott-Raven, Philadelphia
9. Bennett M, O'Brien DP, Phillips JP, Farrell MA (1995) Clinicopathologic observations in 100 consecutive patients with fatal head injury admitted to a neuro- surgical unit. Irish Med J 88:60–62
10. Biller J, Challa VR, Toole JF, Howard VJ (1982) Nonbacterial thrombotic endocarditis. A neurologic perspective of clinicopathologic correlations of 99 patients. Arch Neurol 39:95–98
11. Bogousslavsky J, Barnett HJM, Fox AJ, Hachinski VC, Taylor W for the EC/IC Bypass Study Group (1986) Atherosclerotic disease of the middle cerebral artery. Stroke 17:1112–1120
12. Bogousslavsky J, Cachin C, Regli F, Despland P-A, Van Melle G, Kappenberger L (for the Lausanne Stroke Registry Group) (1991) Cardiac sources of embolism and cerebral infarction–clinical consequences and vascular concomitants: The Lausanne Stroke Registry. Neurology 41:855–859

13. Bogousslavsky J, Regli F, Uske A, Maeder P (1991) Early spontaneous hematoma in cerebral infarct: is primary cerebral hemorrhage overdiagnosed? Neurology 41:837–840
14. Bokemeyer C, Frank B, Brandis A, Weinrich W (1990) Giant aneurysm causing frontal lobe syndrome. J Neurol 237:47–50
15. Bonita R, Thomson S (1985) Subarachnoid hemorrhage: epidemiology, diagnosis, management and outcome. Stroke 16:591–594
16. Bornebroek M, Haan J, Maat-Schieman MLC, van Duinen SG, Roos RAC (1996) Hereditary cerebral hemorrhage with amyloidosis – Dutch type (HCHWA-D): I – A review of clinical, radiologic and genetic aspects. Brain Pathol 6:111–114
17. Bousser M-G, Barnett HJM (1998) Cerebral venous thrombosis. In: Barnett HJM, Mohr JP, Stein BM, Yatsu FM (eds) Stroke pathophysiology, diagnosis, and management. 3rd edition. Churchill Livingstone, NewYork, pp 623–647
18. Brewer DB, Fawcett FJ, Horsfield GI (1968) A necropsy series of non-traumatic cerebral haemorrhages and softenings, with particular reference to heart weight. J Pathol Bacteriol 96:311–320
19. Brierley JB, Excell BJ (1966) The effects of profound systemic hypotension upon the brain of *M. Rhesus*: physiological and pathological observations. Brain 89:269–298
20. Brott T, Thalinger K, Hertzberg V (1986) Hypertension as a risk factor for spontaneous intracerebral hemorrhage. Stroke 17:1078–1083
21. Calabrese LH, Duna GF, Lie JT (1997) Vasculitis in the central nervous system. Arthritis & Rheumatism 40:1189–1201
22. Caplan LR (1993) Stroke A Clinical Approach. 2nd ed. Butterworth-Heinemann, Boston
23. Caplan LR (1998) Should intracranial aneurysms be treated before they rupture? N Engl J Med 339:1774–1775
24. Caplan LR, Amarenco P, Rosengart A, Lafranchise EF, Teal PA, Belkin M et al. (1992) Embolism from vertebral artery origin occlusive disease. Neurology 42:1505–1512
25. Castaigne P, Lhermitte F, Gautier JC, Escourolle R, Derouesne C, Der Agopian P, Popa C (1973) Arterial occlusions in the vertebro-basilar system. A study of 44 patients with postmortem data. Brain 96:133–154
26. Cerebral Embolism Task Force (1989) Cardiogenic brain embolism. The second report of the cerebral embolism task force. Arch Neurol 46:727–743
27. Challa VR, Bell MA, Moody DM (1990) A combined hematoxylin-eosin, alkaline phosphatase and high-resolution microradiographic study of lacunes. Clin Neuropathol 9:196–204
28. Challa VR, Moody DM, Bell MA (1992) The Charcot-Bouchard aneurysm controversy: impact of a new histologic technique. J Neuropathol Exp Neurol 51:264–271
29. Challa VR, Moody DM, Brown WR (1995) Vascular malformations of the central nervous system. J Neuropathol Exp Neurol 54:609–621
30. Cole FM, Yates P (1967) Intracerebral microaneurysms and small cerebrovascular lesions. Brain 90:759–768
31. Conn DL (1989) Update on systemic necrotizing vasculitis. Mayo Clin Proc. 64:535–543
32. Coria F, Rubio I (1996) Cerebral amyloid angiopathies. Neuropathol Appl Neurobiol 22:216–227
33. Costantino A, Vinters HV (1986) A pathologic correlate of the 'steal' phenomenon in a patient with cerebral arteriovenous malformation. Stroke 17:103–106
34. Courville CB (1962) Arterioslcerotic aneurysms of the circle of Willis. Bulletin of the LA. Neurological Society 27:1–13
35. Crooks DA (1991) Pathogenesis and biomechanics of traumatic intracranial haemorrhages. Virchows Archiv A Pathol Anat 418:479–483
36. Davis J van Nostrand WE (1996) Enhanced pathologic properties of Dutch-type mutant amyloid beta-protein. Proc Natl Acad Sci USA 93:2996–3000
37. Decroix JP, Graveleau Ph, Masson M, Cambier J (1986) Infarction in the territory of the anterior choroidal artery. A clinical and cumputerized tomographic study of 16 cases. Brain 109:1071–1085
38. del Zoppo G, Ginis I, Hallenbeck JM, Iadecola C, Wang X, Feuerstein GZ (2000) Inflammation and stroke: putative role for cytokines, adhesion molecules and iNOS in brain response to ischemia. Brain Pathol 10:95–112

39. Devinsky O, Bear D, Volpe BT (1988) Confusional states following posterior cerebral artery infarction. Arch Neurol 45:160–163
40. Dines DE, Burgher LW, Okazaki H (1975) The clinical and pathologic correlation of fat embolism syndrome. Mayo Clin Proc 50:407–411
41. DiNubile MJ (1988) Septic thrombosis of the cavernous sinuses. Arch Neurol 45:567–572
42. Dirnagl U, Iadecola C, Moskowitz MA (1999) Pathobiology of ischaemic stroke: an integrated view. TINS 22:391–397
43. Drapkin AJ (1991) Chronic subdural hematoma: pathophysiological basis for treatment. British J Neurosurg 5:467–473
44. Droste DW, Karl M, Bohle RM, Kaps M (1997) Comparison of ultrasonic and histopathological features of carotid artery stenosis. Neurological Research 19:380–384
45. Einhaupl KM, Villringer A, Meister W, Mehraein S, Garner C, Pellkofer M et al. (1991) Heparin treatment in sinus venous thrombosis. Lancet 338:597–600
46. Ellis RJ, Olichney JM, Thal LJ, Mirra SS, Morris JC, Beekly D, Heyman A (1996) Cerebral amyloid angiopathy in the brains of patients with Alzheimer's disease. The CERAD experience, part XV. Neurology 46:1592–1596
47. Ellison D, Love S, Chimelli L, Harding B, Lowe J, Roberts GW, Vinters HV (1998) Neuropathology. A reference text of CNS pathology, section 3. Mosby International, London
48. Evans JM, Batts KP, Hunder GG (1994) Persistent giant cell arteritis despite corticosteroid treatment. Mayo Clin Proc 69:1060–1061
49. Farrell MA, Gilbert JJ, Kaufmann JCE (1985) Fatal intracranial arterial dissection: clinical pathological correlation. J Neurol Neurosurg Psychiatry 48:111–121
50. Feldenzer JA, Bueche MJ, Venes JL, Gebarski SS (1987) Superior sagittal sinus thrombosis with infarction in sickle cell trait. Stroke 18:656–660
51. Fisher CM (1971) Pathological observations in hypertensive cerebral hemorrhage. J Neuropathol Exp Neurol 30:536–550
52. Fisher CM, Gore I, Okabe N, White PD (1965) Atherosclerosis of the carotid and vertebral arteries–extracranial and intracranial. J Neuropathol Exp Neurol 24:455–476
53. Fisher M (1994) Clinical Atlas of Cerebrovascular Disorders. Mosby-Year Book, London
54. Friede RL (1971) Incidence and distribution of neomembranes of dura mater. J Neurol Neurosurg Psychiatry 34:439–446
55. Furlan AJ (ed) (1987) The Heart and Stroke. Exploring Mutual Cerebrovascular and Cardiovascular Issues. Springer-Verlag, London-Berlin
56. Gacs G, Fox AJ, Barnett HJM, Vinuela F (1983) Occurrence and mechanisms of occlusion of the anterior cerebral artery. Stroke 14:952–959
57. Gan R, Sacco RL, Kargman DE, Roberts JK, Boden-Albala B, Gu Q (1997) Testing the validity of the lacunar hypothesis: The Northern Manhattan Stroke Study experience. Neurology 48:1204–1211
58. Gerber NJ (1984) Giant cell arteritis and its variants. Eur Neurol 23:410–420
59. Ghanchi FD, Dutton GN (1997) Current concepts in giant cell (temporal) arteritis. Survey of Ophthalmology 42:99–123
60. Gil-Nagel A, Dubovsky J, Wilcox KJ, Stewart JM, Anderson VE et al. (1996) Familial cerebral cavernous angioma: a gene localized to a 15-cM interval on chromosome 7q. Ann Neurol 39:807–810
61. Gilbert JJ, Vinters HV (1983) Cerebral amyloid angiopathy: incidence and complications in the aging brain. I. Cerebral hemorrhage. Stroke 14:915–923
62. Gilles C, Brucher JM, Khoubesserian P, Vanderheagan JJ (1984) Cerebral amyloid angiopathy as a cause of multiple intracerebral hemorrhages. Neurology 34:730–735
63. Gillum RF (1988) Stroke in Blacks. Stroke 19:1–9
64. Gordon LK, Levin LH (1998) Visual loss in giant cell arteritis. JAMA 280:385–386
65. Greenberg SM (1998) Cerebral amyloid angiopathy Prospects for clinical diagnosis and treatment. Neurology 51:690–694
66. Greenberg SM, Vonsattel J-PG (1997) Diagnosis of cerebral amyloid angiopathy Sensitivity and specificity of cortical biopsy. Stroke 28:1418–1422
67. Guridi J, Gallego J, Monzon F, Aguilera F (1993) Intracerebral hemorrhage caused by transmural dissection of the anterior cerebral artery. Stroke 24:1400–1402
68. Hachinski V, Norris JW (1985) The Acute Stroke. F.A. Davis, Philadelphia

69. Hart RG (1988) Vertebral artery dissection. Neurology 38:987–989
70. Hart RG, Easton JD (1985) Dissections. Stroke 16:925–927
71. Hayes WT, Bernhardt H, Young JM (1967) Fusiform arteriosclerotic aneurysm of the basilar artery. Five cases including two ruptures. Vasc Surgery 1:171–178
72. Helgason C, Caplan LR, Goodwin J, Hedges T III (1986) Anterior choroidal artery-territory infarction. Report of cases and review. Arch Neurol 43:681–686
73. Hinchey JA, Furlan AJ, Barnett HJM (1998) Cardiogenic brain embolism: incidence, varieties, and treatment. In: Barnett HJM, Mohr JP, Stein BM, Yatsu FM (eds) Stroke pathophysiology, diagnosis, and management. 3rd edition. Churchill Livingstone, New York, pp 1089–1119
74. Hinton DR, Dolan E, Sima AAF (1984) The value of histopathological examination of surgically removed blood clot in determining the etiology of spontaneous intracerebral hemorrhage. Stroke 15:517–520
75. Horowitz M, Purdy P, Unwin H, Carstens G III, Greenlee R, Hise J et al. (1995) Treatment of dural sinus thrombosis using selective catheterization and urokinase. Ann Neurol 38:58–67
76. Huston KA, Hunder GG, Lie JT, Kennedy RH, Elveback LR (1978) Temporal arteritis. A 25-year epidemiologic, clinical, and pathologic study. Ann Intern Med 88:162–167
77. Imakita M, Yutani C, Ishibashi-Ueda H (1993) Giant cell arteritis involving the cerebral artery. Arch Pathol Lab Med 117:729–733
78. Jellinger K (1977) Cerebrovascular amyloidosis with cerebral hemorrhage. J Neurol 214:195–206
79. Jorgensen L, Torvik A (1966) Ischaemic cerebrovascular diseases in an autopsy series. Part 1. Prevalence, location and predisposing factors in verified thrombo-embolic occlusions, and their significance in the pathogenesis of cerebral infarction. J Neurol Sci 3:490–509
80. Jorgensen L, Torvik A (1969) Ischaemic cerebrovascular diseases in an autopsy series. Part 2. Prevalence, location, pathogenesis, and clinical course of cerebral infarcts. J Neurol Sci 9:285–320
81. Kalimo H, Kaste M, Haltia M (1997) Vascular diseases (Chapter 7). In: Graham DI , Lantos PL (eds) Greenfield's neuropathology. 6th edition (vol. 1). Arnold, London, pp 315–396
82. Kamenar E, Burger PC (1980) Cerebral fat embolism: a neuropathological study of a microembolic state. Stroke 11:477–484
83. Kassell NF, Sasaki T, Colohan ART, Nazar G (1985) Cerebral vasospasm following aneurysmal subarachnoid hemorrhage. Stroke 16:562–572
84. Kawai M, Kalaria RN, Cras P, Siedlak SL, Velasco ML, Shelton ER et al. (1993) Degeneration of vascular muscle cells in cerebral amyloid angiopathy of Alzheimer disease. Brain Research 623:142–146
85. Kealy WF (1978) Atheroembolism. J Clin Pathol 31:984–989
86. Kubik CS, Adams RD (1946) Occlusion of the basilar artery– a clinical and pathological study. Brain 69:73–121
87. Lammie AG, Brannan F, Slattery J, Warlow C (1997) Nonhypertensive cerebral small vessel disease. An autopsy study. Stroke 28:2222–2229
88. Levine SR, Kieran S, Puzio K, Feit H, Patel SC, Welch KMA (1987) Cerebral venous thrombosis with lupus anticoagulants. Report of two cases. Stroke 18:801–804
89. Levine SR, Welch KMA (1987) Cocaine and stroke. Stroke 19:779–783
90. Leys D, Lucas C, Henon H, Savoye C, Pasquier F, Pruvo J-P (1996) Ischemic stroke in the elderly: is it necessary to look for a cause? In: Bruno A, Chollet F, Vellas BJ, Albarede JL (eds) Stroke in the elderly. Springer, New York, pp 23–40
91. Little JR, St Louis P, Weinstein M, Dohn DF (1981) Giant fusiform aneurysm of the cerebral arteries. Stroke 12:183–188
92. Maat-Schieman ML, van Duinen SG, Bornebroek M, Haan J, Roos RAC (1996) Hereditary cerebral hemorrhage with amyloidosis – Dutch type (HCHWA-D): II – A review of histopathological aspects. Brain Pathol 6:115–120
93. Mandybur TI (1977) Intracranial hemorrhage caused by metastatic tumors. Neurology 27:650–655
94. Mandybur TI (1986) Cerebral amyloid angiopathy: the vascular pathology and complications. J Neuropathol Exp Neurol 45:79–90

95. Mandybur TI, Bates SRD (1978) Fatal massive intracerebral hemorrhage complicating cerebral amyloid angiopathy. Arch Neurol 35:246–258
96. Manninen HI, Rasanen H, Vanninen RL, Berg M, Hippelainen M et al. (1998) Human carotid arteries: Correlation of intravascular US with angiographic and histpathologic findings. Radiology 206:65–74
97. Martin N, Vinters H (1990) Pathology and grading of intracranial vascular malformations. In: Barrow DL (ed) Intracranial vascular malformations. Amer Assoc of Neurological Surgeons, Park Ridge, Illinois, pp 1–30
98. Masuda J, Ogata J, Yutani C, Miyashita T and Yamaguchi T (1987) Artery-to-artery embolism from a thrombus formed in stenotic middle cerebral artery. Report of an autopsy case. Stroke 18:680–684
99. Masuda J, Tanaka K, Ueda K, Omae T (1988) Autopsy study of incidence and distribution of cerebral amyloid angiopathy in Hisayama, Japan. Stroke 19:205–210
100. Masuda J, Yutani C, Waki R, Ogata J, Kuriyama Y, Yamaguchi T (1992) Histopathological analysis of the mechanisms of intracranial hemorrhage complicating infective endocarditis. Stroke 23:843–850
101. McCormick WF (1966) The pathology of vascular ('arteriovenous') malformations. J Neurosurg 24:807–816
102. McCormick WF, Hardman JM, Boulter TR (1968) Vascular malformations ('angiomas') of the brain, with special reference to those occurring in the posterior fossa J Neurosurg. 28:241–251
103. McCormick WF, Rosenfield DB (1973) Massive brain hemorrhage: a review of 144 cases and an examination of their causes. Stroke 4:946–954
104. Miller Fisher C (1965) Lacunes: small, deep cerebral infarcts. Neurology 15:774–784
105. Miller Fisher C (1978) Ataxic hemiparesis. A pathologic study. Arch Neurol 35:126–128
106. Miller Fisher C (1979) Capsular infarcts. The underlying vascular lesions. Arch Neurol 36:65–73
107. Miller VT (1983) Lacunar stroke. A reassessment. Arch Neurol 40:129–134
108. Mironov A (1995) Classification of spontaneous dural arteriovenous fistulas with regard to their pathogenesis. Acta Radiologica 36:582–592
109. Mody CK, Miller BL, McIntyre HB, Cobb SK, Goldberg MA (1988) Neurologic complications of cocaine abuse. Neurology 38:1189–1193
110. Mohr JP, Kistler JP (1998) Intracranial aneurysms. In: Barnett HJM, Mohr JP, Stein BM, Yatsu FM (eds) Stroke pathophysiology, diagnosis, and management. Third edition. Churchill Livingstone, New York, pp 701–723
111. Mohr JP, Pile-Spellman J, Stein BM (1998) Arteriovenous malformations and other vascular anomalies. In: Barnett HJM, Mohr JP, Stein BM, Yatsu FM (eds) Stroke pathophysiology, diagnosis, and management. 3rd edition. Churchill Livingstone, New York, pp 725–750
112. Mokri B, Houser CW, Sandok BA, Piepgras DG (1988) Spontaneous dissections of the vertebral arteries. Neurology 38:880–885
113. Morgenstern LB, Fox AJ, Sharpe BL, Eliasziw M, Barnett HJM et al. (1997) The risks and benefits of carotid endarterectomy in patients with near occlusion of the carotid artery. Neurology 48:911–915
114. Natte R, de Boer WI, Maat-Schieman MLC, Baelde HJ, Vinters HV, Roos RAC, van Duinen SG (1999) Amyloid beta precursor protein-mRNA is expressed throughout cerebral vessel walls. Brain Research 828:179–183
115. Natte R, Vinters HV, Maat-Schieman MLC, Bornebroek M, Haan J, Roos RAC, van Duinen SG (1998) Microvasculopathy is associated with the number of cerebrovascular lesions in hereditary cerebral hemorrhage with amyloidosis, Dutch type. Stroke 29:1588–1594
116. Navab M, Berliner JA, Watson AD, Hama SY, Territo MC et al. (1996) The Yin and Yang of oxidation in the development of the fatty streak A review based on the 1994 George Lyman Duff Memorial Lecture. Arterioscler Thromb Vasc Biol 16:831–842
117. Nordborg C, Nordborg E, Petursdottir V, LaGuardia J, Mahalingam R, Wellish M, Gilden DH (1998) Search for varicella zoster virus in giant cell arteritis. Ann Neurol 44:413–414
118. Okazaki H, Reagan TJ, Campbell RJ (1979) Clinicopathologic studies of primary cerebral amyloid angiopathy. Mayo Clin Proc. 54:22–31

119. Olafsson E, Hauser WA, Gudmundsson G (1997) A population-based study of prognosis of ruptured cerebral aneurysm: mortality and recurrence of subarachnoid hemorrhage. Neurology 48:1191–1195
120. Olafsson I, Thorsteinsson L, Jensson O (1996) The molecular pathology of hereditary cystatin C amyloid angiopathy causing brain hemorrhage. Brain Pathol 6:121–126
121. Pessin MS, Adelman LS, Barbas NR (1989) Spontaneous intracranial carotid artery dissection. Stroke 20:1100–1103
122. Polymeropoulos MH, Hurko O, Hsu F, Rubenstein J, Basnet S et al. (1997) Linkage of the locus for cerebral cavernous hemangiomas to human chromosome 7q in four families of Mexican-American descent. Neurology 48:752–757
123. Post K, Eckstein H-H, Hoffmann E, Post S, Allenberg JR, Kauffmann GW (1997) Degree of carotid artery stenosis. Comparison of selective and non-selective angiographic findings with surgical specimens. Eur J Radiol 25:9–13
124. Ransohoff J, Derby B, Kricheff I (1971) Spontaneous intracerebral hemorrhage. Clin Neurosurg 18:247–266
125. Resch JA, Okabe N, Loewenson RB, Kimoto K, Katsuki S, Baker AB (1969) Pattern of vessel involvement in cerebral atherosclerosis. A comparative study between a Japanese and Minnesota population. J Atherosclerosis Res 9:239–250
126. Rhodes RH, Madelaire NC, Petrelli M, Cole M, Karaman BA (1995) Primary angiitis and angiopathy of the central nervous system and their relationship to systemic giant cell arteritis. Arch Pathol Lab Med 119:334–349
127. Roach MR, Drake CG (1965) Ruptured cerebral aneurysms caused by microorganisms. N Engl J Med 273:240–244
128. Rorke LB (1992) Anatomical features of the developing brain implicated in pathogenesis of hypoxic-ischemic injury. Brain Pathol 2:211–221
129. Ross R (1999) Atherosclerosis – an inflammatory disease. N Engl J Med 340:115–126
130. Ross R (1993) The pathogenesis of atherosclerosis: a perspective for the 1990s. Nature 362:801–809
131. Sacco RL, Wolf PA, Bharucha NE, Meeks SL, Kannel WB, Charette LJ et al. (1984) Subarachnoid and intracerebral hemorrhage: natural history, prognosis, and precursive factors in the Framingham Study. Neurology 34:847–854
132. Salgado AV, Furlan AJ, Keys TF (1987) Mycotic aneurysm, subarachnoid hemorrhage, and indications for cerebral angiography in infective endocarditis. Stroke 18:1057–1060
133. Save-Soderbergh J, Malmvall B-E, Andersson R, Bengtsson B-A (1986) Giant cell arteritis as a cause of death. Report of nine cases. JAMA 255:493–496
134. Schweitzer JS, Chang BS, Madsen P, Vinuela F, Martin NA, Marroquin CE, Vinters HV (1993) The pathology of arteriovenous malformations of the brain treated by embolotherapy. II. Results of embolization with multiple agents. Neuroradiology 35:468–474
135. Shoji M, Hirai S, Harigaya Y, Kawarabayashi T, Yamaguchi H (1990) The amyloid beta-protein precursor is localized in smooth muscle cells of leptomeningeal vessels. Brain Research 530:113–116
136. Shokunbi MT, Vinters HV, Kaufmann JCE (1988) Fusiform intracranial aneurysms. Clinicopathologic features. Surg Neurol 29:263–270
137. Southwick FS, Richardson EP Jr, MN Swartz (1986) Septic thrombosis of the dural venous sinuses. Medicine 65:82–106
138. Sprung Ch, Collmann H, Kazner E, Duisberg R (1984) Chronic subdural hematoma in geriatric patients – factors affecting prognosis Advances in Neurosurg. 12:204–211
139. Stehbens WE (1972) Pathology of the Cerebral Blood Vessels. C.V. Mosby, St. Louis
140. The International Study of Unruptured Intracranial Aneurysms Investigators (1998) Unruptured intracranial aneurysms – risk of rupture and risks of surgical intervention. N Engl J Med 339:1725–1733
141. Thomas WE (1992) Brain macrophages: evaluation of microglia and their functions. Brain Research Reviews 17:61–74
142. Torvik A (1984) The pathogenesis of watershed infarcts in the brain. Stroke 15:221–223
143. Torvik A, Jorgensen L (1964) Thrombotic and embolic occlusions of the carotid arteries in an autopsy material. Part 1. Prevalence, location and associated diseases. J Neurol Sci 1:24–39

144. Torvik A, Jorgensen L (1966) Thrombotic and embolic occlusions of the carotid arteries in an autopsy series. Part 2. Cerebral lesions and clinical course. J Neurol Sci 3:410–432
145. Tuszynski MH, Petito CK, Levy DE (1989) Risk factors and clinical manifestations of pathologically verified lacunar infarctions. Stroke 20:990–999
146. Ueda K, Hasuo Y, Kiyohara Y, Wada J, Kawano H et al. (1988) Intracerebral hemorrhage in a Japanese community, Hisayama: incidence, changing pattern during long-term follow-up, and related factors. Stroke 19:48–52
147. Usher BW (1993) Cardiac valvular disease and stroke. Neurologic Clinics 11:391–398
148. Vinters HV (1987) Cerebral amyloid angiopathy– a critical review. Stroke 18:311–324
149. Vinters HV (1991) Interactions between the heart and brain. In: Silver MD (ed) Cardiovascular pathology. 2nd edition. Churchill Livingstone, New York, pp 1029–1071
150. Vinters HV (1997) Pathology of cervical and intracranial atherosclerosis and fibromuscular dysplasia. In: Batjer HH (ed) Cerebrovascular disease. Lippincott-Raven, Philadelphia, pp 41–51
151. Vinters HV (1998) Cerebral amyloid angiopathy. In: Barnett HJM, Mohr JP, Stein BM, Yatsu FM (eds) Stroke pathophysiology, diagnosis, and management. 3rd edition. Churchill Livingstone, New York, pp 945–962
152. Vinters HV (1998) Alzheimer's disease: a neuropathologic perspective. Curr Diagn Pathol 5:109–117
153. Vinters HV (2000) Cerebral microvascular and macrovascular disease in the aging brain; similarities and differences. In: Verbeek MM, de Waal RMW, Vinters HV (eds) Cerebral amyloid angiopathy in Alzheimer's disease and related disorders. Kluwer, Dordrecht, pp 59–78
154. Vinters HV, Anders KH (1990) Neuropathology of AIDS. CRC Press, Boca Raton, Florida, pp 229
155. Vinters HV, Duckwiler GR (1992) Intracranial hemorrhage in the normotensive elderly patient. Neuroimaging Clin N America 2:153–169
156. Vinters HV, Farrell MA, Mischel PS, Anders KH (1998) Diagnostic Neuropathology. Marcel Dekker, New York, pp 51–171
157. Vinters HV, Gilbert JJ (1983) Cerebral amyloid angiopathy: incidence and complications in the aging brain. II. The distribution of amyloid vascular changes. Stroke 14:924–928
158. Vinters HV, Kaufmann JCE, Drake CG (1983) 'Foreign' particles in encephalic vascular malformations. Arch Neurol 40:221–225
159. Vinters HV, Lundie MJ, Kaufmann JCE (1986) Long-term pathological follow-up of cerebral arteriovenous malformations treated by embolization with bucrylate. N Engl J Med 314:477–483
160. Vinters HV, Natte R, Maat-Schieman MLC, van Duinen SG, Hegeman-Kleinn I, Welling-Graafland C, et al. (1998) Secondary microvascular degeneration in amyloid angiopathy of patients with hereditary cerebral hemorrhage with amyloidosis, Dutch type (HCHWA-D). Acta Neuropathol 95:235–244
161. Vinters HV, Secor DL, Read SL, Frazee JG, Tomiyasu U et al. (1994) The microvasculature in brain biopsy specimens from patients with Alzheimer's disease: an immunohistochemical and ultrastructural study. Ultrastruct Pathol 18:333–348
162. Vinters HV, Vonsattel J-PG (2000) Neuropathologic features and grading of Alzheimer-related and sporadic CAA. In: Verbeek MM, de Waal RMW, Vinters HV (eds) Cerebral amyloid angiopathy in Alzheimer's disease and related disorders. Kluwer, Dordrecht, pp 137–155
163. Vinters HV, Wang ZZ, Secor DL (1996) Brain parenchymal and microvascular amyloid in Alzheimer's disease. Brain Pathol 6:179–195
164. Vonsattel JPG, Myers RH, Hedley-Whyte ET, Ropper AH, Bird ED, Richardson EP Jr (1991) Cerebral amyloid angiopathy without and with cerebral hemorrhages: a comparative histological study. Ann Neurol 30:637–649
165. Wang ZZ, Jensson O, Thorsteinsson L, Vinters HV (1997) Microvascular degeneration in hereditary cystatin C amyloid angiopathy of the brain. APMIS 105:41–47
166. Wang ZZ, Natte R, Berliner JA, van Duinen SG, Vinters HV (2000) Toxicity of Dutch (E22Q) and Flemish (A21G) mutant amyloid beta proteins to human cerebral microvessel and aortic smooth muscle cells. Stroke 31:534–538

167. Waterston JA, Brown MM, Butler P, Swash M (1990) Small deep cerebral infarcts associated with occlusive internal carotid artery disease. A hemodynamic phenomenon? Arch Neurol 47:953–957
168. Weisberg LA (1988) Diagnostic classification of stroke, especially lacunes. Stroke 19:1071–1073
169. Weaver JP, Fisher M (1994) Subarachnoid hemorrhage: an update of pathogenesis, diagnosis and management. J Neurol Sci 125:119–131
170. Wechsler B, Vidailhet M, Piette JC, Bousser MG, Dell Isola B, Bletry O, Godeau P (1992) Cerebral venous thrombosis in Behçet's disease: clinical study and long-term follow-up of 25 cases. Neurology 42:614–618
171. Whetsell WO Jr. (1996) Current concepts of excitotoxicity. J Neuropathol Exp Neurol 55:1–13
172. Wilkinson IMS, Russell RWR (1972) Arteries of the head and neck in giant cell arteritis. A pathological study to show the pattern of arterial involvement. Arch Neurol 27:378–391
173. Yong WH, Robert ME, Secor DL, Kleikamp TJ, Vinters HV (1992) Cerebral hemorrhage with biopsy-proved amyloid angiopathy. Arch Neurol 49:51–58

# Head Injury in Routine and Forensic Pathological Practice

J. F. Geddes, H. L. Whitwell



## 1 Introduction

In recent years, head injury has lost its Cinderella status in the neuroscience world, as advances in the understanding of the cellular pathology have opened up the very real possibility of therapeutic intervention. For pathologists, a direct consequence of this has been that not only can much more of the tissue damage resulting from trauma now be appreciated on light microscopy, thanks to the development of immunocytochemical markers, but also there are often greater expectations of the autopsy and brain examination in a head injury case. This chapter describes a modern approach to head injury for non-neuropathologists, then addresses the specific problem of axonal injury, and finally tackles a rather specialist subject about which there is very little published information – namely, non-accidental head injury in infants.

## 2 Neuropathological Aspects of the Autopsy in Head Injury

Head injury may be a leading cause of death and morbidity, but the pathological investigation of such cases has traditionally often been cursory, limited to the

Current Topics in Pathology, Vol. 95
S. Love (Ed.): Neuropathology

documentation of scalp bruises, skull fractures, intracranial haematomas and brain swelling. The practice of many pathologists in a case of head injury is to establish a cause of death, and not to examine the brain further once this has been done. However, with greater knowledge of the cellular processes that occur in trauma, and the availability of markers of traumatic injury, such an approach is no longer adequate. Whatever its aetiology, head injury is always an unnatural cause of death, and it is rare that a pathologist has all the necessary information at postmortem to enable him or her to predict questions that are likely to be asked at a later date, at least some of which might only be answered by looking at sections of the brain. Lawyers are familiar with the vocabulary of neuropathology, if not the science underlying it, and their understanding, at least in most criminal cases, is that the brain should be properly examined. That their expectations of such an examination may often be wildly unrealistic is irrelevant; in many instances the histology of the brain, if properly done, can contribute to the interpretation of a head injury. For that reason alone, in every case of head injury the pathologist should decide whether to seek the coroner's consent for the brain to be retained and fixed intact for later examination, and be aware that if it is not, there is a possibility that potentially useful material will be irretrievably lost. As little as a week's fixation, especially if the brain is put in a large container and cut in half after a few days to allow the formalin to enter the ventricular cavities, produces much better results than blocks cut from an unfixed brain.

A counsel of perfection is to have a full history of the incident that caused the fatal head injury, and to see any X-rays, especially CT scans, before starting the autopsy. In practice, the 'history' usually comprises a sentence or two, and it is only at a later stage that further details, clinical notes and copies of scans become available. Consider in advance how macroscopic findings are to be recorded. Photographs are ideal, but remember that photographs taken with digital cameras are not acceptable for legal proceedings in some countries. A set of standard line drawings of the body, head, skull and brain, on which macroscopic findings can be recorded, is another way in which pathology can be documented, and these may of course be disclosable as evidence in court at a later date, as may all the notes made at the time of autopsy. All external injuries should be noted, as should internal injuries found in the general postmortem – e.g. extensive blood loss, long bone fractures, damage to the lungs – as these may turn out to be relevant to the findings in the brain.

## 2.1 External Examination

Subscalp bruising, skull fractures, membrane haemorrhages (extradural, subdural) should all be measured and described, and photographed where possible. The volume of any haematoma must be estimated, and the dura carefully examined for evidence of previous subdural bleeding, in the form of subdural membranes. The brain should then be carefully removed and weighed, and the weight recorded. A significant increase in brain weight, calculated from standard tables [17] means that there is likely to have been raised intracranial pressure; evidence of grooving and haemorrhage in one or both medial temporal lobes, or necrosis of the cerebellar tonsils will provide useful supporting evidence. (Beware of diagnosing raised intracranial pressure without adequate grounds for doing so – for example, the foramen magnum is extremely variable in diameter, and in many normal brains the cerebellar tonsils can appear deeply grooved and moulded, but they will be firm, not necrotic.) After removal of the brain, strip the dura from the base of the skull to check for fractures. These too should be photographed or drawn on a diagram.

Before the brain is fixed, it should be studied externally. Apart from swelling, is there subarachnoid haemorrhage? This is usually relatively trivial, and often related to fractures. However, if there is a quantity of blood in the basal cisterns, other possibilities have to be excluded. Has the blood in the subarachnoid space come from a primary intraventricular haemorrhage, or is it the result of bleeding from one of the arteries on the surface of the brain? An attempt should be made to answer this before the brain is fixed, as once it is immersed in formalin, the blood will become solid and difficult to dissect from the vessels. Any subarachnoid blood at the base should be carefully washed off, and the basal arteries exposed by blunt dissection, because it is, of course, always possible for a patient who has had a spontaneous subarachnoid haemorrhage to collapse and injure his head. If no aneurysm or other vascular anomaly is found, it is possible that the subarachnoid bleeding is traumatic in origin, in which case the posterior circulation, particularly the basilar and vertebral arteries, should be examined carefully. Arterial rupture, pseudoaneurysm formation and dissection, both intracranial and extracranial, are all well described after head and neck injury [14, 16, 44, 67, 80, 84] and may be responsible for either subarachnoid haemorrhage or cerebral infarction (Fig. 1). The intracranial vertebral and basilar arteries should be dissected off the base of the brain in a single piece and examined under a dissecting microscope.

The extracranial vertebral arteries can be examined at the time of autopsy [10], but by far the easiest way is to remove a block of foramen magnum and cervical spine whole, with the cervical cord inside, and examine it after fixation [26]. The vertebral arteries can then be dissected out of the bony foramina quite easily with a pair of small rongeurs or curved heavy pattern wire cutting scissors, and then cut across transversely and serially embedded for histology. Examination of the part of the internal carotid that passes through the base of the skull may necessitate removal of a block of skull base, which will have to be decalcified before the artery can be exposed.

Finally, the presence of contusions should be noted before the brain is fixed, and their relationship to fractures and other signs of impact ascertained and described.

An external examination such as this may well reveal a cause of death. However, ideally the brain should be still be suspended by the basilar artery in formalin, as soon as possible after removal from the body. All the dura should also be preserved and fixed with the brain.

## 2.2 Internal Examination

Standard neuropathological practice is to suspend a brain in formalin and, ideally, fix it for at least a month. While this is the time necessary for most brains to become

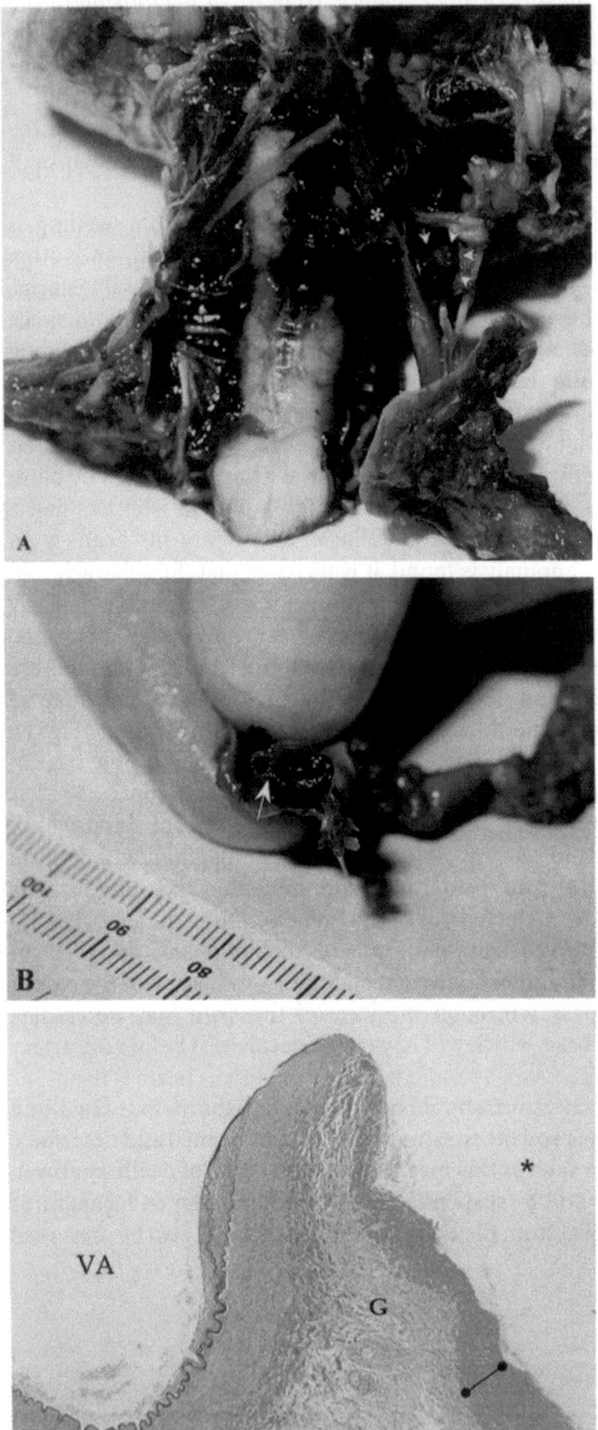
A
B
100
90
80
C
VA
G
*

properly fixed, a brain can be cut earlier than this, if necessary. However, the enforced interval before a brain can be cut means that by the time it is ready, further details of the head injury, and scans, should be available. Perhaps the single most useful piece of information to obtain before continuing is the survival time after injury, as this may significantly influence both the interpretation of the macroscopic findings and the approach to block-taking. Before cutting, one should be satisfied that the external appearances have been adequately documented and described. If, as is increasingly common, the relatives have requested the brain to be returned to them after it has been examined, it is particularly important to be certain that an adequate neuropathological record has been preserved.

The brain is usually sliced in the coronal plane but any approach that yields anatomically identifiable slices is acceptable. The internal examination will reveal the full extent of the macroscopic pathology, and once the brain slices are laid out, one should consider carefully whether the external and internal findings together are compatible with the history and clinical details. Recommended detailed descriptions of the pathology of head injury can be found in *Greenfield's Neuropathology* [37] or other neuropathology texts. A useful reference that considers clinical aspects and mechanisms in conjunction with the radiological and pathological findings in head injury is *Imaging of Head Trauma*, by A.E. Gean [25]. In some situations, the distribution of lesions may be of considerable help in interpreting the circumstances of an injury – a classic example being the occipital fracture with frontotemporal 'contre-coup' contusions that typically result from a fall on the back of the head. Equally, the brain of a patient who has been in prolonged coma which is macroscopically normal or shows apparently trivial lesions can be expected to have widespread histological damage [6, 39, 49, 62].

**Fig. 1 A–C.** A young man suffered a head injury as a result of which he lost consciousness briefly. He was discharged from hospital, but returned the following day, complaining of headache. Investigations were negative, but he continued to complain of pains in the head and neck over the next few days, and died suddenly just over a week after the injury. At postmortem there was an extensive basal subarachnoid haemorrhage, the source of the bleeding being a ruptured pseudoaneurysm on the left vertebral artery. **A** The hindbrain and vessels with the extracranial vertebral arteries attached, seen at autopsy. *Asterisk* marks the left vertebral artery, and *four small arrows* outline the pseudoaneurysm. **B** The vertebral artery has been cut across through the dilatation, and a double lumen is seen. The smaller, on the *left*, is the vertebral artery, the larger is the false aneurysm. *Arrow* indicates the communication between the two. A section at this point is shown below. **C** The vertebral artery (*VA*) is on the *left*, the actual site of rupture being at the *top* of the picture, with the aneurysm (*asterisked*) on the *right*. Its wall is composed of granulation tissue (*G*) and a thick layer of fibrin, indicated by the *heavy line*. (Case reproduced by kind permission of Dr. Hugh White)

## 2.3 Histology in Head Injury

It is our practice to take a set of large of representative blocks of all regions from any brain that is destined to be returned to the body for burial, to ensure that tissue is available should histology be required at a later date. In many other cases of head injury, however, there will be other specific reasons why microscopy is required. The most usual are: (1) to 'age' lesions; (2) to look for vascular pathology; (3) to assess diffuse brain injury; (4) to look for evidence of previous trauma; (5) to exclude underlying pathology which may have aggravated the effects of (or indeed have caused) the head injury. The selection of blocks will depend on what one is looking for, but in most of the instances just cited the brain should be widely sampled.

### 2.3.1 Ageing Lesions

The principal reason for trying to 'age' pathology (in practice, usually a subdural haematoma, a vascular lesion or damage to axons), is to estimate the timing of an incident for medicolegal purposes. This is a potential minefield and a prudent pathologist will only undertake to give an opinion on dating after a very thorough examination and wide tissue sampling. Even when such an opinion is given, the report should convey the limitations of dating from histological criteria. In the case of subdural haemorrhages, the temporal evolution of the process of organisation was well described in the 1930s by Munro and Merritt, who studied histological changes in 47 subdural haemorrhages of known ages [64]; most modern tables published [42, 43, 53, 55] are based on their work. There are drawbacks to using this otherwise thorough study to pinpoint the time of injury, however: the principal ones are that there were very few subjects – sometimes only one – in some of the survival groups studied, and there is not enough information in the paper about the normal variation at any survival time. Several samples of dura should be processed for histology, both dura with blood adherent as well as apparently normal areas: it is surprising how often a piece of dura that looks normal at a cursory glance is found to have organising haemorrhage when looked at under the microscope. Perls, reticulin, HVG stains and immunohistochemistry for microglia may all be helpful to demonstrate the extent of the cellular reaction to the haemorrhage and so the stage of organisation.

Dating of vascular lesions – haemorrhages and areas of infarction – can be attempted by comparing the findings to information in a standard neuropathology text (e.g. Davis and Robertson's *Textbook of Neuropathology* [24]). Once again, neither individual variation nor the effects of treatment on the evolution of such processes have been explored. And similarly, while traumatic axonal damage is known to evolve [27, 37], there are simply not enough data in the literature to permit more than a very approximate estimate of timing – words such as 'a few days' or 'a few weeks' are always preferable to attempts at more precise dating.

### 2.3.2 Vascular Pathology

Microscopy will be needed to confirm the presence of vascular rupture, dissection or antemortem thrombus. Two examples indicate the use of sampling of vessels

- A young man died of raised intracranial pressure caused by a large middle cerebral artery territory infarct 36 h after an assault. He was found to have suffered a traumatic dissection of his internal carotid artery: the base of the skull was removed and decalcified, the artery dissected out and serially embedded for microscopy. Two areas of dissection with occlusive thrombus were found just above the roof of the cavernous sinus.
- A 65-year-old woman with unstable hypertension was involved in a domestic argument during which she received a trivial blow to the head. She died from the effects of a huge parenchymal haemorrhage in the basal ganglia, 10 h after the incident. There was no subscalp bruising or other evidence of head injury, and careful sampling showed extensive severe degenerative changes in parenchymal arterioles, typical of systemic hypertension. The prosecution argued that she had had a spontaneous hypertensive bleed, provoked by the circumstances of the fight.

### 2.3.3 Diffuse Brain Damage

'Diffuse brain injury' is a term coined by clinicians to describe head-injured patients who have global disruption of neurological function without a lesion (or lesions) on CT scan that would account for their clinical state. The phrase implies widespread structural damage, which neuropathologically is likely to be either traumatic or hypoxic/ischaemic in aetiology – or indeed, as often happens, both together. A search for such damage becomes an issue particularly where there is very little macroscopic evidence of trauma, and must be based on a study of samples taken from appropriate areas of the brain (see below, and Table 1). The

**Table 1.** Minimum set of blocks recommended for assessing axonal injury

1. Corpus callosum and parasagittal anterior frontal white matter
2. Corpus callosum and parasagittal posterior frontal white matter
3. Deep grey matter to include posterior limb of the internal capsule
4. Cerebellar hemisphere
5. Midbrain (to include decussation of superior cerebellar peduncle)
6. Pons (to include superior or middle cerebellar peduncles)

Suggested also:

7. Temporal lobe (to include hippocampus)
8. Splenium of the corpus callosum

And, in non-accidental infant head injury:

9. Lower pons and medulla
10. All the upper cervical cord segments

If blocks are taken to fit on standard size [3 × 1 inch (7.62 × 2.54 cm)] slides, the number of blocks taken should be doubled.

question of sampling for and interpreting diffuse axonal damage is discussed below; in the case of hypoxia-ischaemia, a series of blocks of frontal, temporal, parietal and occipital cortex (including 'watershed' regions between different arterial territories), the hippocampus, deep grey matter and cerebellum, should establish whether or not a significant amount of such damage was present.

### 2.3.4 Evidence of Previous Head Injury

Tell-tale signs of previous trauma to the head are occasionally encountered in head injury victims, chronic subdural membranes being the most common. Contusions, which with increasing survival become orange-pigmented areas of superficial cortical atrophy, classically in the orbital and inferolateral temporal gyri, are a relatively common incidental finding at postmortem (Fig. 2). Signs of previously raised intracranial pressure (haemorrhagic or pigmented necrotic lesions in the parahippocampal gyri, in the parasagittal white matter adjacent to the cingulum, and in the visual cortex, for example) might represent the sequelae of an earlier

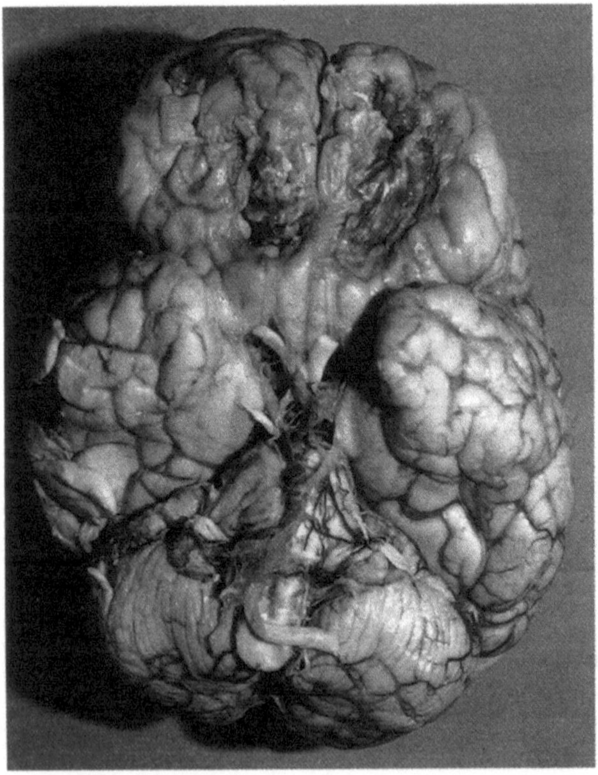

**Fig. 2.** Old contusions, the residua of a head injury 1 year before death, appear as pigmented atrophic areas on the base of both frontal lobes

severe head injury. In yet other cases, sections of hemispheric white matter, immunostained for a microglial antigen, show clusters of microglial cells and, on occasion, evidence of secondary long-tract degeneration in the brain stem. In many cases these microglial 'nodules' may well be the residua of an old head injury, but microglial clusters are not only seen in trauma and so cannot in isolation be taken as evidence of such. In fact, in the absence of either a history of earlier trauma or macroscopic signs such as a subdural membrane or old contusions, it is unwise to assume they are traumatic, because they can also be found scattered in the white matter, without other diagnostic features, after fat embolism, after an episode of global hypoxia, and in HIV encephalitis, to give just a few examples.

## 3 Traumatic Axonal Injury

All the evidence currently available suggests that while axons may be injured at the time of head injury, in most cases the process takes many hours, or even days, to be completed. It is believed that axonal damage occurs in virtually all head injuries in which there is significant movement of the brain inside the skull, the amount of axonal damage depending entirely on the severity and direction of this movement. As methods of detecting white matter damage have become more sensitive, it has become clear that there is a wide neuropathological spectrum of traumatic axonal injury (TAI), while experimental work has shown that there is a corresponding clinical spectrum of disability after head injury which correlates well with the pathology. Cases of documented mild head injury, of course, rarely come to a neuropathologist [8, 38, 70, 72], but recent work on experimental models suggests that in its mildest forms, traumatic damage to axons is probably completely reversible [59, 81] and is the neuropathological substrate of various concussion syndromes [32]. At the other end of the spectrum, where TAI is severe and damage widespread, the patient is unconscious from the time of the head injury, and is left vegetative or severely disabled after recovery from coma; this is the clinicopathological syndrome known as 'diffuse axonal injury' (DAI) [2–5]. In DAI the damage is by definition very widespread, involving the brain stem as well as the hemispheres.

### 3.1 Sampling for TAI

It is important to note that while the clinical features of DAI are well recognised, there is little or no information available at present about the clinical features of lesser degrees of traumatic damage to axons. From a practical point of view, therefore, the only useful outcome of an attempt to diagnose axonal injury is that the presence of the most severe form – DAI – can be either confirmed or excluded. Mild degrees of traumatic axonal damage, for example axonal swellings scattered through the hemispheric white matter but not in the brain stem, can merely be noted as confirmation that there has been a head injury. Despite the fact that the distribution and amount of axonal damage will differ widely from one head injury to another, there are certain sites in the brain which are particularly vulnerable. These include white matter bundles such as the corpus callosum and the internal capsule, the parasagittal white matter of the hemispheres, and – in more severe cases – the cerebellar white matter and cerebellar peduncles in the brain stem [2, 37, 65], and so these are the first sites that should be sampled (Table 1).

The blocks should be as large as the laboratory can handle: the smaller the blocks have to be, the more of them should be taken. We recommend that a minimum set of blocks should include two samples of corpus callosum, one of which should be the splenium, together with adjacent parasagittal white matter; one block of the posterior limb of the internal capsule; one block of cerebellar hemispheric white matter with middle cerebellar peduncle; and at least two of the upper brain stem, preferably to include the superior and middle cerebellar peduncles. However, if blocks are small – i.e. for the routine 3 × 1-inch slides in use in general histopathology – many more should be taken. The more the brain is sampled, the better the chance of detecting any white matter damage and of estimating its extent [27]. All blocks should be taken to avoid obvious areas of haemorrhage and infarction, which also cause damage to axons.

### 3.2 Detecting Axonal Damage

After about 12–18 h survival, traumatic axonal damage can be detected by conventional stains such as haematoxylin and eosin (H&E) or silver impregnations for axons. Where survival is shorter, a more sensitive indicator of damage is required. Current practice is to use immunohistochemistry to demonstrate a protein which normally moves down axons in undetectable quantities but which becomes detectable when it accumulates at the site of injury because axonal transport has been interrupted. While theoretically a number of such 'markers' would be suitable for this purpose, the most widely used in routine neuropathological practice is $\beta$-amyloid precursor protein ($\beta$APP) [33, 78]. There is now considerable experience of the use of this antibody in diagnosis [9, 27, 34]. Derangement of axonal transport can be detected with anti-$\beta$APP at least as early as 2 h after injury [61], which is considerably sooner than it can be demonstrated with routine stains, and earlier than other histological features, particularly the changes of hypoxia-ischaemia, are detectable. A small study of the evolution of staining patterns in DAI has shown that after approximately 1 week, axonal bulbs fail to stain for $\beta$APP, although adjacent axons still stain strongly [27]. After about 1 month to 6 weeks' survival after injury, our experience is that $\beta$APP expression disappears; small granular clumps of immunoreactivity may occasionally be seen in the white matter. After survival of about 1 week, immunocytochemistry for microglia, with an antibody to an epitope such as CD68 (PG-M1), is a useful adjunct to $\beta$APP. We have documented aggregation of microglia round axonal bulbs as early as 5 days, with microglial clusters (stars) first appearing at 10/11 days. By 2 weeks' survival, microglial stars are present in considerable numbers in cases of DAI, but as survival increases they tend to be obscured by the large numbers of lipid-laden macrophages in long tracts which mark the start of secondary 'wallerian' degeneration [27]. Note that these timings should be considered a very rough guide only: the process is an ongoing one and, from all the evidence available, probably not uniform in its evolution in axons of different sizes [27, 46, 60]. This fact means that estimation of the age of an injury from the size of the axonal bulbs [83] is not likely to be accurate either. A final caveat is that all timings in the literature are derived entirely from adult work and there is no information about the evolution of axonal pathology in infants or very young children.

## 3.3 Problems in Interpretation

The ability to detect histological changes with immunocytochemistry at very short survival, well before they could possibly be demonstrated by any of the more routinely used stains, may create problems for the interpretation of pathology. Axonal damage demonstrated by βAPP expression is not necessarily traumatic: a number of different pathological processes can injure axons sufficiently to interfere with intracellular transport, and so cause detectable βAPP accumulation. Damaged axons can be seen at the edges of a haemorrhage or infarct, but other less-obvious pathological situations in which βAPP immunoreactivity has demonstrated axonal involvement include HIV encephalitis, multiple sclerosis, and in gunshot injuries, at sites distant from the bullet track [15, 23, 31, 35, 51, 63]. In practical terms, in closed head injury the most challenging differential diagnosis is global hypoxic-ischaemic damage. While this is more usually thought of as affecting neuronal cell bodies, the use of immunocytochemistry for axonally transported proteins such as βAPP in cases of hypoxic-ischaemic encephalopathy reveals that axons may also be directly damaged [1, 51, 78]. In support of this idea, other workers have shown that white matter is particularly susceptible to hypoxic-ischaemic conditions [79]. This can pose serious diagnostic difficulties in many head injuries, where brain swelling and terminal ischaemia and hypoxia are exceptionally common. The situation is made more difficult by the fact that when there is brain swelling and internal herniation, blood vessels are compressed, notably pericallosal arteries and perforators from the circle of Willis, which leads to ischaemic white matter damage in very much the same distribution as that of traumatic axonal injury [28, 77]. The result is that in cases of short survival it is frequently impossible to know how to interpret βAPP expression. In such cases, the histology report should be quite honest about this. As a general rule, we find that hypoxic-ischaemic white matter damage tends to result in linear or geographic foci βAPP positivity, sometimes around vessels, while traumatic damage, though often affecting fascicles, tends to manifest as single or scattered axons expressing βAPP, but the distinction is not always clear cut. Some examples are illustrated in Fig. 3 (see also Fig. 6). One reason that large blocks are preferable is that it is sometimes easier to interpret such βAPP expression after scanning a large field at low power. With increasing survival after head injury, the distinction between hypoxic and traumatic damage is easier to make: cellular changes such as neuronal nuclear pyknosis and cytoplasmic eosinophilia can be detected, and the correct diagnosis made. When there has been sufficient survival after injury for axonal bulbs to be detectable on H&E (12–18 h), any significant areas of axonal immunoreactivity without bulb formation are likely to have been produced by terminal hypoxia secondary to raised intracranial pressure, not the initial head injury.

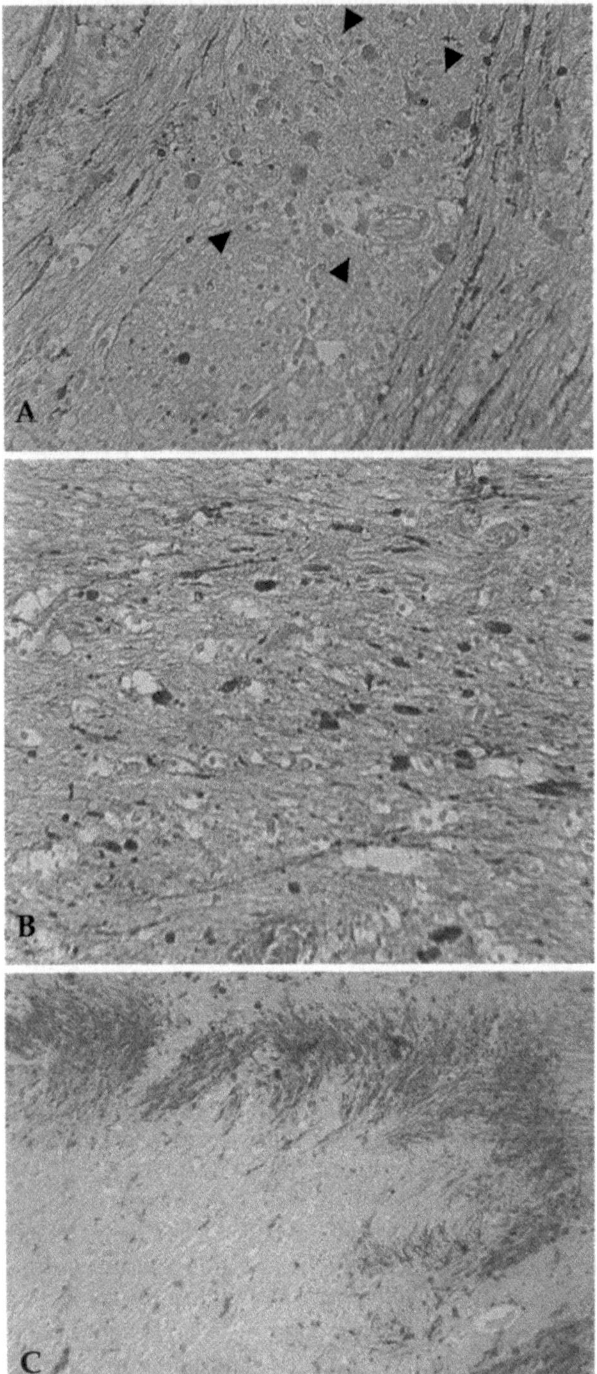
A
B
C

### 3.4 Axonal Pathology and Clinicopathological Correlations

Of course, the primary reason for undertaking any histology in head injury is to relate the neuropathological findings to the circumstances of the injury and/or the patient's subsequent clinical course. This may be in answer to questions posed by a number of different groups – typically, the coroner, the police, defence lawyers or clinicians. Most such questions, especially those of the "which blow killed him?" variety, cannot be answered by neuropathological examination alone. The expectations are often high, and one may find that enormous significance is placed on a particular microscopic finding, through a basic lack of understanding of neuropathology. For example, confusion has been created by the misuse of the term 'DAI' to cover axonal injury of any sort, particularly in the forensic literature, and compounded by case reports quoted in court which are inadequately documented neuropathologically. In many ways, it would be much simpler if the term 'DAI' could be abandoned, in favour of phrases that describe the presumed aetiology – e.g. 'widespread traumatic/hypoxic/hypoglycaemic axonal injury', which would avoid any ambiguities. However, the concept of DAI is used by clinicians, for whom it has considerable relevance. In our practice, we use 'DAI' in the sense in which it was originally defined – namely, severe traumatic axonal damage in a widespread distribution in both the hemispheres and the brain stem. We usually add the word 'traumatic', in order to emphasise that we are talking about diffuse traumatic axonal injury, rather than diffuse axonal injury caused by anything else. DAI thus defined means that the head injury was of a severity to have caused immediate loss of consciousness and prolonged coma. Unfortunately, that is about all one can say, because despite the fact that experimental work under controlled situations shows that accelerations of high magnitude, with or without deceleration, are necessary to produce DAI, there is no way that one can be sure from the neuropathology exactly how the head injury might have been caused [28].

## 4 Non-Accidental Head Injury in Children

While older victims of abuse tend to die of extracranial injuries, head injury is the principal cause of death in infants who suffer non-accidental injury (NAI). Given the frequency with which neuropathologists tend nowadays to become involved in fatal cases of head injury in which NAI is suspected, it is quite surprising to discover that the neuropathology of inflicted head injury in children is far from

**Fig. 3A–C.** Severe brain swelling, vascular compromise and βAPP immunohistochemistry. **A** Immunoreactive axons in both transverse and descending bundles, and cytoplasmic βAPP staining in neurons (*between arrowheads*), all resulting from ischaemia of the ventral pons, caused by cerebral oedema and raised intracranial pressure. **B** Axonal bulbs round an area of established infarction (i.e. detectable on H&E and other stains) in the ventral part of the posterior limb of the internal capsule. From a patient with raised intracranial pressure and transtentorial herniation. **C** The typical geographic immunoreactivity produced by ischaemia, seen here in the central white matter established and that there is very little reliable neuropathological information on the subject in the literature. A paper by LINDENBERG and FREYTAG in 1969 described 'contusional tears' in a small series of young infants who had suffered non-accidental head injury with impact [56], and since then few neuropathological reports have been published [12, 36, 41, 77, 82]. The largest series contains only 14 cases, and none has attempted detailed clinicopathological correlation. Most lack full information, particularly of potentially relevant clinical factors that might affect interpretation of pathology. This lack of reliable data has meant that for medicolegal purposes opinions have had in many instances to be based on what is known about adult head injury, despite many reasons why the biomechanics of the two should be fundamentally different. Reviews of NAI have tended to compound the confusion by reiterating the neuropathology of adult trauma [11, 13, 54]. We have studied a large series of inflicted head injury in children in order to provide neuropathological data, and have demonstrated that age-related patterns of injury can be detected, with infants (i.e. children up to 1 year old) showing rather different clinicopathological pictures from children over 1 year old, who tend have neuropathology more akin to that seen in adults [29, 30].

## 4.1 Neuropathological Aspects of the Autopsy in NAI Cases

A description of the procedure for an autopsy in a case of suspected child abuse is beyond the scope of this chapter; accounts can be found in paediatric pathology texts [50, 68]. Where possible, the prosector should have details of the story given by the carer at the time of the child's presentation, as well as the findings of paramedics and hospital staff involved in resuscitation and treatment. In a large proportion of infant cases there is a history of apnoea or respiratory collapse: descriptions such as the baby "went blue" or "stopped breathing" are extremely common, and in many cases are supported both by the accounts of ambulance staff and by the CT scan on arrival at hospital, which frequently shows a swollen hypoxic brain and little else. Others are said to have been accidentally dropped or to have fallen from a height or down stairs – every effort should be made to match the injuries found at postmortem to the scenario that is said to have occurred.

Extracranial injuries are frequent in NAI. In infants these are most frequently rib fractures, often multiple, which may on radiological and histological criteria predate the head injury from which the child died. In older children, thoracic and abdominal injuries, often serious, are more common. Bony injuries should be assessed by a radiological skeletal survey performed before the autopsy, but bruising and other injuries should be sought, and may of course be helpful in assessing the mechanism of injury. The approach to examination of the scalp and skull is the same as for adult head injury, and all abnormalities should be photographed at every stage. The scalp should be carefully examined externally and internally for bruising, and the pattern of bruising related, if possible, to the possible types of injury, whether associated with finger marks, slap marks or other forms of impact. The state of the fontanelles should be recorded. Skull fractures are common in inflicted head injury, particularly in infants – in our series of 53 cases, 43% of infants (<1 year old) had one or more skull fractures, compared to 19% of those over

1 year of age. The biomechanics of skull fracture in infant head injury have been investigated by DUHAIME and her colleagues [18] and reviewed by BROWN and MINNS [11], who also discuss the features that are more characteristic of non-accidental skull fractures.

Although skull fractures are a frequent feature of NAI in the very young, extra-dural haemorrhages are distinctly rare. The factors that militate against extradural bleeding include the compliance of the infant skull, relative mobility of the middle meningeal artery in infants, adherence of dura to the skull in early life, and the predominantly posterior distribution of skull fractures in NAI [19]. Subdural haemorrhage, which occurs when veins crossing the subdural space are torn, is extremely common: in our own series, 84% of the infant cases had subdural bleeding. This bleeding is often also posteriorly sited [18] and covers both hemispheres, but unlike adult head injury, rarely requires neurosurgical evacuation (Fig. 4). Characteristically, the amount of blood involved is scanty [19] - indeed, may not show up on neuroimaging [22, 45]. In postmortem reports, words such as 'thin film' are commonly used to describe the bleeding. Not infrequently, there is evidence of an earlier subdural haemorrhage. For this reason, several samples of dura should always be taken for histology; even macroscopically normal dura may prove to have organising haemorrhage adherent to it [75]. However, the presence of subdural membranes or haemosiderin staining in the setting of an acute head injury may not necessarily be evidence of previous NAI, and must be interpreted very cautiously. Subdural haemorrhage has been detected in utero, in one case resolving by the time of delivery [7, 40, 52]. There are also descriptions in the literature of subdural haemorrhage occurring shortly after birth; these have been variously attributed to mode of delivery [58, 71], to the presence of coagulopathies [21, 73], and to septicaemia [66]. Such cases suggest that if cranial ultrasound or CT scanning were routinely performed on all neonates, the incidence of perinatal subdural bleeding might be found to be higher. Because of this possibility, it is better to be agnostic about the cause of old subdural bleeding where there are no unexplained other injuries to suggest an earlier episode of trauma.

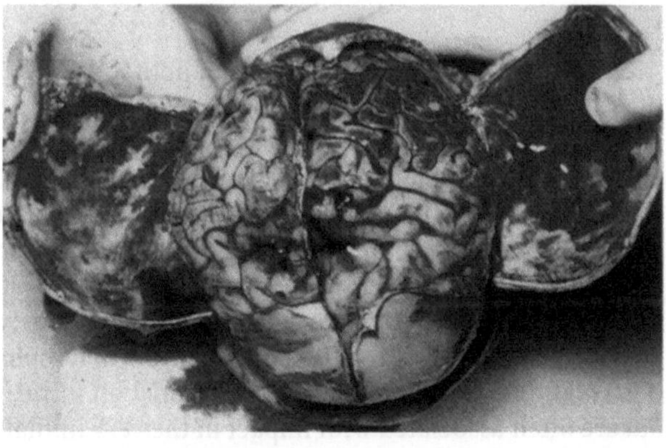

**Fig. 4.** The film of subdural haemorrhage, spread over both hemispheres of a swollen brain, which is commonly seen in infant NAI cases at postmortem. The bleeding may not have been detected by scanning when the child was alive

In our experience, subarachnoid haemorrhage is seldom clinically significant, but is associated with fractures or sometimes with subdural bleeding. Contusions, the impact lesions seen so frequently in older head injury cases, are rare in infants. The principal abnormality of the brain at autopsy is an increase in weight, which may be considerable in relation to the expected size for the age of the child. Note that despite pronounced brain swelling and raised intracranial pressure there is seldom naked-eye evidence of transtentorial or transforaminal herniation in infants, because the skull retains some capacity to expand. Accurate scales are always essential for weighing the very small brains, as an increase of 100 g or so may not be detected on machines used to weigh adult organs. Once weighed, the brain should be suspended in formalin for fixation, ideally with the dura still attached or in the pot.

There have been suggestions in the recent literature that in very young infants damage to the craniocervical junction may be a crucial factor in determining outcome after injury [41, 48]. Reports of bleeding into paraspinal muscles and of extradural haemorrhage at the cervicomedullary junction, even spinal cord lesions, have highlighted the fact that this region is vulnerable [41, 45, 55, 76]. With this in mind, the craniocervical junction should be very carefully dissected at postmortem, ideally from behind. Epidural bleeding can be sought, and the cord then removed in its dural sheath and fixed. Finally, both the eyes should be removed and fixed for specialist examination by an ophthalmic pathologist, because full histological examination may detect bleeding that has been missed clinically. Retinal haemorrhages are of course commonly seen in cases of NAI [19], although, despite a recent consensus statement from a working party set up by the Royal College of Ophthalmologists [69], their significance and pathogenesis is far from clear in every case. The literature on retinal haemorrhages should be read with caution, and a golden rule is never to interpret intraocular bleeding in a case in isolation – that is, without first studying a report on the neuropathological and general autopsy findings.

## 4.2 Examination of the Fixed Brain and Spinal Cord in NAI

An infant's brain is sliced after fixation in the same way as that of an adult, though the soft swollen brain of a young subject who has been ventilated may not fix well. In NAI cases, slicing seldom reveals any further macroscopic pathology apart from compression of the lateral ventricles due to brain swelling. Parenchymal haemorrhages may occur, but in our experience are uncommon. Contusional tears, traumatic lesions seen only in the brains of infants a few months old [56], appear as slits in the hemispheric white matter, often close to the grey-white matter junction. They may look artefactual, but under the microscope bleeding into the tissue tear and reaction by astrocytes, microglia and macrophages proves that they are indeed real. Such tears, which can be detected on ultrasound [47], are not common but are often associated with impact in the very immature brain (Fig. 5).

So when should blocks be taken? We believe that all areas of the brain should be sampled in all cases, even in those where the child was supposedly found dead. Our experience of NAI is that many of the infants said not to have survived show

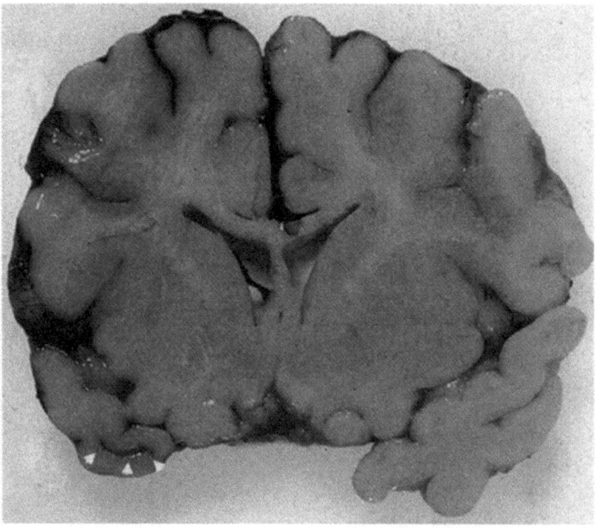

**Fig. 5.** The *arrowheads* indicate a contusional tear at the grey-white matter junction at one temporal pole, in the brain of a 4-month-old girl who survived 11 days after a head injury. The slit-like lesions can appear artefactual, but histology will show bleeding and a cellular reaction

histological changes suggesting that they did in fact live some hours or longer after a cerebral insult [29]. A set of blocks taken from all regions – anterior and posterior frontal lobes, both with corpus callosum; parietal lobe; temporal lobe with hippocampus; deep grey matter with insula; midbrain, pons and medulla; several cervical, thoracic and lumbar cord segments – will provide the best chance of detecting microscopic pathology, and of assessing its extent. The stains we use are similar to those used in adult head injury, namely H&E and immunohistochemistry for $\beta$APP, with Perls and a microglial immunostain (e.g. for CD68/PG-M1) where indicated. As with adults, distinguishing between hypoxic-ischaemic and traumatic damage with immunohistochemistry for $\beta$APP in cases of very short survival may be problematic. Some typical vascular patterns of immunoreactivity taken from a series of NAI cases are illustrated in Fig. 6 (see also Fig. 3). When the axonal injury has been present long enough for bulbs to be detectable on H&E the distinction is easier, because by that time changes of hypoxia or infarction will also be readily detectable.

There is no doubt that in fatal cases of inflicted head injury, infants clinically suffer severe diffuse brain damage. They are almost always collapsed and unresponsive by the time the ambulance arrives, and remain in coma on ventilation until death, which is usually rapid – in our series, the median survival of 53 children with head injury was 1 day. The question is, what is the neuropathological substrate of coma in these children? The assumption has always been that it is traumatic brain damage, but in fact there is surprisingly little evidence to support this. In 1987 Vowles et al. published a study of ten infants and claimed to have found DAI in six [82]. This study was done before the use of immunohistochemistry had revealed the full spectrum of traumatic axonal damage, and critical reading of their findings reveals that the authors were not in fact describing DAI

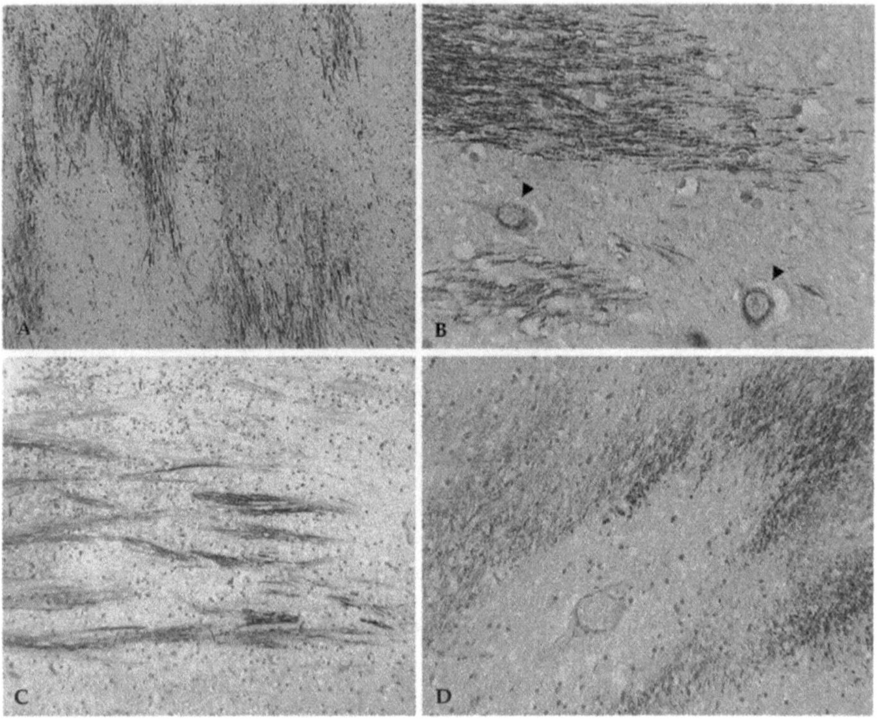

**Fig. 6 A–D.** Patterns of βAPP immunoreactivity in NAI cases, interpreted as vascular, seen in white matter (**A,D**) in the deep grey matter (**B**) and in the pontine base (**C**). **A** Geographic staining, outlining areas of ischaemia in the centrum semiovale; **B** Bundles of diffusely reactive axons running through the putamen. The two neurons in the lower half of the field (*arrowheads*) also show cytoplasmic expression of βAPP; **C** Olivocerebellar fibres just to one side of the midline in the medulla, in a grossly swollen brain; **D** Perivascular staining. Very often, as shown here, the swathes of immunoreactive axons have few or no bulbs

but lesser degrees of axonal damage, which may or may not have been traumatic. The paper, which has been widely quoted, remained the only study until 1998, when SHANNON et al. used βAPP immunocytochemistry on the brains of 14 children believed to have been shaken, with seven hypoxic-ischaemic cases as controls. They found similar types of axonal staining in both groups, assumed to be ischaemic, and immunoreactivity in the cervical nerve roots, which was only present in the NAI group. This was the first demonstration of axonal damage localised to the upper cervical spine and the authors suggested that the damage might have been the result of stretch to that region.

A subsequent report by GLECKMAN et al. claimed to have detected DAI in five cases of 'shaken baby syndrome' with βAPP immunohistochemistry [36]. However, the pictures that accompany the report show patterns of βAPP immunoreactivity that we consider to be typical of ischaemic injury and many neuropathological details are missing from the account. We have discussed this paper further in relation to our own study [30], as our experience is different from that of GLECKMAN and his colleagues. We have found DAI to be rare (2/37 infant cases, and only

**Fig. 7.** Fresh blood in the epidural space at the top of the spinal cord, in an infant believed to have been shaken

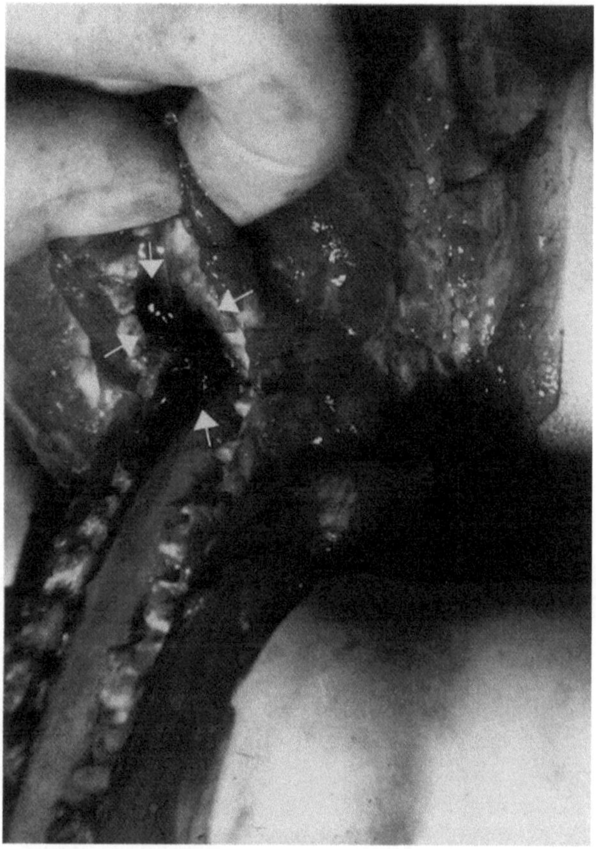

3 in the whole series of 53 cases). In addition, a significant proportion of the infants (13/37) were shown to have either macroscopic or microscopic damage at the craniocervical junction, sometimes both: epidural bleeding (see Fig. 7), βAPP immunopositivity in cervical cord roots and axonal damage confined to the corticospinal tracts in the lower pons and medulla (8 cases, see Fig. 8). This last is a striking finding, reported in adult hyperextension injury [28, 57, 74] but not previously in NAI. The severity of the damage in terms of the number of immunoreactive axons varies enormously from case to case, but we believe this long tract distribution to be the result of stretch injury to the neuraxis caused by hyperextension of the neck. Such injury must be particularly easy to inflict, given the inherently unstable anatomy of the head and the neck in the infant. We believe that in many cases damage at the craniocervical junction causes apnoea, as others have suggested [48], which in turn results in global hypoxic brain damage and secondary brain swelling. In the vast majority of cases the microscopic pathology responsible for these children being in coma is not DAI but hypoxic-ischaemic damage. Thirty of the 37 infants in our series died as a result of raised intracranial pressure associated with severe widespread neuronal and, often, axonal hypoxia-ischaemia. Our findings suggest that in many cases of inflicted infant head injury

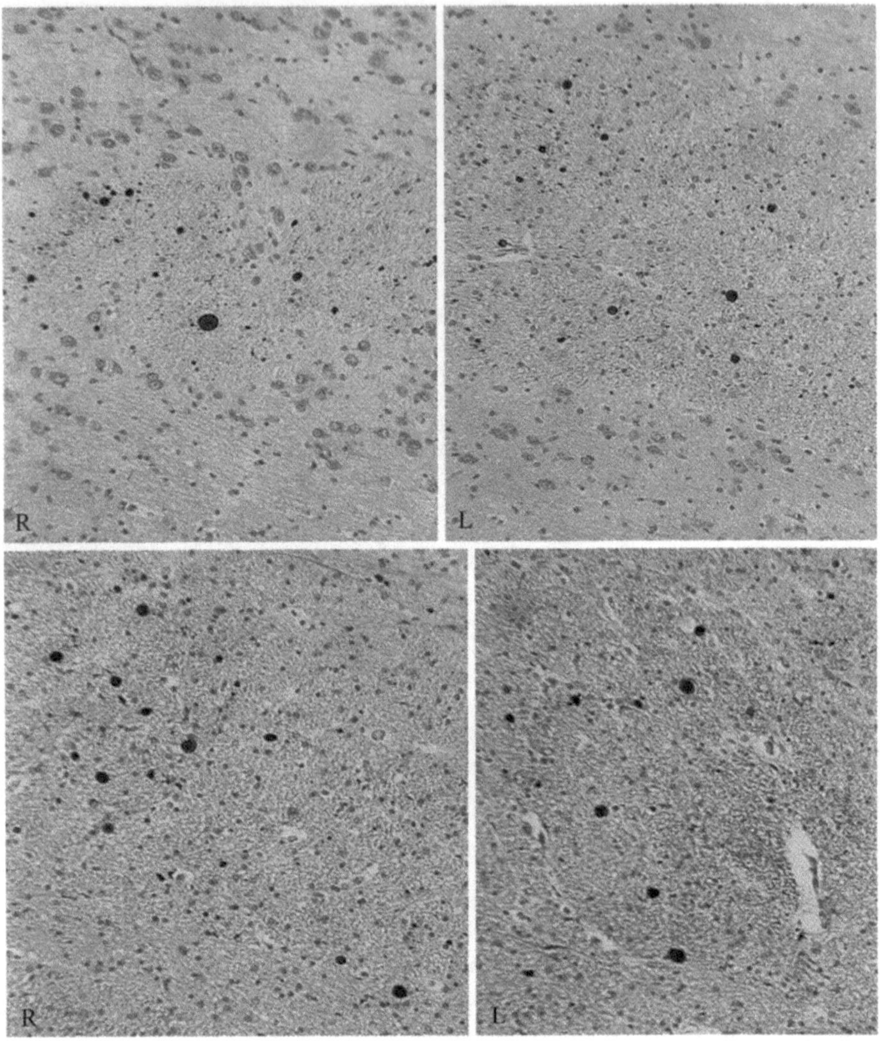


**Fig. 8.** Low power view of axonal swellings in the descending tracts in the pons (*above*) and pyramids (*below*) of a 3-week-old child (anti-βAPP; *R*, right; *L*, left)

the traumatic damage is slight, even survivable; what is not survivable is the brain swelling.

If DAI is a relative rarity, it is possible (as has been suggested by Duhaime [20]) that shaking does not produce the high degrees of angular/rotational acceleration necessary to cause it. If so, then perhaps the mode of injury need not necessarily be the "violent shaking" so often confidently alleged in expert reports and, indeed, in court. Data on how different people shake infants of different weights – and indeed, anatomical infant models that might be informative in this context – are sorely lacking. Certainly, there is seldom anything in the neuropathology of such cases, apart from impact injuries, that would enable a pathologist to give an opinion on the degree of force involved in the injury. The tearing of subdural veins would merely reflect movement of the brain in an arc about the fulcrum at the top of the neck. In NAI work it is important to appreciate that without either a confession or a witness to the injury the conclusion that it was inflicted cannot, and should not, be made by one person alone. Clinical identification of retinal haemorrhages or the discovery at autopsy of an unexpected subdural bleed may raise the question of NAI, but neither finding is diagnostic of child abuse. It is critical that the findings of paramedics, paediatricians, forensic, ophthalmic and neuropathologists should be taken together to ensure as high a degree of certainty as possible before any allegations are made.

**Acknowledgements.** The authors are grateful for the help of Allan Hackshaw, Georgina Lindop and Geoff Vowles, without whom this chapter could not have been written.

## References

1. Abou-Hamden A, Blumbergs PC, Scott G, Manavis J, Wainwright H, Jones N, McLean J (1997) Axonal injury in falls. J Neurotrauma 14:699–713
2. Adams JH, Doyle D, Ford I, Gennarelli TA, Graham DI, McLellan DR (1989) Diffuse axonal injury in head injury: definition, diagnosis and grading. Histopathology 15:49–59
3. Adams JH, Doyle D, Graham DI, Lawrence AE, McLellan DR (1984) Diffuse axonal injury in head injuries caused by a fall. Lancet 2:1420–1422
4. Adams JH, Doyle D, Graham DI, Lawrence AE, McLellan DR (1985) Microscopic diffuse axonal injury in cases of head injury. Med Sci Law 25:265–269
5. Adams JH, Graham DI, Gennarelli TA, Maxwell WL (1991) Diffuse axonal injury in non-missile head injury. J Neurol Neurosurg Psychiatry 54:481–483
6. Adams JH, Jennett B, McLellan DR, Murray LS, Graham DI (1999) The neuropathology of the vegetative state after head injury. J Clin Pathol 52:804–806
7. Barozzino T, Sgro M, Toi A, Akouri H, Wilson S, Yeo E, Blaser S, Chitayat D (1998) Fetal bilateral subdural haemorrhages. Prenatal diagnosis and spontaneous resolution by time of delivery. Prenat Diagn 18:496–503
8. Blumbergs PC, Scott G, Manavis J, Wainwright H, Simpson DA, McLean AJ (1994) Staining of amyloid precursor protein to study axonal damage in mild head injury. Lancet 344:1055–1056
9. Blumbergs PC, Scott G, Manavis J, Wainwright H, Simpson DA, McLean AJ (1995) Topography of axonal injury as defined by amyloid precursor protein and the sector scoring method in mild and severe closed head injury. J Neurotrauma 12:565–572
10. Bromilow A, Burns J (1985) Technique for removal of the vertebral arteries. J Clin Pathol 38:1400–1402
11. Brown JK, Minns RA (1993) Non-accidental head injury, with particular reference to whiplash shaking injury and medico-legal aspects. Dev Med Child Neurol 35:849–869
12. Calder IM, Hill I, Scholtz CL (1984) Primary brain trauma in non-accidental injury. J Clin Pathol 37:1095–1100
13. David TJ (1999) Shaken baby (shaken impact) syndrome: non-accidental head injury in infancy. J Roy Soc Med 92:556–561
14. De Caro R, Munari PF, Parenti A (1998) Middle cerebral artery thrombosis following blunt head trauma. Clin Neuropathol 17:1–5
15. De Stefano N, Matthews PM, Fu L, Narayanan S, Stanley J, Francis GS, Antel JP, Arnold DL (1998) Axonal damage correlates with disability in patients with relapsing-remitting multiple sclerosis. Results of a longitudinal magnetic resonance spectroscopy study. Brain 121:1469–1477
16. Deck JH, Jagadha V (1986) Fatal subarachnoid hemorrhage due to traumatic rupture of the vertebral artery. Arch Pathol Lab Med 110:489–493

17. Dekaban AS, Sadowsky D (1978) Changes in brain weights during the span of human life: relation of brain weights to body heights and body weights. Ann Neurol 4:345–356
18. Duhaime AC, Alario AJ, Lewander WJ, Schut L, Sutton LN, Seidl TS, Nudelman S, Budenz D, Hertle R, Tsiaras W et al. (1992) Head injury in very young children: mechanisms, injury types, and ophthalmologic findings in 100 hospitalized patients younger than 2 years of age. Pediatrics 90:179–185
19. Duhaime AC, Christian CW, Rorke LB, Zimmerman RA (1998) Nonaccidental head injury in infants–the "shaken-baby syndrome". N Engl J Med 338:1822–1829
20. Duhaime AC, Gennarelli TA, Thibault LE, Bruce DA, Margulies SS, Wiser R (1987) The shaken baby syndrome. A clinical, pathological, and biomechanical study. J Neurosurg 66:409–415
21. Ehrenforth S, Klarmann D, Zabel B, Scharrer I, Kreuz W (1998) Severe factor V deficiency presenting as subdural haematoma in the newborn [letter]. Eur J Pediatr 157:1032
22. Feldman KW, Weinberger E, Milstein JM, Fligner CL (1997) Cervical spine MRI in abused infants. Child Abuse Negl 21:199–205
23. Ferguson B, Matyszak MK, Esiri MM, Perry VH (1997) Axonal damage in acute multiple sclerosis lesions. Brain 120:393–399
24. Garcia JH, Anderson M (1997) Circulatory disorders and their effects on the brain. In: Davis RL, Robertson DM (eds) Textbook of neuropathology. Williams and Wilkins, Baltimore, pp 715–822
25. Gean AD (1994) Imaging of Head Trauma. Raven Press, New York
26. Geddes JF, Gonzalez AG (1991) Examination of spinal cord in diseases of the craniocervical junction and high cervical spine. J Clin Pathol 44:170–172
27. Geddes JF, Vowles GH, Beer TW, Ellison DW (1997) The diagnosis of diffuse axonal injury: implications for forensic practice. Neuropathol Appl Neurobiol 23:339–347
28. Geddes JF, Whitwell HL, Graham DI (2000) Traumatic axonal injury: practical issues for diagnosis in medicolegal cases. Neuropathol Appl Neurobiol 26:105–116
29. Geddes JF, Hackshaw AK, Vowles GH, Nickols CD, Whitwell HL (2001) Neuropathology of inflicted head injury in children. 1: Patterns of brain damage. Brain (in press)
30. Geddes JF, Vowles GH, Hackshaw AK, Nickols CD, Scott IS, Whitwell HL (2001) Neuropathology of inflicted head injury in children. 2: Microscopic brain injury in infants. Brain (in press)
31. Gehrmann J, Banati RB, Cuzner ML, Kreutzberg GW, Newcombe J (1995) Amyloid precursor protein (APP) expression in multiple sclerosis lesions. Glia 15:141–151
32. Gennarelli TA, Thibault LE, Graham DI (1998) Diffuse axonal injury: an important form of traumatic brain damage. Neuroscientist 4:202–215
33. Gentleman SM, Nash MJ, Sweeting CJ, Graham DI, Roberts GW (1993) Beta-amyloid precursor protein (beta APP) as a marker for axonal injury after head injury. Neurosci Lett 160:139–144
34. Gentleman SM, Roberts GW, Gennarelli TA, Maxwell WL, Adams JH, Kerr S, Graham DI (1995) Axonal injury: a universal consequence of fatal closed head injury? Acta Neuropathol 89:537–543
35. Giometto B, An SF, Groves M, Scaravilli T, Geddes JF, Miller R, Tavolato B, Beckett AA, Scaravilli F (1997) Accumulation of beta-amyloid precursor protein in HIV encephalitis: relationship with neuropsychological abnormalities. Ann Neurol 42:34–40
36. Gleckman AM, Bell MD, Evans RJ, Smith TW (1999) Diffuse axonal injury in infants with nonaccidental craniocerebral trauma: enhanced detection by beta-amyloid precursor protein immunohistochemical staining. Arch Pathol Lab Med 123:146–151
37. Graham DI, Gennarelli TA (1996) Trauma. In: Graham DI, Lantos PL (eds) Greenfield's neuropathology. 1. Arnold, London, pp 197–262
38. Graham DI, Lawrence AE, Adams JH, Doyle D, McLellan D, Gennarelli TA (1989) Pathology of mild head injury. In: Hoff JT, Anderson T, Cole T (eds) Mild to moderate head injury. Blackwell Scientific, Boston, pp 63–75
39. Graham DI, McLellan D, Adams JH, Doyle D, Kerr A, Murray LS (1983) The neuropathology of the vegetative state and severe disability after non-missile head injury. Acta Neurochir Supp 32:65–67
40. Green PM, Wilson H, Romaniuk C, May P, Welch CR (1999) Idiopathic intracranial haemorrhage in the fetus. Fetal Diagn Ther 14:275–278

41. Hadley MN, Sonntag VK, Rekate HL, Murphy A (1989) The infant whiplash-shake injury syndrome: a clinical and pathological study. Neurosurgery 24:536–540
42. Hardman JM (1979) The pathology of traumatic brain injuries. In: Thompson RA, Green JR (eds) Complications of nervous system Trauma. Adv Neurol 22. Raven Press, New York, pp 15–50
43. Hardman JM (1997) Cerebrospinal trauma. In: Davis RL, Robertson DM (eds) Textbook of neuropathology. Williams & Wilkins, Baltimore, pp 1199
44. Harland WA, Pitts JF, Watson AA (1983) Subarachnoid haemorrhage due to upper cervical trauma. J Clin Pathol 36:1335–1341
45. Hart BL, Dudley MH, Zumwalt RE (1996) Postmortem cranial MRI and autopsy correlation in suspected child abuse. Am J Forensic Med Pathol 17:217–224
46. Jafari SS, Nielson M, Graham DI, Maxwell WL (1998) Axonal cytoskeletal changes after nondisruptive axonal injury. II. Intermediate sized axons. J Neurotrauma 15:955–966
47. Jaspan T, Narborough G, Punt JA, Lowe J (1992) Cerebral contusional tears as a marker of child abuse–detection by cranial sonography. Pediatr Radiol 22:237–245
48. Johnson DL, Boal D, Baule R (1995) Role of apnea in nonaccidental head injury. Pediatr Neurosurg 23:305–310
49. Kinney HC, Samuels MA (1994) Neuropathology of the persistent vegetative state. A review. J Neuropathol Exp Neurol 53:548–558
50. Knight B (1989) The autopsy in the non-accidental injury syndrome. In: Mason JK (ed) Paediatric forensic medicine and pathology. Chapman & Hall Medical, London, pp 269–287
51. Koszyca B, Blumbergs PC, Manavis J, Wainwright H, James R, Gilbert J, Jones N, Reilly PL (1998) Widespread axonal injury in gunshot wounds to the head using amyloid precursor protein as a marker. J Neurotrauma 15:675–683
52. Lafont M, Lamarque M, Daussac E (1999) [Favorable outcome of a subdural hematoma diagnosed in utero]. Arch Pediatr 6:962–965
53. Leetsma J (1995) Forensic neuropathology. In: Duckett S (ed) Pediatric neuropathology. Williams & Wilkins, Baltimore, pp 243–283
54. Leetsma JE (1988) Neuropathology of child abuse. In: Forensic neuropathology. Raven Press, New York, pp 333–356
55. Leetsma JE (1997) Forensic neuropathology. In: Garcia JH (ed) neuropathology: The Diagnostic Approach. Mosby, St Louis, pp 518
56. Lindenberg R, Freytag E (1969) Morphology of brain lesions from blunt trauma in early infancy. Arch Pathol 87:298–305
57. Lindenberg R, Freytag E (1970) Brainstem lesions characteristic of traumatic hyperextension of the head. Arch Pathol 90:509–515
58. Liu HY, Huang LT, Lui CC (1998) Vacuum extraction delivery complicated with acute subdural hematoma and cerebral infarction: report of one case. Chung-Hua Min Kuo Hsiao Erh Ko i Hsueh Hui Tsa Chih 39:119–122
59. Maxwell WL, Islam MN, Graham DI, Gennarelli TA (1994) A qualitative and quantitative analysis of the response of the retinal ganglion cell soma after stretch injury to the adult guinea-pig optic nerve. J Neurocytol 23:379–392
60. Maxwell WL, Povlishock JT, Graham DI (1997) A mechanistic analysis of nondisruptive axonal injury: a review. J Neurotrauma 14:419–440
61. McKenzie KJ, McLellan DR, Gentleman SM, Maxwell WL, Gennarelli TA, Graham DI (1996) Is beta-APP a marker of axonal damage in short-surviving head injury? Acta Neuropathol 92:608–613
62. McLellan DR, Adams JH, Graham DI, Kerr AE, Teasdale GM (1986) The structural basis of the vegetative state and prolonged coma after non-missile head injury. In: Papo I, Cohadon F, Massarotti M (eds) Le coma traumatique. Liviana Editrice, Padova, pp 165–185
63. Meyerhoff DJ, MacKay S, Constans JM, Norman D, Van Dyke C, Fein G, Weiner MW (1994) Axonal injury and membrane alterations in Alzheimer's disease suggested by in vivo proton magnetic resonance spectroscopic imaging. Ann Neurol 36:40–47
64. Munro D, Merritt HH (1936) Surgical pathology of subdural hematoma. Arch Neurol Psychiatry 35:64–78

65. Ng HK, Mahaliyana RD, Poon WS (1994) The pathological spectrum of diffuse axonal injury in blunt head trauma: assessment with axon and myelin strains. Clin Neurol Neurosurg 96:24–31
66. Ng PC, Fok TF, Lee CH, Wong W, Cheung KL (1998) Massive subdural haematoma: an unusual complication of septicaemia in preterm very low birthweight infants. J Pediatr Child Health 34:296–298
67. Opeskin K, Burke MP (1998) Vertebral artery trauma. Am J Forensic Med Pathol 19:206–217
68. Ophoven JJ (1997) Pediatric forensic pathology. In: Gilbert-Barness E (ed) Potter's pathology of the fetus and infant. 2. Mosby, St Louis, pp 1582–1624
69. Ophthalmology Child Abuse Working Party (1999) Child abuse and the eye. Eye 13:3–10
70. Oppenheimer DR (1968) Microscopic lesions in the brain following head injury. J Neurol Neurosurg Psychiatry 31:299–306
71. Perrin RG, Rutka JT, Drake JM, Meltzer H, Hellman J, Jay V, Hoffman HJ, Humphreys RP (1997) Management and outcomes of posterior fossa subdural hematomas in neonates. Neurosurgery 40:1190–1199; discussion 1199–1200
72. Pilz P (1983) Axonal injury in head injury. Acta Neurochir Suppl 32:119–123
73. Renzulli P, Tuchschmid P, Eich G, Fanconi S, Schwobel MG (1998) Early vitamin K deficiency bleeding after maternal phenobarbital intake: management of massive intracranial haemorrhage by minimal surgical intervention. Eur J Pediatr 157:663–665
74. Riggs JE, Schochet SS (1995) Spastic quadriparesis, dysarthria, and dysphagia following cervical hyperextension: a traumatic pontomedullary syndrome. Milit Med 160:94–95
75. Rogers CB, Itabashi HH, Tomiyasu U, Heuser ET (1998) Subdural neomembranes and sudden infant death syndrome. J Forensic Sci 43:375–376
76. Saternus K, Kernbach-Wighton G, Oehmichen M (2000) The shaking trauma in infants – kinetic chains. Forensic Sci Int 109:203–213
77. Shannon P, Smith CR, Deck J, Ang LC, Ho M, Becker L (1998) Axonal injury and the neuropathology of shaken baby syndrome. Acta Neuropathol 95:625–631
78. Sherriff FE, Bridges LR, Sivaloganathan S (1994) Early detection of axonal injury after human head trauma using immunocytochemistry for beta-amyloid precursor protein. Acta Neuropathol 87:55–62
79. Stys PK (1998) Anoxic and ischemic injury of myelinated axons in CNS white matter: from mechanistic concepts to therapeutics. J Cereb Blood Flow Metab 18:2–25
80. Tatsuno Y, Lindenberg R (1974) Basal subarachnoid hematomas as sole intracranial traumatic lesions. Arch Pathol 97:211–215
81. Tomei G, Spagnoli D, Ducati A, Landi A, Villani R, Fumagalli G, Sala C, Gennarelli TA (1990) Morphology and neurophysiology of focal axonal injury experimentally induced in the guinea pig optic nerve. Acta Neuropathol 80:506–513
82. Vowles GH, Scholtz CL, Cameron JM (1987) Diffuse axonal injury in early infancy. J Clin Pathol 40:185–189
83. Wilkinson AE, Bridges LR, Sivaloganathan S (1999) Correlation of survival time with size of axonal swellings in diffuse axonal injury. Acta Neuropathol 98:197–202
84. Willis BK (1995) Vertebral and basilar artery injuries. In: Carter LP, Spetzler RF (eds) Neurovascular surgery. McGraw-Hill, New York, pp 1313–1336

# Sudden Unexplained Death in Adults

M. Black, D. I. Graham



## 1 Introduction

Forensic medicine and neuropathology not infrequently come together in the investigation of cases of sudden death, which in a small but significant number of instances is due to intracranial pathology rather than cardiovascular disease. Clinical information may help to provide the cause of an unexpected death but may be absent in circumstances that are unexplained.

Current Topics in Pathology, Vol. 95
S. Love (Ed.): Neuropathology

## 1.1 Definition of Sudden Unexplained Death in Adults

Sudden unexpected or unexplained natural deaths comprise the vast majority of deaths encountered in the practice of forensic pathologists in the United Kingdom. The percentage of cases investigated by individual pathologists varies, but in England and Wales, approximately 80% of cases reported to the coroner will be natural deaths. In Scotland the number of cases reported to the Procurator Fiscal system, and which undergo postmortem examination where death is due to natural causes, will be slightly less. In the Department of Forensic Medicine at the University of Glasgow, approximately 60% of the workload of about 1,500–2,000 deaths per annum comprise such deaths.

The definition of sudden unexpected or unexplained death is not entirely straightforward nor are the two necessarily always interchangeable. The definition of "sudden" is also open to interpretation. Mason defines sudden death "as unexpected death following so rapidly from the onset of symptoms that the cause of death could not be certified with confidence by a medical practitioner familiar with the patient" [50]. Whilst the World Health Organization accepts a limit of 24 h between the onset of symptoms and death (cited by Knight [37]) this is considered too long an interval for many practitioners and pathologists and a much shorter time interval of within a few hours of apparently good health [68] or of 1 h is preferred [37]. This is a separate category of death from those that remain unexplained after full postmortem examination including further investigations, e.g. toxicology and histology. For the purposes of this paper we would interpret 'unexplained' as meaning unexplained at the time of death and 'sudden' as dying within 1 h of onset of symptoms or where the deceased was found dead unexpectedly.

## 1.2 Database

The Department of Forensic Medicine and Science at the University of Glasgow provides a postmortem examination service for the former region of Strathclyde in Scotland, the population of which is approximately 2.7 million. The department examines virtually all cases of suspicious deaths within this region and also a significant proportion of natural, suicidal and accidental deaths. The records of the department have been reviewed for deaths involving epilepsy and subarachnoid haemorrhage. These cases could be retrieved only if these or related terms were mentioned in the cause of death. For cases investigated by the department where the brain was retained for further examination after fixation, this was carried out by the University Department of Neuropathology at the Institute of Neurological Sciences, Southern General Hospital, Glasgow.

The Department of Neuropathology provides specialist services for the cognate disciplines of neurology and neurosurgery and acts as a tertiary reference centre for most of the hospitals in central and western parts of Scotland, including the city of Glasgow. This forms the basis of some two thirds of the 800–900 specimens referred to the department for examination each year. The additional one third consists of material referred for medico-legal purposes, which is the major source of the cases falling within the definition of sudden unexplained death in adults and is the basis of some of the findings described in this chapter.

In our experience, the most common causes of death in these circumstances are associated with epilepsy, trauma, intracranial haemorrhage and acute bacterial meningitis.

## 2 Sudden Unexplained Death in Epilepsy

Epilepsy is well recognised as being associated with sudden unexpected death as a result of trauma or drowning. In addition, however, it has long been associated with an increased risk of death other than from these causes [31, 38]. In the past, these deaths were often attributed to either asphyxia or status epilepticus [24, 85]. It is now, however, recognised that individuals with epilepsy are at an increased risk of sudden unexpected death (SUDEP) that is not attributable to either of these causes [21, 74]. There is a large number of publications looking at the incidence of these unexpected deaths in different populations groups, e.g. in specific hospitals [46, 56, 80, 85] or in the general population with epilepsy [21, 42, 67, 73] and this is reflected in rates which can vary from 0.4–1.35/1,000 person years [73] to 4.9/1,000 person years [46], but all agree that there is a significantly increased risk of sudden death in epilepsy [58]. Ficker et al. [21] gave a risk approximately times 24 that of the general population and Leestma et al. [42] reported a prevalence of SUDEP of 1/370 to 1/1,110 epileptics/year with a risk of 1/200 for people with severe epilepsy.

### 2.1 Definition of SUDEP

In 1996 a workshop on sudden unexpected death and epilepsy agreed the definition of SUDEP as "that of a sudden unexpected witnessed or unwitnessed non-traumatic and non-drowning death in patients with epilepsy with or without evidence of a seizure and excluding documented status epilepticus where necropsy does not reveal a toxicological or anatomical cause for death" [54].

### 2.2 Risk Factors

A number of risk factors for such deaths have been identified and include being a young adult, male, early onset of epilepsy, poor seizure control, multiple drug therapy, a history of generalised tonic/clonic seizures, treatment non-compliance/low levels of anticonvulsant drugs on postmortem testing, alcoholism, unwitnessed seizures and body position [36, 41–43, 56, 73]. Information about the circumstances of death is often difficult to obtain. Death is, however, often preceded by witnessed fits, these comprising 67% of cases in the series of Kloster and Engelskjon [36], 50% in the study by Leestma et al. [42] and 64% in the study of Nashef [54], and in many cases death seemed to occur whilst the person was asleep, such cases comprising between 40%–50% according to LEESTMA et al. [41], 60% of cases according to KLOSTER and ENGELSKJON [36] and 79% in the study of SCHWENDER and TRONCOSO [66].

### 2.3 Autopsy Investigation

The investigation of these deaths is variable, in some series only a minority having had a postmortem examination [46]. In addition, whilst the value of postmortem toxicology remains debatable [9], and analysis shows that the postmortem levels of anticonvulsants are commonly subtherapeutic or negative [36, 41, 42, 74], toxicological examination is not always carried out. In addition, despite a significant proportion showing abnormalities [24, 41, 42, 75], the brain is often not formally examined by a neuropathologist.

A retrospective review of cases from the Department of Forensic Medicine and Science during the years 1991–1996 showed that a relatively constant percentage of deaths was attributed to epilepsy (0.7%–1.8% of all cases). Of this total of 131 cases, 119 had a history of epilepsy with male subjects accounting for 84 cases (2:1 male:female) and a wide age range at death of 3–74 years, but with the majority of deaths occurring in the 30- to 40-year age group. Information about the frequency of seizures or exact type of epilepsy was not always available, although 43% had a history of alcohol abuse. In approximately one-third of the cases, information about the circumstances of the death was not available. In another one-third the deceased had had a witnessed seizure before death and in almost 50% of cases the circumstances suggested that the patient had died in his or her sleep.

Postmortem examination in our series was carried out in virtually all cases. Abnormalities that may have been associated with a seizure were bruising of the tongue, recorded in 17%, and petechial haemorrhages in the mucous membranes, in 7.6%. The brain was submitted for formal neuropathology in 41 of the 131 cases (31.3%). In keeping with previous findings [36], there were abnormalities in two-thirds of the cases, most commonly comprising evidence of recent or old contusional damage (Fig. 1), alcohol abuse, or hypoxic damage. In 3 cases, Ammon's horn sclerosis was seen (Fig. 2). When the brain was cut unfixed at the time of postmortem examination, abnormalities were noted in only 8 of 90 cases. Postmortem toxicology was performed in 101 of the cases and of the 81 cases in which the results could be obtained, only 65 were tested for anticonvulsants. In these cases analysis was negative in 35%, and subtherapeutic levels were identified in the majority of the remaining cases.

The cause of death as certified by the pathologist was extremely variable. The majority of deaths were certified as being due either to epileptic seizure or epilepsy. In a small number of cases death was ascribed to status epilepticus or asphyxia. This variety of terminology can be confusing, particularly when in some instances the basis for implicating a seizure or asphyxia is not clearly apparent from the information available [9, 46]. It is also misleading and potentially distressing to the relatives of the deceased [29]. Indeed it is possible, given that deaths from epilepsy essentially result in a negative postmortem examination, that these deaths may be underestimated as, if an additional pathological abnormality is found at post-

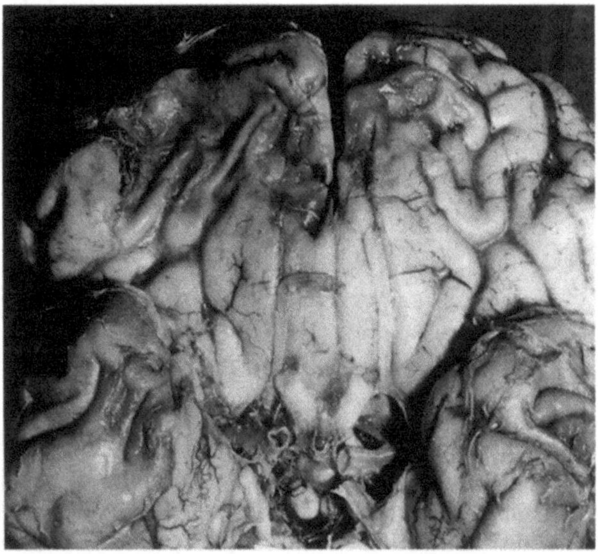

**Fig. 1.** Old contusions in the frontal and temporal lobes. They comprise surface defects, the margins of which were scarred and orange-brown in colour

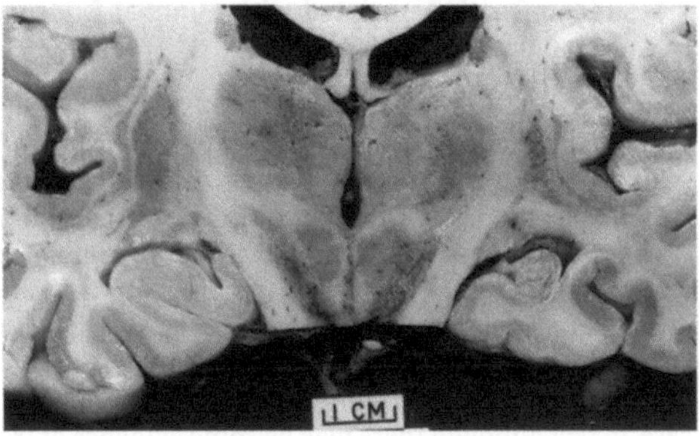


**Fig. 2.** Sclerosis of Ammon's horn. There is asymmetry of the hippocampi, the right being smaller than the left

mortem examination (e.g. coronary artery atheroma), in the absence of any clear circumstantial evidence such as witnessed seizures, the cause of death may well be ascribed to a pathology other than epilepsy. This may be both reasonable and pragmatic given that the reported incidence of ischaemic heart disease is increased in patients with epilepsy [6]. The 1996 workshop recommends that if a death remains unexplained after a full autopsy including toxicology and examination of the heart, it should be certified as witnessed or unwitnessed sudden unexpected death/epilepsy.

### 2.4 Mechanisms of Death Associated with Epilepsy

The circumstantial evidence is consistent with the current view that death associated with epilepsy is seizure related. Animal experiments have shown hypoventilation and death to be associated with seizures [33], and central apnoea is known to occur in epileptic seizures [55, 81]. The common occurrence of pulmonary oedema at autopsy is in keeping with this. Other theories include seizure-associated cardiac arrhythmia [55] or arrhythmia associated with anti-epileptic drug withdrawal [35].

## 3 Sudden Death Associated with Trauma

The principal neuropathological findings are diverse and range from a brain that may appear to be relatively normal, to one with massive subarachnoid haemorrhage or multiple petechial haemorrhages. Whereas there is an observable abnormality in the latter two that at least provide a structural basis for instantaneous death, the former makes it difficult to achieve a satisfactory clinicopathological correlation.

### 3.1 Sudden Death Associated with Minimal Evidence of Traumatic Brain Injury

In our experience there are several cases per year in which the circumstances associated with death strongly suggest trauma as being the most important contributing factor. Thus, there may be both external and internal evidence of trauma with some injuries to the thoracic and abdominal cavities but insufficient in amount and severity to provide a satisfactory explanation for death, or indeed evidence of trauma may be confined to the head. Under these circumstances there is a reasonable expectation that the cause of death may lie within the skull and that examination of a fixed brain might provide the answer. All too often this is not the case, in that although there may be some evidence of trauma with a small subdural haematoma and minimal surface contusions, slicing of the brain fails to reveal any evidence of internal damage even in the form of haemorrhages either parenchymatous or intraventricular. Therefore, uncertainties remain about the exact mechanism of death. Even after exhaustive histological studies uncertainties may remain. The failure to identify specific structural changes, no doubt, reflects the speed with which death has occurred. Clearly, under these circumstances there are limitations even of modern techniques and perhaps there is a reluctance to accept that a sudden death after trauma may be a consequence of massive neurochemical or autonomic dysfunction in the absence of identifiable structural change.

## 3.2 Traumatic Intraventricular Haemorrhage

Variable amounts of recent haemorrhage within the ventricular system are commonly found, either as an isolated finding or in association with multiple haemorrhages principally within midline structures (see below). The source of the haemorrhage may be difficult to determine but has been attributed to tearing of small blood vessels in the walls of the ventricular system, including the interventricular septum, and in the choroid plexus [28, 44]. In addition, the deformation of central portions of the brain may sufficiently dilate the ventricular system to cause the rupture of small blood vessels beneath the ependyma [87]. Sometimes, it is due to the extension of midline haemorrhages into the ventricular system, or is evidence of diffuse brain damage [14] and therefore part of the continuum between diffuse vascular injury and diffuse axonal injury [83, 86].

Experimental evidence in support of damage to the choroid plexus as one source of intraventricular haemorrhage has been provided in the model of acceleration–deceleration in non-human primates [51, 52].

## 3.3 Traumatic Subarachnoid Haemorrhage

Some bleeding into the subarachnoid space is probably the most common finding after head injury. It is usually minor and of little clinical significance. Larger amounts may occur, usually in association with cortical contusions, but occasionally the subarachnoid haemorrhage is massive and is the principal finding in cases of sudden unexplained death [10, 30].

This entity is said to occur typically in a "young, healthy, but intoxicated man who receives a minor blow, immediately collapses and dies within minutes" [16, 78]. Certainly most subjects are male and have been involved in moderate levels of violence with blunt impact injury to the lateral or posterolateral aspect of the neck, demonstrable at autopsy after appropriate dissection [13]. In one case [25], however, traumatic subarachnoid haemorrhage resulted from violently jerking the head to avoid a blow. Although immediate collapse is the norm, there have been documented instances in which death has been delayed by up to 60 min post injury [40]. In cases where death has occurred rapidly, there are usually considerable amounts of subarachnoid haemorrhage in the posterior fossa; rarely is this associated with actual damage to the brain stem [12, 45, 72]. Some studies have demonstrated fractures of the transverse process of the upper cervical spine at the same level as the arterial injury in a significant number of cases [12, 25, 78]. The site of damage to the vasculature remains uncertain, but it is generally accepted that in over two-thirds of the cases a tear occurs in the vertebral artery either in its intracranial or extracranial course [11, 19, 40]. Indeed, the vulnerability of the vertebral artery has been attributed to a decrease in the amount of elastic fibres between the extracranial and intracranial segments [84]. Johnson et al. [32] demonstrated an abnormal course of the vertebral artery in its upper cervical part in 5 of 20 dissections and postulated that subjects with this loop deficiency may be more susceptible to such trauma.

Difficulty remains in identifying the source of haemorrhage at autopsy, further compounded by the possible occurrence of artefactual tears during the course of examination. A number of techniques have been described to identify the site of vascular rupture [8]. These include en bloc removal of the hind brain and upper cervical spinal cord and block dissection or suboccipital exposure of the neck combined with defleshing or postmortem angiography [78]. Another technique that yields good results involves the cannulation of the proximal vertebral arteries in the neck and flushing normal saline through them whilst inspecting the anterior brain stem surface for escaping water, the calvaria having been previously removed.

The mechanisms of death remain somewhat controversial, and there is debate as to the role of alcohol and its contribution to head injury. Figures in the literature show intoxication with alcohol in 40% – 100% of cases [79], and it is suggested that violent jerking of the head and neck in such cases may be due to slow protective responses [37]. The vasodilatory role of alcohol is also unclear. However, alcohol intoxication is a common finding in any violent death. Other theories include the effects of direct trauma [13], characterised by the triad of massive basal subarachnoid haemorrhage, the absence of a ruptured saccular aneurysm or vascular malformation, and the demonstration of blunt force injury to the lateral or ipsilateral portion of the neck. Other authors have invoked hyperextension with some rotation and/or flexion of the neck.

## 3.4 Diffuse Vascular Injury

The forensic pathologist not infrequently undertakes an autopsy on a patient who has died rapidly, usually with features of external trauma but without obvious abnormality of the brain externally. There may be multiple injuries to the skeleton, chest and abdomen, so that an intracranial cause of death is not sought. However, even after autopsy, uncertainties may remain, and consideration is given to whether or not the cause of death can be attributed to intracranial pathology. Under these circumstances neuropathological examination after a period of fixation is likely to show multiple petechial haemorrhages throughout the brain, especially in the brain stem (Fig. 3a) and in the white matter of the anterior parts of the frontal (Fig. 3b) and temporal lobes adjacent to the thalamus. This type of acute vascular injury has been reported previously in patients who have died instantaneously. It has been suggested that such petechial haemorrhages are indicative of damage of a type and distribution that is incompatible with life [70, 76]. The hindbrain haemorrhages have been referred to in the past as primary brain stem haemorrhages [76], but in the experience of others it has been considered that they are more appropriately considered as a primary type of diffuse brain damage in view of their wide distribution throughout the cerebral hemispheres as well as in the brain stem [1].

While it is undoubtedly true that patients with this pattern of multiple petechial haemorrhages in the brain die either instantaneously or within a few minutes, increasing experience has shown that a number of patients with this type of vascular pathology survive the initial injury only to die some hours later. This suggests that

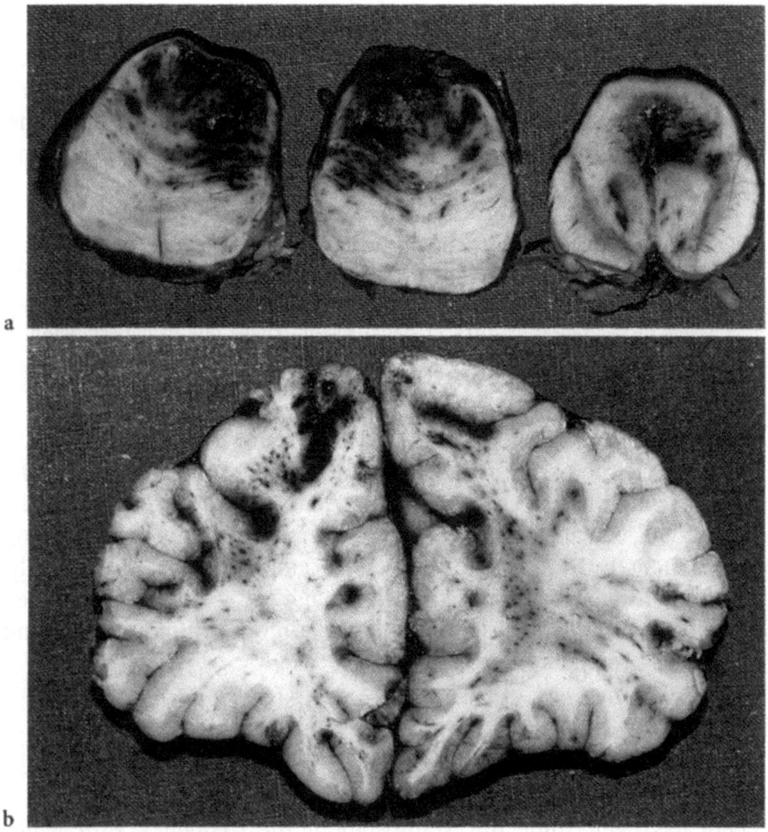

Fig. 3 a, b. Diffuse vascular injury. There are multiple small haemorrhages in the: a dorsal parts of the rostral brain stem; b white matter of the frontal lobes

there is likely to be a spectrum of damage characterised by multiple small haemorrhages in the brain and that diffuse vascular injury (DVI) is unlikely to be an all-or-none phenomenon. Further, it is becoming increasingly apparent that there is a continuum between the pattern of brain haemorrhages seen in DVI and the pattern of haemorrhages associated with diffuse axonal injury (DAI). Previous studies have shown grade 3 DAI, with haemorrhages in the corpus callosum and dorsolateral quadrant of the upper brain stem, to be the most severe end of the spectrum of DAI [2, 7], previously called shearing injury [61, 69, 86]. This is the most severe form of all of the diffuse types of brain injury and occurs predominantly after motor vehicle accidents [5], although not exclusively so [3, 26]. In those patients who die within 1 h of injury and have DVI, it is not possible to identify damage to axons and therefore, by definition, a diagnosis of even the most severe form of DAI is not possible. However, experience has shown that those patients who survive and have the same pattern of petechial haemorrhages do, after some 2–3 h survival, manifest evidence of diffuse axonal injury (K. J. McKenzie, personal communication).

# 4 Sudden Death Due to Non-Traumatic Intracranial Haemorrhage

Sudden death may occur as a result of rapid bleeding into any one or more of the intracranial compartments, viz. subdural, subarachnoid, or intraventricular spaces, or into brain substance. The causes vary depending upon the age of the individual and the anatomical location of the haemorrhage. The principal causes are given in Table 1.

**Table 1.** Principal causes of non-traumatic intracranial haemorrhage

| |
|---|
| 1. Rupture of saccular aneurysm |
| 2. Massive intracerebral or intracerebellar haemorrhage due to hypertension, vascular malformation, blood dyscrasia, sickle cell disease and tumour strokes |

In most instances there is bleeding into more than one intracranial compartment. For example, rupture of saccular aneurysm may be associated with a subdural haematoma, bleeding into the subarachnoid space and an intracerebral haematoma, which in the course of expanding may in turn rupture into the ventricular system. In contrast, a primary intracerebral haematoma is rarely associated with a subdural haematoma although it may occasionally present at the surface and be associated with subarachnoid bleeding; more commonly, it extends medially into the ventricular system.

## 4.1 Sudden Death from Ruptured Saccular Aneurysm

There has been some uncertainty about the frequency with which ruptured intracranial saccular aneurysms are associated with either instantaneous or very rapid death. Early medicolegal literature [18, 22] based on surveys of large numbers of patients who died prior to or on arriving at a hospital, records that 60% of the patients died immediately after rupture of the aneurysm. The mean age was 46 years and at autopsy there was massive subarachnoid haemorrhage in 96% of the cases, subdural haemorrhage in 22% and intracerebral haemorrhage in 43%. Patients with saccular aneurysms of the posterior part of the circle of Willis or the internal carotid artery showed a greater tendency to die at the time of rupture than those with aneurysms arising at other sites [22].

A community-based study of ruptured intracranial saccular aneurysms was undertaken by Crawford and Sarner [15]. In this study it was possible to scrutinise the records of the Neurosurgical Unit at St George's Hospital at Atkinson and Morleys Hospital, Wimbledon, UK and the cases of sudden death reported to the appropriate coroner. Based on a census of 1.1 million people, there was a population of 913,000 under the age of 60 years. In the years 1962 and 1963 from the study area, there were 280 deaths certified as due to cerebrovascular disease, of which 78 were due to a ruptured intracranial saccular aneurysm. The estimated number of patients under the age of 60 years with a ruptured intracranial saccular aneurysm who died either at home or before reaching hospital was 57. Somewhat similar figures were found in a study undertaken at the Mayo Clinic [62]. In the 30-

year study period, 129 residents of Rochester had a lumbar puncture-confirmed subarachnoid haemorrhage due to either rupture or presumed rupture of an intracranial saccular aneurysm. Ten patients (8%) died rapidly before receiving medical attention. A subsequent study in the same population [65] analysed 136 cases of confirmed subarachnoid haemorrhage due to rupture of an intracranial saccular aneurysm of which 11 were reported as sudden death. In discussion,

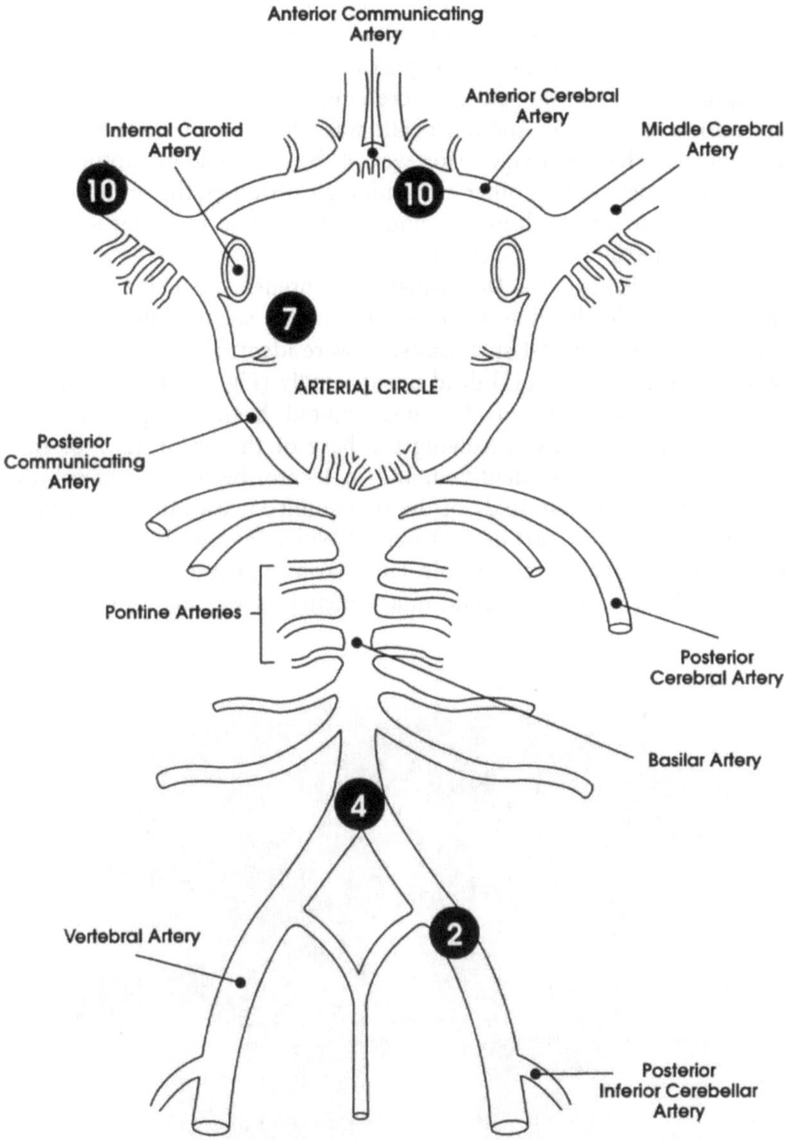


Fig. 4. Origin of saccular aneurysms in 33 cases of sudden death due to non-traumatic subarachnoid haemorrhage

particular emphasis was placed on the high fatality rate in patients with ruptured saccular aneurysms arising from the posterior circulation. A few hospital-based studies have also suggested a somewhat higher mortality for rupture of posterior circulation saccular aneurysms [34, 63] whereas others have failed to detect any differences in outcome [57, 60, 71, 77].

The frequency of posterior circulation saccular aneurysms has been variably reported as between 5% and 10% of all intracranial aneurysms [20, 34, 63], whereas in some referral-based medical centres the frequency of posterior circulation aneurysms may approach 20% [64, 71]. The under-representation of posterior circulation aneurysms in most other series of patients with subarachnoid haemorrhage may be explained, in part, by the high early mortality associated with a rupture prior to the patient receiving medical attention. In the study of Schievink et al. [65], sudden death was recorded in 10% of all aneurysmal subarachnoid haemorrhages. However, of the cases due to rupture of a posterior circulation aneurysm in other epidemiological studies, the proportion of patients succumbing to subarachnoid haemorrhage prior to reaching medical attention ranged from 3%–17% [15, 48, 82].

The case files of the Department of Forensic Medicine and Science were reviewed for deaths due to a non-traumatic subarachnoid haemorrhage in the years 1995–1998. Of such cases, 41 were identified where death was sudden or the deceased was found dead unexpectedly (Fig. 4). In the majority of these cases, the distribution of the subarachnoid haemorrhage was described as mainly basal or diffuse involving the base of the brain. In 7 of the 41 cases an aneurysm was not identified, and in 1 case the haemorrhage was due to a vascular malformation. In 27 of the remaining 33 cases the ruptured aneurysms arose in the anterior part of the Circle of Willis. In only six deaths were posterior circulation aneurysms responsible. The distribution of the aneurysms is illustrated in Fig. 4. In five cases a second intact aneurysm was identified. It would there-

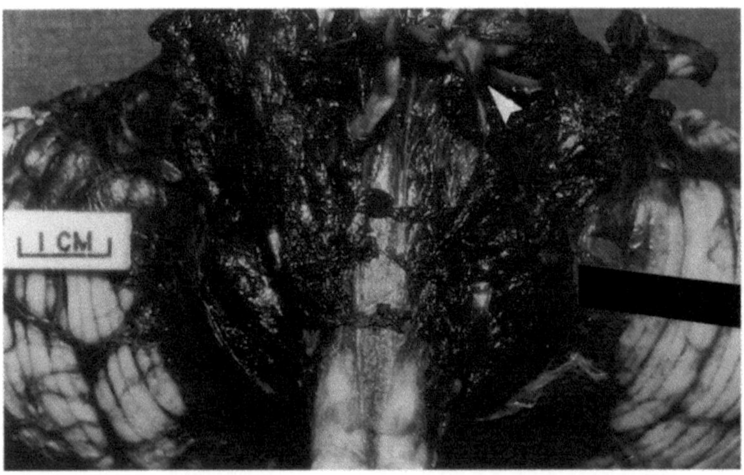


**Fig. 5.** Massive posterior fossa subarachnoid haemorrhage. Dissection revealed a ruptured saccular aneurysm arising from the vertebral artery (*arrow*)

fore seem that the frequency with which massive subarachnoid haemorrhage has been attributed to saccular aneurysms arising from either the anterior or posterior part of the Circle of Willis can be explained by case selection and referral patterns.

At autopsy the diagnosis of massive subarachnoid haemorrhage is self-evident (Fig. 5). However, because of the large amounts of freshly formed blood clot, it is often difficult to locate the saccular aneurysm unless the brain is examined when fresh. The subarachnoid membrane should be removed with forceps and the ventral surface of the brain washed with isotonic saline. Even with the use of a dissecting microscope it may not be possible to identify the source of the subarachnoid haemorrhage in between 5%–10% of cases, raising the possibility that the source in these cases is a small saccular aneurysm which has been obliterated by the rupture of the blood vessel.

## 4.2 Intracerebral Haemorrhage

Massive haemorrhage into brain substance is characterised clinically by an abrupt onset and rapid evolution (Fig. 6). It occurs particularly in middle-aged men with a known history of hypertension. In one study [23], 393 cases of intracerebral haemorrhage were studied in a medicolegal practice of which 40% originated within the basal ganglia, 16% in the pons, 15% in the thalamus, 12% in the cerebellum and 10% in the cerebral white matter. In three-quarters of the cases the

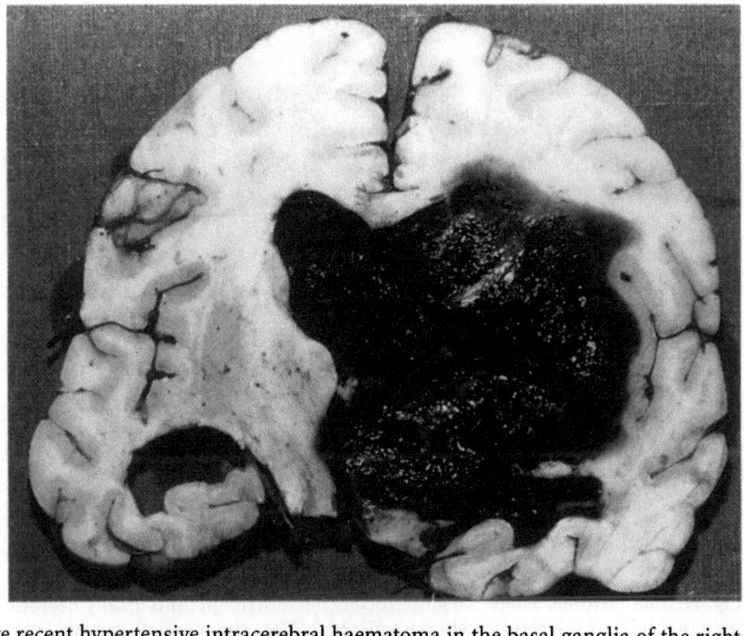

**Fig. 6.** Massive recent hypertensive intracerebral haematoma in the basal ganglia of the right cerebral hemisphere with extension into the ventricular system

intracerebral haematoma had ruptured into the ventricular system, 15% had presented at the surface within the subarachnoid space, and in 6% there was an associated subdural haematoma. In 35% of the cases the individuals were found dead or were dead on arrival at a hospital.

The great majority of large intracerebral haematomas occur in association with hypertension or in the elderly. There are occasional examples that are due to rupture of a vascular malformation or in association with a blood dyscrasia, sickle cell disease, or anti-thrombotic therapy. There are also a small number of cases on record where there has been massive haemorrhage into a pre-existing tumour (see below).

## 5 Sudden Death Due to Brain Tumours

Intracranial tumours are said to account for 8% of non-traumatic intracerebral haemorrhage, in about half of which it may be the first manifestation [47, 49], and in a small proportion of which the patient may die very rapidly. Among the primary brain tumours, glioblastoma (Fig. 7) predominates [17]. Other tumours that have been reported to present in this way include oligodendroglioma, medulloblastoma, lymphoma, teratoma and pituitary adenoma (with apoplexy). Of the metastatic intracranial tumours, bronchial carcinoma, choriocarcinoma and melanoma are the most likely to cause rapid death due to haemorrhage.

Colloid cysts of the third ventricle are also associated with acute neurological deterioration and sudden death (Fig. 8) in adults [59].

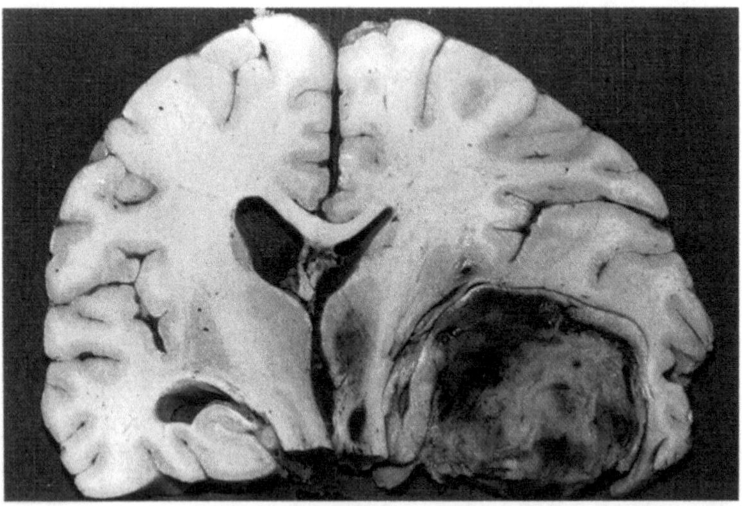

**Fig. 7.** Glioblastoma. There is a large, focally haemorrhagic, and focally necrotic tumour in the temporal lobe of the right cerebral hemisphere. Note the mass effect with internal herniation, asymmetry of the ventricles, and a shift of the midline structures

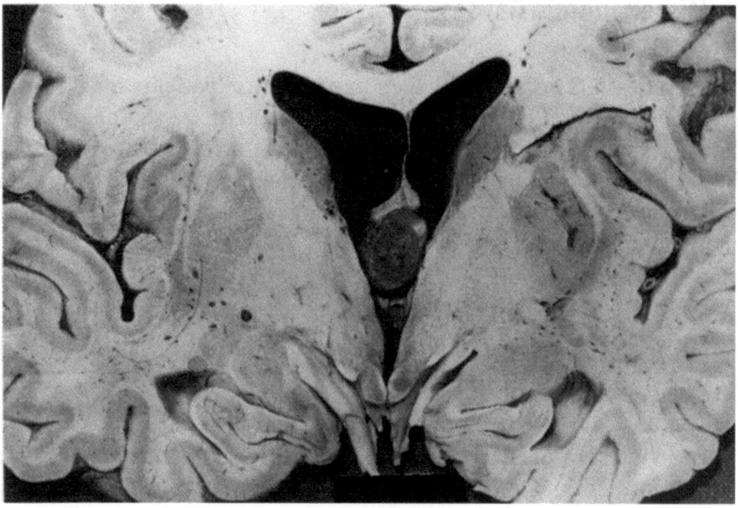

**Fig. 8.** Colloid cyst. The cyst has plugged the third ventricle causing acute obstructive hydrocephalus

## 6 Sudden Death Due to Intracranial Infection

Although intracranial infection occurs most frequently in children, there are nevertheless examples in adults of sudden unexplained deaths due to either acute bacterial meningitis or in association with a large cerebral abscess. In adulthood the acute bacterial meningitis is almost invariably secondary to a bacteraemia and is most commonly due to pneumococci or meningococci. At autopsy the brain may be markedly swollen and the sulci filled by a cloudy, pale, yellow-green exudate which, in meningococcal meningitis may be so slight as to be difficult to identify at autopsy. Acute bacterial meningitis is frequently associated with social and economic deprivation and alcohol abuse, and is commonly associated with pneumonia, a compromised immune system and an absence of the spleen. It is usually possible to culture pneumococcus from samples taken postmortem, but this less likely to be successful in the case of meningococcal meningitis, although the diagnosis may be suspected if there is other evidence of meningococcal disease such as petechial haemorrhages and purpura of the mucous membranes and skin, and haemorrhagic necrosis of the adrenal glands.

Chronic suppurative otitis media or occasionally long-standing infection of other sinuses may be forerunners of a brain abscess. Usually chronic, the abscess has a grey and rather translucent capsule with its effective size often increased by brain swelling. An abscess therefore acts as an intracranial expanding lesion. Additional complications are rupture of the abscess into the ventricular system to produce an acute purulent ventriculitis or rupture into the subarachnoid space to produce acute purulent meningitis. Review of the department's archive identifies two cases of sudden unexplained death from brain abscess, both in heroin addicts. Apparently symptoms had been masked by the drug habit and failure of the Health Care Services to recognise the potential importance of a discharging ear. Death in both instances was associated with mass effect and acute purulent meningitis.

## 7 Miscellaneous Causes

Sudden death is occasionally seen in psychiatric patients most commonly chronic schizophrenics on phenothiazine in whom there are therapeutic or high but not lethal levels. Death in these cases has been attributed to cardiac arrhythmias, hyperthermia, hypotension with development of tachycardia and cardiovascular collapse, respiratory dyskinesia, laryngeal-pharyngeal dystonias, neuroleptic malignant syndrome and seizures [39].

## 8 Principal Mechanisms of Sudden Unexplained Death in Patients with an Intracranial Mass Lesion

With an intracranial mass lesion there are three main mechanisms, viz. a rapid rise in the intracranial pressure (ICP), acute obstructive hydrocephalus and intracranial haemorrhage.

### 8.1 Intracranial Expanding Lesions

After the fontanelles have closed in infancy, the intracranial contents, comprising brain (about 70% of the intracranial volume), cerebrospinal fluid (about 15%) and blood (about 15%), are enclosed in the rigid confines of the bone of the base of the skull and calvaria. Any increase in the volume of one of these compartments will, unless compensated for by a corresponding reduction in the volume of the other component parts, lead to an increase in ICP [53].

The most common cause of a raised ICP in clinical practice is an intracranial expanding mass which, as a result of distortion and herniation of the brain (see below), leads to impaction of brain tissue in the tentorial opening or the foramen magnum (Fig. 9). This results in the development of a pressure gradient between the supratentorial and infratentorial compartments of the skull, or between the intracranial and spinal subarachnoid spaces. Such a gradient leads to rapid deterioration of the patient's clinical state. The situation is different in infants when an increase in the volume of the intracranial contents results in bulging of the fontanelles and separation of the sutures, leading to enlargement of the skull.

A wide variety of pathological processes may present as intracranial expanding (space occupying) lesions. However, although the location of the lesion is important in the ultimate rise in ICP, it is not so much its nature but the rapidity with which it enlarges that determines the ultimate fate of the patient. Thus when a lesion expands rapidly compensatory mechanisms are exhausted quickly and the ICP soon increases. This is more likely to happen sooner in the young patient than in the older age group, in whom there may be some pre-existing cerebral atrophy and therefore an increased volume of CSF in the ventricles and subarachnoid space.

Because of the intrinsic compensatory mechanisms by which the total volume of the intracranial contents does not necessarily increase as soon as an expanding

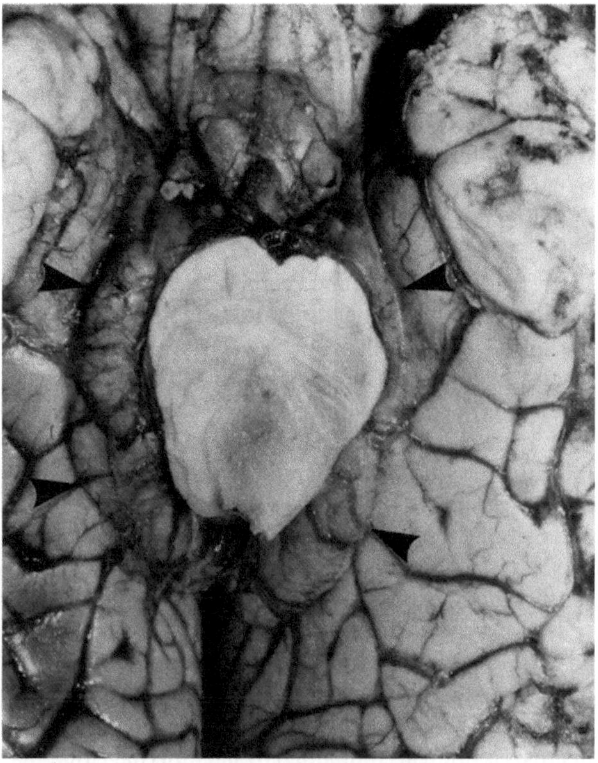

**Fig. 9.** Raised intracranial pressure. There are bilateral tentorial herniae (*arrows*) and haemorrhagic discolouration of the brain stem

lesion develops, distortion and displacement of the brain usually precede any clinically significant increase in ICP. Were it not for this spatial compensation the addition of a very small extra volume of fluid or tissue in the intracranial cavity would produce an abrupt and rapidly fatal increase in ICP.

The widespread introduction of continuous monitoring of ICP during life has established that various types of pressure wave (i.e. transient increases of ICP) are common in patients in whom there is an intracranial expanding lesion and that pressure gradients between intracranial compartments and the spinal subarachnoid space are of great importance. The skull is divided into three compartments, two supratentorial and one infratentorial by the dura mater. The falx cerebri separates the cerebral hemispheres and the tentorium cerebelli separates the cerebral hemispheres from the cerebellum and essentially surrounds the midbrain – the tentorial opening. In normal circumstances the supratentorial spaces, the infratentorial space and the spinal subarachnoid space, are in continuity via the tentorial opening and the foramen magnum, respectively. The normal upper limit of ICP is about 2.7 kPa (20 mmHg). A moderately elevated ICP is between 2.7 kPa and 5.4 kPa (20–40 mmHg); a level greater than 5.4 kPa (40 mmHg) must be considered high.

## 8.2 Supratentorial Expanding Lesions

As the lesion expands, the surface of the brain is pressed against the unyielding dura, gyri are flattened, sulci are narrowed and the CSF is displaced from the subarachnoid space and the surface of the brain becomes dry. The ventricle on the side of the lesion becomes reduced in size and there is a lateral shift in the midline structures. There is frequently enlargement of the contralateral ventricle because of obliteration of the interventricular foramen.

The next stage is the appearance of internal herniae, i.e. displacement of brain tissue from one intracranial compartment to another. For example, a supracallosal hernia occurs when the ipsilateral cingulate gyrus herniates under the free edge of the falx. The pericallosal arteries are selectively displaced from the mid-line. A small wedge of pressure necrosis may occur in the cortex of the cingulate gyrus where it is in contact with the falx.

A tentorial hernia occurs when there is displacement of the uncus and the medial part of the ipsilateral parahippocampal gyrus through the tentorial opening (Fig. 10). The medial part of the temporal lobe pushes towards the midline and over the free edge of the tentorium. The midbrain is narrowed in its transverse axis. The aqueduct is compressed and the contralateral cerebral peduncle is pushed against the opposite free edge of the tentorium. This may be sufficiently severe to cause infarction (the Kernohan lesion) in the peduncle. The nerve then becomes angled over the artery, and if herniation is severe there may be haemorrhage into it. As the hernia enlarges, it produces a groove on the upper surface of the adjacent cerebellar hemisphere. As with the supracallosal hernia, a wedge of pressure necrosis is often accompanied by haemorrhage that may occur along the line of the groove in the parahippocampal gyrus. If there is no haemorrhage, the wedge of pressure necrosis may be identifiable only microscopically [4]. Clinicopathological studies of patients in whom the ICP has been continuously monitored during life have established that when the increase in ICP has been produced by a supra-

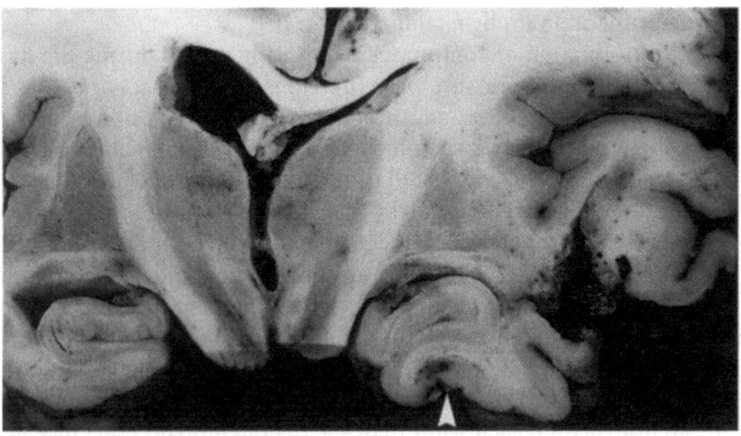

**Fig. 10.** Raised intracranial pressure. There is haemorrhagic pressure necrosis along the line of a tentorial hernia (*arrow*)

tentorial expanding lesion there is always pressure necrosis in the parahippocampal gyrus when the ICP exceeds 5.4 kPa (40 mmHg). A tentorial hernia may also produce selective compression of the posterior cerebral artery, but rarely in acute unexplained death due to a high ICP is there evidence of infarction in the medial occipital cortex. Haemorrhage and infarction in the midbrain and pons occur mainly adjacent to the midline in the tegmentum of the midbrain and in the tegmental and basal parts of the rostral pons [27].

A tonsillar hernia, i.e. downward displacement of the cerebellar tonsils through the foramen magnum, can occur in association with a supratentorial expanding lesion because of transmission of a high ICP from the supratentorial to the infratentorial compartment. The tentorium cerebelli is displaced downwards and the upper surface of each cerebellar hemisphere becomes concave. The volume of the posterior cranial fossa is reduced and a tonsillar hernia develops. Herniation can only be said to be present if there is impaction of the tonsils in the foramen magnum producing a depression on the ventral surface of the medulla where it is being compressed against the foramen magnum or if there is necrosis of the tips of the tonsils.

When brain swelling is diffuse and bilateral, ventricles become small but remain symmetrical and there is no lateral shift of the midline structures. Tentorial herniae may occur but they are usually relatively small and often bilateral, the size depending on the rate of brain swelling and the size of the tentorial opening. Caudal displacement of the diencephalon and the brain stem will be more severe than with the unilateral expanding lesion.

## 8.3 Infratentorial Expanding Lesions

When the lesion is not in the midline, the aqueduct and fourth ventricle are compressed and displaced to the other side. Tonsillar herniation is more severe than with supratentorial expanding lesions. When there is a severe tonsillar hernia, the posterior inferior cerebellar arteries may be so compressed that infarction occurs in the inferior part of one or both cerebellar hemispheres.

A common association with an infratentorial expanding lesion is the increase in the size of the lateral ventricles – hydrocephalus.

Herniation of the cerebellum may also occur in an upward direction through the tentorial opening: a so-called reversed tentorial hernia.

Raised ICP is also a feature of diffuse bleeding into the subarachnoid space, as from a ruptured saccular aneurysm. The elevation of ICP may be such that the cerebral circulation ceases. A somewhat similar sequence of events may be seen in patients dying from purulent meningococcal meningitis. Because of the wide distribution of the disease process throughout the subarachnoid space, the features that normally accompany the unilateral intracranial mass lesion are not seen. However, that the death can be attributed to raised ICP can usually be surmised from the large amounts of haemorrhage and/or exudate within the subarachnoid space, obliteration of the sulcal and folial pattern of the cerebral and cerebellar hemispheres, and on section, uniform dilatation of the ventricular system.

## 8.4 Acute Obstructive Hydrocephalus

The CSF has a volume of about 120 ml and is exchanged some three to five times per day. The term hydrocephalus means an increased volume of CSF within the cranial cavity. In internal hydrocephalus, the increased volume of CSF is within the ventricular system; the hydrocephalus is said to be communicating if CSF can flow freely from the ventricular system to the subarachnoid space and non-communicating if it cannot.

In obstructive hydrocephalus it is the site of the lesion rather than its nature that is of critical importance. A small lesion in a sensitive site adjacent to a ventricular foramen, the aqueduct or the midbrain, may be of much greater significance than a large expanding lesion in a frontal or occipital lobe. The abnormality, however, need not be adjacent to the ventricular system, since any process such as previous meningitis or subarachnoid haemorrhage that results in obliteration of subarachnoid space – particularly at the level of the tentorial opening – will obstruct the free flow of CSF. It is also clear that the rapid development of hydrocephalus is a particular risk of lesions in the infratentorial compartment of the skull.

In essence the ventricular system proximal to the obstruction enlarges. If there is obstruction of an interventricular foramen (Monro) one lateral ventricle enlarges; if it is in the third ventricle or the aqueduct both lateral ventricles enlarge; if it is at the exit foramina of the fourth ventricle due to some previous inflammatory process the entire ventricular system enlarges; if the obstruction is in the subarachnoid space at the level of the tentorium, again the entire ventricular system enlarges – on this occasion the hydrocephalus is communicating in type.

## 8.5 Intracranial Haemorrhage

Several mechanisms are thought to be operating here. If the haemorrhage is massive, whether intracerebral or subarachnoid, there is a rapid rise in ICP, the cerebral circulation ceases and death may ensue. Under these circumstances, as described above, the conventional features of shift, distortion, internal herniation and secondary haemorrhage in the brain stem may either be incompletely formed or absent.

When death is virtually instantaneous the mechanism remains uncertain, although several processes may be responsible. The sudden enveloping of the brain stem by blood from a ruptured saccular aneurysm may, for example, cause an autonomic discharge with resulting dysrhythmia or cardiac arrest, severe ischaemia of the brain stem from the induction of intense vasospasm, or a rapid rise in ICP and a marked reduction in the cerebral perfusion pressure. Such mechanisms can be inferred in those patients in whom it is possible to perform a computed tomography (CT) scan either during or immediately after an intracranial bleed from which there is an absence of a mass effect from a localised haematoma. In those patients who have large bleeds in the immediate vicinity of the ventricular system and particularly within the posterior fossa, there may be an element of acute obstructive hydrocephalus.

**Acknowledgements.** Particular thanks to Mrs. Mary Roche for secretarial assistance and Prof. P. Vanezis and Dr. C. Smith for helpful comments.

## References


1. Adams JH (1992) Head injury. In: Adams JH, Duchen LW (eds) Greenfield's neuropathology, 5th edn. Edward Arnold, London, pp 106–152
2. Adams JH, Doyle D, Ford I, Gennarelli TA, Graham DI, McLellan DR (1989) Diffuse axonal injury in head injury: definition, diagnosis and grading. Histopathology 15:49–59
3. Adams JH, Doyle D, Graham DI, Lawrence AE, McLellan DR (1984) Diffuse axonal injury in head injuries caused by a fall. Lancet 2:1420–1421
4. Adams JH, Graham DI (1976) The relationship between ventricular fluid pressure and the neuropathology of raised intracranial pressure. Neuropathol Appl Neurobiol 2: 323–332
5. Adams JH, Graham DI, Murray LS, Scott G (1982) Diffuse axonal injury due to non-missile head injury in humans: an analysis of 45 cases. Ann. Neurology 12:557–563
6. Annegers JF, Hauser WA, Shirts SB (1984) Heart disease mortality and morbidity in patients with epilepsy. Epilepsia 25(6):699–704
7. Blumbergs PC, Jones NR, North JB (1989) Diffuse axonal injury in head trauma. J Neurol Neurosurg Psychiat. 52:838–841
8. Bromilow A, Burns J (1985) Technique for removal of the vertebral arteries. J Clin Pathol 38:1400–02
9. Brown SW, Mawar GE, Lawler W, Taylor DC, Shorvon S, Betts TA, Noronha MJ et al. (1990) Sudden death and epilepsy. Lancet (letters) 335:606–607
10. Cameron JM, Mant AK (1972) Fatal subarachnoid haemorrhage associated with cervical trauma. Med Sci Law 12:66–70
11. Coast GC, McGhee DJ (1984) Traumatic subarachnoid haemorrhage: an alternative source. J Clin Pathol 37:1245–1248
12. Contostavlos DL (1971) Massive subarachnoid haemorrhage due to laceration of the vertebral artery associated with fracture of the transverse process of the atlas. J Forensic Sci 16:40–56
13. Contostavlos DL (1995) Isolated basilar subarachnoid haemorrhage: an observer's 25 year re-evaluation of the pathogenic possibilities. Forensic Sci Int 73:61–74
14. Cordobes F, de la Fuente M, Lobato RD, Roger R, Perez C, Millan JM, Bargena A et al. (1983) Intraventricular haemorrhage in severe head injury. J Neurosurgery 58:217–222
15. Crawford MD, Sarner M (1965) Ruptured intracranial aneurysms: community study. Lancet ii 1254–1257
16. Deck JH, Jagadha V (1986) Fatal subarachnoid haemorrhage due to traumatic rupture of the vertebral artery. Arch Pathol Lab Med 110:489–493
17. DiMaio SJ, Dimaio VJM, Kirkpatrick J (1980) Sudden death due to primary intracranial neoplasm. Am J Forensic Med Pathol 1:29–46
18. Dinning TAR, Falconer MA (1953) Sudden or unexpected natural death due to ruptured intracranial aneurysms: survey of 250 forensic cases. Lancet 2:799–801
19. Dowling G, Currie B (1988) Traumatic basal subarachnoid haemorrhage. Amer J Forensic Med Pathol 9:23–31
20. Drake CG (1979) The treatment of aneurysms of the posterior circulation. Clin Neurosurg 26:96–144
21. Ficker DM, So EL, Shen WK, Annegers JF, O'Brien PC, Cascino GD, Belau PG (1998) Population-based study of the incidence of sudden unexplained death in epilepsy. Neurology 51:1270–1274
22. Freytag E (1966) Fatal rupture of intracranial aneurysms. Arch Pathol 81:418–424
23. Freytag E (1968) Fatal hypertensive intracerebral haematomas. J Neurol Neurosurg Psychiat 31:616–620
24. Freytag E, Lindenberg R (1964) 294 medicolegal autopsies on epileptics. Arch Pathol 78:274–286
25. Gee DJ (1982) Traumatic subarachnoid haemorrhage. Proceedings of the 12th Congress of the International Academy of Forensic and Social Medicine. Egermann, Vienna, pp 495–498
26. Gennarelli TA (1983) Head injury in man and experimental animals – clinical aspects. Acta Neurochirug Suppl 32:1–13

27. Graham DI, Lawrence AE, Adams JH, Doyle D, McLellan DR (1987) Brain damage in non-missile head injury secondary to a high intracranial pressure. Neuropathol Appl Neurobiol 13:209–217
28. Grcevic N (1983) Traumatic tears to the tela choriodia: a hitherto unrecognised cause of post-traumatic hydrocephalus. Acta Neurochirug Suppl. 32:79–85
29. Hanna J (1997) Epilepsy and sudden death: a personal view. Epilepsia 38 [suppl 11]: S3–S5
30. Harland WA, Pitts JF, Watson AA (1983) Subarachnoid haemorrhage due to upper cervical trauma. J Clin Pathol 36:1335–1341
31. Hirsch CS, Martin DL (1971) Unexpected death in young epileptics. Neurology 21:682–689
32. Johnson CP, Scraggs M, How T, Burns J (1995) A necropsy and histomorphometric study of abnormalities in the course of the vertebral artery associated with ossified syloinoid ligaments. J Clin Pathol 48:637–640
33. Johnston SC, Horn JK, Valente J, Simon RP (1995) The role of hypoventilation in a sheep model of epileptic sudden death. Ann Neurol 37:531–537
34. Kassell NF, Torner JC, Haley EC, Jane JA, Adams HP, Kongable GL (1990) The International Cooperative Study on the Timing of Aneurysm Surgery. Part 1: Overall management results. J Neurosurg 73:18–36
35. Kenneback G, Ericson M, Tomson J, Bergfeldt L (1997) Changes in arrhythmia profile and heart rate variability during abrupt withdrawal of anti-epileptic drugs. Implications for sudden death. Seizure 6:369–375
36. Kloster R, Engelskjon T (1999) Sudden unexpected death in epilepsy (SUDEP): a clinical perspective and a search for risk factors. J Neurol Neurosurg Psychiatry 67:439–444
37. Knight B (1996) Forensic pathology, 2nd edn. Edward Arnold, London
38. Krohn W (1963) Causes of death among epileptics. Epilepsia 4:315–321
39. Laposata EA, Hale P, Poklis A (1988) Evaluation of sudden death in psychiatric patients with special reference to phenothiazine therapy: forensic pathology. J Forensic Sci 33:432–440
40. Leadbetter S (1994) Extracranial vertebral artery injury – evolution of a pathological illusion? Forensic Sci Int 67:33–40
41. Leestma JE, Teas SS, Hughes JR, Kalelkar MB (1985) Sudden epilepsy deaths and the forensic pathologist. Am J Forensic Med Pathol 6(3):215–218
42. Leestma JE, Walczak T, Hughes JR, Kalelkar MB, Teas SS (1989) A prospective study on sudden unexpected death in epilepsy. Ann Neurol 26:195–203
43. Lhatoo SD, Langan Y, Sander JWAS (1999) Sudden and unexpected death in epilepsy. Postgrad Med J 75:706–709
44. Lindenberg R (1971) Trauma of meninges and brain. In: Minckler J (ed) Pathology of the nervous system, vol 2. McGraw Hill, New York, pp 1705–1765
45. Lindenberg R, Freytag E (1970) Brainstem lesions characteristic of traumatic hyperextension of the head. Arch Pathol 90:509–515
46. Lip GYM, Brodie MJ (1992) Sudden death in epilepsy: an avoidable outcome. J R Gy Soc Med 1992 85:609–611
47. Little JR, Dial B, Belanger G, Carpenter S (1979) Brain haemorrhage from intracranial tumour. Stroke 10:283–288
48. Ljunggren B, Saveland H, Brandt L, Zygmunt S (1985) Early operation and overall outcome in aneurysmal subarachnoid haemorrhage. J Neurosurg 62:547–551
49. Mandybur TI (1977) Intracranial haemorrhage caused by metastatic tumours. Neurology 27:650–655
50. Mason JK (1995) Forensic medicine for lawyers, 3rd edn. Butterworths, London, Dublin, Edinburgh
51. Maxwell WL, Hardy IG, Watt C, McGadey J, Graham DI, Adams JH, Gennarelli TA (1992) Changes in the choroid plexus, responses by intrinsic epiplexus cells and recruitment from monocytes after experimental head acceleration injury in the non-human primate. Acta Neuropathol 84:78–84
52. Maxwell WL, Whitfield PC, Suzen B, Graham DI, Adams JH, Watt C, Gennarelli TA (1992) The cerebrovascular response to experimental lateral head acceleration. Acta Neuropathol 84:289–296

53. Miller JD, Ironside JW (1997) Raised intracranial pressure, oedema and hydrocephalus. In: Graham DI, Lantos PL (eds) Greenfield's neuropathology, 6th edn. Arnold, London, pp 157–195
54. Nashef L (1997) Sudden unexpected death in epilepsy: terminology and definitions. Epilepsia 38 [suppl 11]: S6–S8
55. Nashef L, Walker F, Allen P, Sander JWAS, Shorvon SD, Fish DR (1996) Apnoea and bradycardia during epileptic seizures: relation to sudden death in epilepsy. J Neurol Neurosurg Psychiatry 60:297–300
56. Nilsson L, Farahmand BY, Persson P-G, Thibilin I, Tomson T (1999) Risk factors for sudden unexpected death in epilepsy: a case-control study. Lancet 353:888–893
57. Nishioka H (1966) Report on the co-operative study of intracranial aneurysms and subarachnoid haemorrhage. Section VII, Part 1: Evaluation of the conservative management of ruptured intracranial aneurysms. J Neurosurg 25:574–592
58. O'Donoghue MF, Sander JW (1997) The mortality associated with epilepsy, with particular reference to sudden unexpected death: a review. Epilepsia 38 [suppl 11]: S15–S19
59. Opeskin K, Anderson RM, Lee KA (1993) Colloid cyst of the third ventricle as a cause of acute neurological deterioration and sudden death. J Paediat Child Health 29:476–477
60. Peerless SJ, Drake CC (1990) Management of aneurysm of the posterior circulation. In: Youmans JR (ed) Neurosurgical surgery: a comprehensive reference guide to the management of aneurysmal problems, 3rd edn, vol 3. WB Saunders, Philadelphia, pp 1764–1800
61. Peerless SJ, Rewcastle NB (1967) Shear injuries of the brain. Canad Med Assoc 96:577–582
62. Phillips LH, Whisnant JP, O'Fallon WM, Sundt TM (1980) The unchanging pattern of subarachnoid haemorrhage in a community. Neurology 30:1034–1040
63. Rasmussen P. Bosch H, Haase J et al. (1980) Intracranial saccular aneurysms: results of treatment in 851 patients. Acta Neurochirur 53:1–17
64. Schievink WI, Van Der Werf DJM, Hageman LM, Dreissen JJ (1988) Referral pattern of patients with aneurysmal subarachnoid hemorrhage. Surg Neurol 29:367–371
65. Schievink WI, Wijdicks EFM, Piepgras DG, Chu C-P, O'Fallon M, Whisnant JP (1995) The poor prognosis of ruptured intracranial aneurysms of the posterior circulation. J Neurosurg 82:791–795
66. Schwender LA, Troncoso JC (1986) Evaluation of sudden death in epilepsy. AM J Forensic Med Pathol 7(4):283–287
67. Sillanpau ML, Koskenvuo MJ (1994) Population-based mortality of persons with epilepsy. Epilepsia 35(7):18
68. Simpson K (1947) Pathology of sudden death. Lancet: 745–747
69. Strich SJ (1961) Shearing of nerve fibres as a cause of brain damage due to head injury. Lancet 2:443–448
70. Strich SJ (1976) Cerebral trauma. In: Blackwood W, Corsellis JA (eds) Greenfield's neuropathology. 3rd edition. Edward Arnold, London, pp 327–360
71. Sundt TM, Kobayashi S, Fode NC, Whisnant JP (1982) Results and complications of surgical management of 809 intracranial aneurysms in 722 cases. J Neurosurg 56:753–765
72. Tatsuno Y, Lindenberg R (1974) Basal subarachnoid haematomas as sole intracranial traumatic lesions. Arch Pathol 97:211–215
73. Tennis P, Cole TB, Annegers JF, Leestma JE, McNutt M, Rajput A (1995) Cohort study of incidence of sudden unexplained death in persons with seizure disorder treated with antiepileptic drugs in Saskatchewan, Canada. Epilepsia 36(1):29–36
74. Terrence CF, Wisotzskey HM, Perper JA (1975) Unexpected, unexplained death in epileptic patients. Neurology 25:594–598
75. Thom M (1997) Neuropathologic findings in post-mortem studies of sudden death in epilepsy. Epilepsia 38 [suppl 11]: 532–534
76. Tomlinson BE (1970) Brain-stem lesions after head injury. J Clin Pathol 23: Suppls (R Coll Pathol) 4:154–165
77. Troupp H (1971) The natural history of aneurysms of the basilar bifurcation. Acta Neurol Sciences 47:350–356
78. Vanezis P (1984) Vertebral artery trauma: a post-mortem study. MD Thesis, University of Bristol
79. Vanezis P (1989) Pathology of neck injury. Butterworths, London

80. VanParijs JAP, deHaan GJ, Mantel R, Meüer P (1994) Mortality in the outpatient population of a Dutch epilepsy centre. Epilepsia 35 [suppl 7]: 18
81. Walker F, Fish DR (1997) Recording respiratory parameters in patients with epilepsy. Epilepsia 39(11):S31–S42
82. Wiebers DO, Whisnant JP, O'Fallon WM (1981) The natural history of unruptured intracranial aneurysms. N Engl J Med 304:696–698
83. Wilberger JE, Ruthfus WE, Tabas J, Goldbere AL, Deeb ZI (1990) Acute tissue tear haemorrhages of the brain: computed tomography and clinicopathological correlations. Neurosurgery 27:208–213
84. Wilkinson IM (1972) The vertebral artery. Extracranial and intracranial structure. Arch Neurol 27:392–396
85. Zielinski JJ (1974) Epilepsy and mortality rate and cause of death. Epilepsia 15:191–201
86. Zimmerman RA, Larissa T, Gilaniuk LT, Gennarelli TA (1978) Computed tomography of shearing injuries of the cerebral white matter. Radiology 127:393–396
87. Zuccarello M, Iavicoli R, Pardatscher K, Cervellini P, Fiore D, Minerino S, Gerosa M (1981) Post-traumatic intraventricular haemorrhages. Acta Neurochir 55:283–293

# The Pathological Diagnosis of Neurodegenerative Diseases Causing Dementia

J. Lowe



## 1 Introduction and Background

Understanding the pathological cause of disease is a fundamental goal in all areas of medicine. An understanding of what is going wrong allows a rational approach to developing preventive and therapeutic interventions. In the pathological characterisation of diseases associated with dementia there have been great advances in understanding that, in the long term, promise insights leading to therapy.

Current Topics in Pathology, Vol. 95
S. Love (Ed.): Neuropathology

Three main factors have lead to this position:

- Multi-disciplinary longitudinal studies of patients with cognitive abnormality involving psychology, psychiatry, neurology, imaging, neuropathology, cell biology and genetics
- Development and wide adoption of new pathological techniques for visualisation of pathological changes in the brain, especially immunohistochemical techniques
- Development of cell biological techniques able to associate disease with specific proteins and their genes

Establishing a pathological cause for a clinically diagnosed dementia syndrome has never been more important.

- The clinical diagnosis of neurodegenerative processes is inaccurate. About 25% of clinical diagnoses are not confirmed pathologically, and accurate diagnostic feedback is being sought for purposes of audit and epidemiology [5, 25, 35].
- Many neurodegenerative diseases are familial, and it is important to obtain pathological confirmation of the nature of disease for the purpose of genetic counselling.
- The recent publicity surrounding Creutzfeldt-Jakob disease and its possible relation to bovine spongiform encephalopathy has highlighted public concerns over the cause of dementia as well as health and safety concerns over the transmissibility of these diseases at autopsy. An increased requirement for pathological ascertainment of the cause of dementia is likely as part of public health surveillance [11, 22, 38, 54, 65, 67].

This overview will present an essentially practical approach to diagnosis of the neurodegenerative and vascular causes of dementia with appropriate background information on the main diseases and their pathology. It is intended mainly for non-specialist pathologists but, it is hoped, may also be informative for neuropathologists.

## 2 Clinical Features of Dementia Syndromes

It is important to realise the implications of a clinical diagnosis of dementia. Dementia has been clinically defined as an impairment of previously attained occupational or social functioning due to development of acquired and persistent memory impairment associated with impairment of intellectual function, in the presence of normal consciousness, in one or more of the following domains:

- Language
- Visuospatial skills
- Emotion or personality
- Cognition

The fact that a patient had previously attained an appropriate degree of occupational and social functioning separates a dementia syndrome from mental retardation. The requirement for involvement of multiple domains of cognitive function separates dementia from so-called focal neurobehavioural disorders, for example isolated loss of recent memory (amnesia) due to bilateral hippocampal damage or an isolated language disorder such as expressive dysphasia due to a localised cerebral infarct. The presence of multiple cognitive deficits implies involvement of multiple cortical areas.

- Disease of the medial temporal lobe, hippocampus, amygdala and limbic system leads to disorders of memory and hallucinations.
- Disease of the temporal neocortex is associated with receptive dysphasia and automatisms.
- Disease of the frontal lobes produces abnormalities in behaviour and is a major feature of the group of frontal lobe dementias. Typical abnormalities include impairment of: judgement, abstract reasoning, strategic planning, emotional restraint and control of appetite and continence.
- Disease of the parietal lobe causes impairment of visuospatial skills and interferes with integration of sensory inputs, leading to sensory agnosias and apraxias.
- Disease of the occipital lobe leads to failure of visual sensory systems.

There are two main clinical patterns of dementia:

- Temporoparietal dementias begin with impairment of memory and dysfunction of the temporal lobes. Patients later develop parietal lobe dysfunction, characterised by dysphasias and dyspraxias.
- Frontotemporal dementias usually begin with behavioural disturbances of frontal lobe type (see above). Patients later develop temporal lobe dysfunction, manifested by memory disturbance. Typically, parietal lobe function is preserved.

The diseases causing cortical pathology may also affect subcortical structures and lead to other neurological signs, the most common of which is the movement disorder, parkinsonism.

## 3 The Main Causes of Dementia

Many conditions can result in a dementia syndrome.

### Neurodegenerative Diseases

- Common
  - Alzheimer's disease
  - Dementia with Lewy bodies
- Less common
  - Dementia of frontal type – with motor neuron disease (MND) inclusions or ubiquitin-immunopositive neurites
  - Dementia of frontal type – no inclusions
  - Tangle-only dementia
  - Huntington's disease
  - Progressive supranuclear palsy
  - Corticobasal degeneration

- Uncommon
  - Pick's disease
  - Multiple system atrophy
- Rare
  - Multi-system degenerations
  - Chromosome 17-linked dementia

**Cerebrovascular Disease**

- Multi-infarct dementia, ischaemic white matter degeneration (Binswanger's disease) or hippocampal sclerosis
  - Atherosclerotic
  - Arteriolosclerotic
  - Vasculitic (several causes)
  - Amyloid angiopathy
  - Cerebral autosomal dominant arteriopathy with subcortical infarction and leukoencephalopathy (CADASIL)

**Hydrocephalus**

- CSF resorption abnormality
- Obstruction in CSF pathways

**Toxic, Metabolic and Nutritional Disorders**

- Drug-induced
- Chronic alcoholism
- Chronic hepatic encephalopathy
- Vitamin deficiency (thiamine, B12, niacin)
- Hypothyroidism
- Neurometabolic storage diseases
- Mitochondrial cytopathy
- Hypocalcaemia
- Hypoglycaemia

**Demyelinating Diseases**

- Multiple sclerosis
- Leukodystrophies

**Head Injury**

- Diffuse or focal brain damage
- Subdural haematoma
- Dementia pugilistica

**Prion Disease**

- Creutzfeldt-Jakob disease
- Kuru
- Gerstmann-Straüssler-Scheinker syndrome
- Fatal familial insomnia
- Variant Creutzfeldt-Jakob disease

**Infective Disorders**

- Human immunodeficiency virus infection
- Whipple's disease
- Neurosyphilis
- Herpes simplex virus encephalitis

**Neoplasia**

- Paraneoplastic encephalitis
- Primary and secondary tumours

## 3.1 Alzheimer's Disease

### 3.1.1 Incidence and Classification

Alzheimer's disease (AD) is the most common cause of dementia and increases in incidence with age. AD accounts for between 50 % and 75 % of all cases of dementia. It is possible to divide cases into five main groups, each of which tends to be associated with distinct molecular genetic abnormalities.

- Sporadic late-onset AD (commonest)
- Familial late-onset AD (uncommon)
- Familial early-onset AD (rare)
- Associated with Down's syndrome
- Associated with other degenerative disease

Familial Alzheimer's disease probably represents about 10 % of all cases.

### 3.1.2 Pathological Features of Alzheimer's Disease

The brain is smaller than normal in AD and brain weight is reduced. There is shrinkage of gyri and widening of sulci of the cerebral hemispheres, most evident in the medial temporal regions (particularly the hippocampus) but also affecting frontal and parietal regions (Fig. 1). The occipital lobe and the motor cortex are generally spared. Slicing of the brain reveals reduction in the thickness of the cerebral cortex, due to loss of both neurons and neuronal cell processes. The amount of

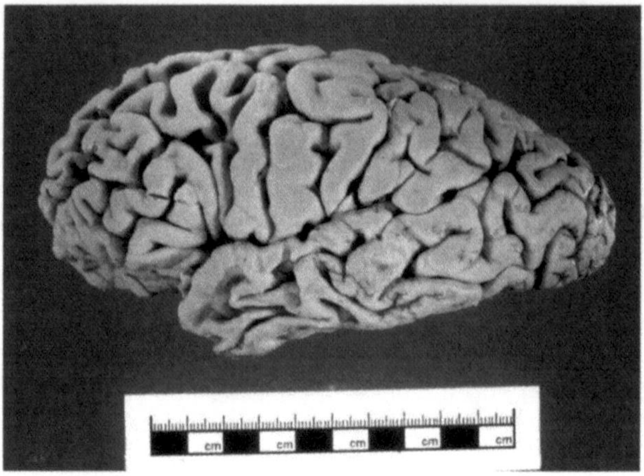

**Fig. 1.** Alzheimer's disease. Note atrophy especially in lower part of temporal lobe

white matter is reduced, with dilatation of the ventricular system, especially the inferior horn of the lateral ventricles. In the midbrain, the substantia nigra shows normal pigmentation, and this is an important distinction from cases of dementia with Lewy bodies, discussed later.

Histologically, AD is associated with several abnormalities, none of which is pathognomonic [32, 49].

- Deposition amyloid in the brain, as plaques. The amyloid is composed A$\beta$ peptide, derived by proteolytic breakdown of a normal neuronal membrane protein called amyloid precursor protein (APP) (Fig. 2).
- Intraneuronal filamentous inclusions termed neurofibrillary tangles, the main constituent of these being the microtubule-binding protein, tau protein, present in an abnormally phosphorylated form (Fig. 3).
- Accumulation of tau protein in distorted nerve cell processes termed dystrophic neurites and neuropil threads.
- Neuronal and synaptic loss (~50%) from the cerebral cortex.
- Microvacuolation, often termed status spongiosus, occurs in the neocortex in areas of neuronal loss. This is usually most severe in the outer cortical layers and is of a coarse pattern, in contrast to the fine vacuoles seen in prion disease.
- Amyloid is often deposited in cerebral arteries (congophilic angiopathy) (Fig. 4).
- Granulovacuolar degeneration may be seen in neurons.
- Hirano bodies are seen with increased frequency in neurons.
- Astrocytic gliosis occurs in the neocortex. This is best detected by immunohistochemical staining for glial fibrillary acidic protein (GFAP).

These changes may be seen in the brains of cognitively normal elderly individuals in low density or restricted distribution. The diagnosis of AD is based on the collective presence of lesions in high density in a patient with clinical dementia. AD is believed to develop in a predictable manner, which has been documented and divided into several stages. Six stages in the development of AD pathology have been condensed into three main stages, based on the work of Braak and Braak.

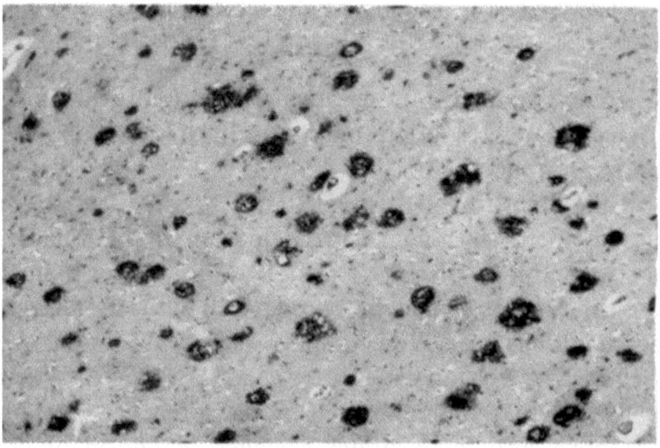

**Fig. 2.** Cerebral cortex showing plaques in Alzheimer's disease. Silver stain - Garvey

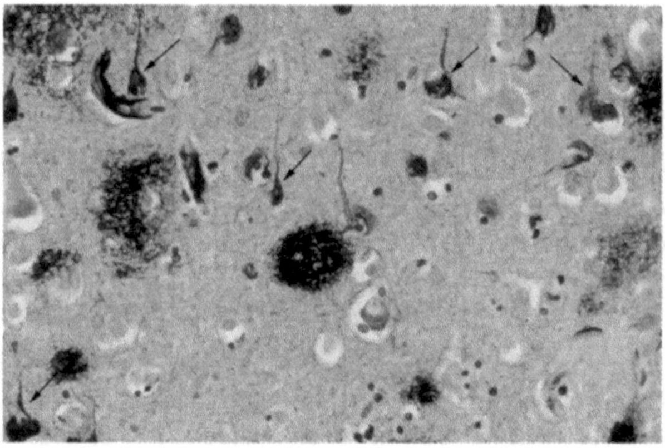

**Fig. 3.** Cerebral cortex showing tangles (*arrows*) in Alzheimer's disease as well as plaques in the cerebral cortex. Silver stain - Garvey

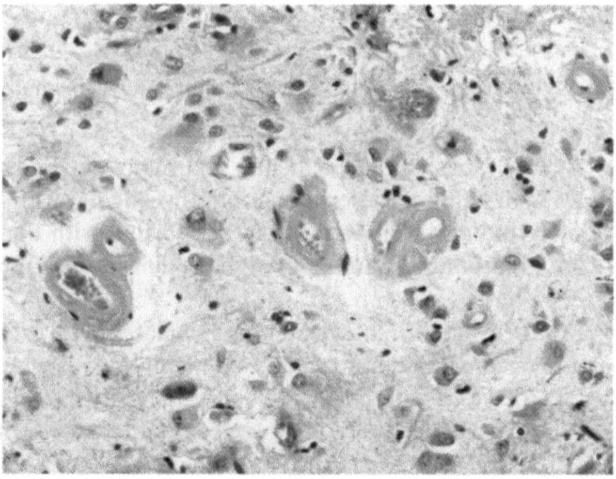

**Fig. 4.** Thick-walled, amyloid-laden vessels in the cortex in Alzheimer's disease. These would stain with Congo red

### 3.1.3 Pathological Diagnostic Criteria for Alzheimer's Disease

There are problems in making a pathological diagnosis of AD because the histological changes overlap those seen in the normal elderly population and are not pathognomonic [13].

Guidelines for the histological diagnosis of AD have been adapted from those used by neuropathologists participating in the Consortium to Establish a Registry for Alzheimer's Disease (CERAD) [50]. A semi-quantitative assessment of histological changes is made by comparison with standard reference diagrams. This assessment has been shown to have good reproducibility between different workers.

The NIA Reagan criteria for diagnosis for AD may also be used. This scheme places increased importance on the presence of neurofibrillary tangles in the diagnosis and incorporates a staged evolution of tangle pathology in the assessment [53].

### 3.1.4 Molecular Pathology of Alzheimer's Disease

Molecular investigation has now revealed several genes with a central role in AD pathogenesis. AD has been divided into four genetic subtypes [59, 61].

- AD1: mutations in the amyloid precursor gene on chromosome 21
- AD2: associated with the APOE4 allele on chromosome 19
- AD3: mutation in the presenilin 1 gene on chromosome 14
- AD4: mutation in the presenilin 2 gene on chromosome 1

Neurochemical analysis of brains has shown widespread transmitter defects in the brains of patients with AD. There is a marked loss of acetylcholine from the cerebral cortex in AD. This has been related to loss of neurons from the nucleus basalis of Meynert (one of the basal forebrain nuclei), which is the major cholinergic input nucleus to the cerebral cortex. Treatments which augment cholinergic transmission are licensed for use in AD [20].

### 3.1.5 Problems in the Pathological Diagnosis of Alzheimer's Disease

- A patient has clinical dementia and many amyloid plaques but absent or rare NFT on histological examination. Investigation in such cases has shown that such findings are nearly always associated with the presence of cortical Lewy bodies. Immunostaining for alpha synuclein or ubiquitin is indicated to detect Lewy bodies [23, 42].
- A patient has clinical dementia associated with large numbers of NFT in the hippocampal and entorhinal regions in the absence of plaques. This has been regarded as a distinct form of dementia termed tangle-only dementia. There are overlaps with the pathology seen in patients with other tau-protein disorders [33, 34, 51, 63].

- A patient has clinical dementia and clinical features of cerebrovascular disease. Pathological examination shows plaques, tangles and evidence of cerebrovascular disease. A diagnosis of mixed dementia may be considered [24].
- Histological lesions as seen in AD may be found in restricted distribution or low density in cognitively normal elderly patients. There is some evidence that this may represent an early, pre-clinical stage of AD, and had such a patient lived for a longer time, clinical disease would have developed with advance of the pathology [1, 13, 27].

## 3.2 Dementia with Lewy Bodies

### 3.2.1 Clinical Features and Incidence

Dementia with Lewy bodies (DLB) emerged as a common form of dementia in most clinical series in the late 1980s. Studies showed that in hospital-based practice, this condition accounted for between 10% and 25% of all cases of dementia, making it the second commonest pathological cause of dementia after AD. Community-based studies suggest that DLB probably has a lower incidence amongst patients with dementia who are managed in the community. DLB is a temporoparietal dementia. The core clinical features that suggest a diagnosis of DLB are early hallucinations, memory loss and some motor features of Parkinson's disease. Patients may present with frequent falls, recognised as being present with a higher incidence than in patients with AD. Importantly, patients with DLB exhibit abnormal sensitivity to neuroleptic drugs, which may precipitate a fatal reaction [8, 26, 39, 46–48].

Clinical features which suggest a diagnosis of DLB have been proposed:

1. The central requirement is progressive cognitive decline of sufficient magnitude to interfere with normal social or occupational function. Prominent or persistent memory impairment may not necessarily occur in the early stages but is usually evident with progression. Deficits on tests of attention and frontal-subcortical skills and visuospatial ability may be especially prominent.
2. Two of the following are required for a probable and one for a possible diagnosis of dementia with Lewy bodies:
   - Fluctuating cognition with pronounced variations in attention and alertness
   - Recurrent visual hallucinations which are typically well-formed and detailed
   - Spontaneous motor features of parkinsonism
3. Features supportive of the diagnosis are:
   - Repeated falls
   - Syncope or transient loss of consciousness
   - Neuroleptic sensitivity
   - Systematised delusions
   - Hallucinations in other modalities
4. A diagnosis of dementia with Lewy bodies is less likely in the presence of:
   - Stroke disease, evident as focal neurological signs or on brain imaging
   - Evidence on physical examination and investigation of any physical illness or other brain disorder sufficient to account for the clinical picture

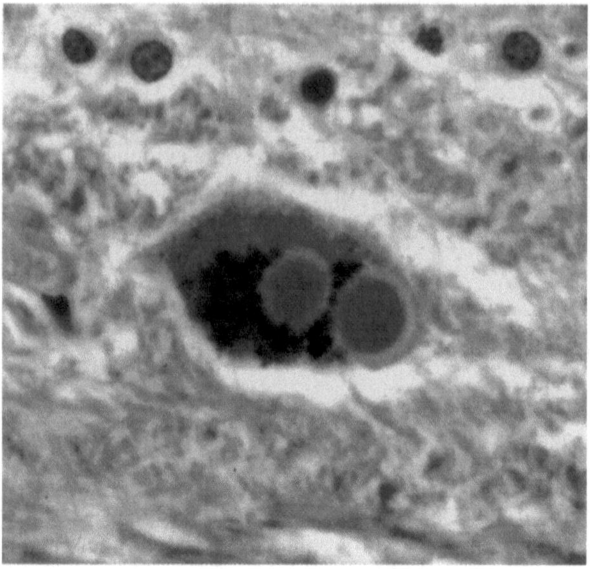

**Fig. 5.** Two Lewy bodies in a neuron in the substantia nigra (Haematoxylin and eosin stain)

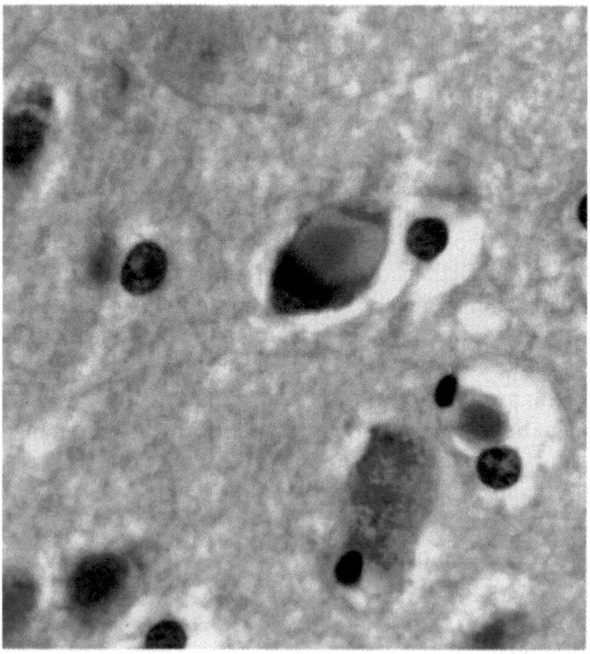

**Fig. 6.** A cortical Lewy body in a small cortical neuron (Haematoxylin and eosin stain)

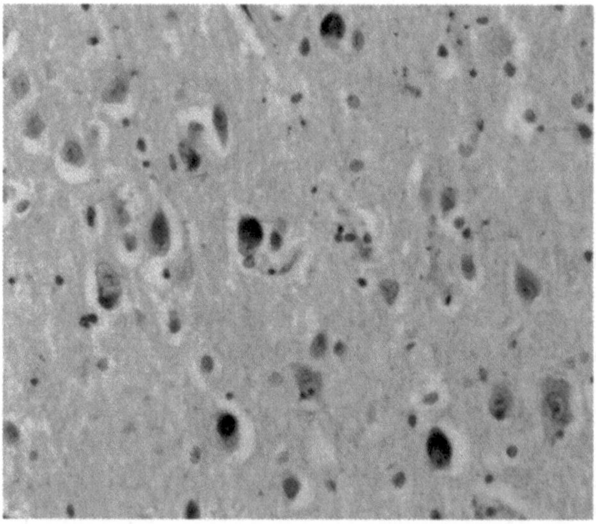

**Fig. 7.** Cortical Lewy bodies immunostained with anti-ubiquitin

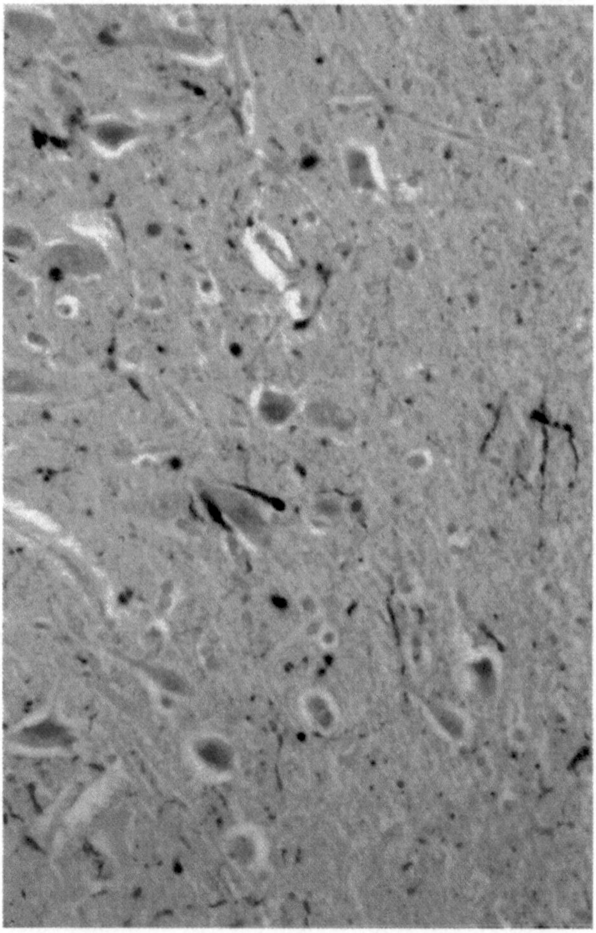

**Fig. 8.** Neurites detected with anti-ubiquitin in Lewy body disease

### 3.2.2 Macroscopic and Histological Features of Dementia with Lewy Bodies

The macroscopic appearances of the brain are similar to those seen in Alzheimer's disease, although typically brains are not as severely atrophic. An important suggestive finding is pallor of the substantia nigra in the midbrain, reflecting cell loss from the substantia nigra.

Histological changes identical to those in idiopathic Parkinson's disease are seen in the substantia nigra: there is loss of pigmented neurons, and classical Lewy bodies are seen some of the pigmented neurons that remain (Fig. 5). Cortical Lewy bodies can be seen in cortical neurons on haematoxylin and eosin (H&E) staining (Fig. 6). They are best demonstrated by immunochemical staining for alpha synuclein or ubiquitin (Figs. 7, 8). In addition to cortical and brain-stem Lewy bodies, immunohistochemistry using anti alpha synuclein or ubiquitin reveals the presence of abnormal neurites (termed Lewy neurites) in cortical and sub-cortical regions. These abnormalities of neurites are believed to contribute to the neurological dysfunction. Most patients also have histological features of plaques and tangles in the cortex, identical to those in AD. Spongiform change, virtually identical to that seen in Creutzfeldt-Jakob disease (CJD), can be found in a restricted distribution in the medial temporal lobe structures [48].

### 3.2.3 Diagnostic Criteria for Dementia with Lewy Bodies

Diagnostic criteria for pathological assessment of dementia with Lewy bodies have been published (Newcastle criteria) and are recommended for detailed assessment [48]. Three patterns of disease are recognised:

- Brain stem: Lewy bodies restricted to brain stem nuclei
- Transitional: cortical Lewy bodies seen in limbic cortical regions
- Necortical: cortical Lewy bodies seen extensively in neocortex

### 3.2.4 Problems in the Diagnosis of Dementia with Lewy Bodies

Some patients with DLB have a rapid clinical course and myoclonus, suggesting a clinical diagnosis of CJD. The presence of spongiform change in such cases should not be confused with that seen in CJD. Detection of Lewy pathology with anti-alpha synuclein, and absence of prion protein (PrP) immunostaining are helpful in confirming the correct pathological diagnosis [48].

In patients with clinical parkinsonism who develop dementia, Lewy body pathology may not be evident, reflecting the fact that there are other causes of parkinsonism with dementia, including cerebrovascular disease with lacunar infarction and white matter degeneration, progressive supranuclear palsy (PSP) and corticobasal degeneration (CBD). Tau immunohistochemistry will reveal PSP and CBD pathology in suspected [16, 63] cases.

## 3.3 Frontotemporal Dementias

Patients who present with progressive frontal lobe dysfunction (that may later be followed by evidence of temporal lobe disturbance) can be grouped together as having a frontotemporal dementia. This clinical syndrome has been increasingly recognised over the last decade and is believed to account for about 10% of all cases of dementia. This syndrome is still under-diagnosed and other labels are frequently applied. There are several well-defined pathological causes of this syndrome, amongst which is classical Pick's disease. Immunohistochemical assessment of brain is essential in establishing a diagnosis [4, 21, 41, 45].

### 3.3.1 Clinical Features of Frontotemporal Dementias

In contrast to patients with AD, parietal and even temporal lobe function is usually preserved until late in the disease. The main clinical features of disease are behavioural, including loss of insight, disinhibited behaviour, apathy, dietary fads and symptomatic alcoholism. As disease progresses, memory problems develop, reflecting temporal lobe disease.

### 3.3.2 Pathological Features of Frontotemporal Dementias

Macroscopically, most cases show severe frontotemporal atrophy, although in some cases little atrophy is noted macroscopically. Neuronal loss is seen from the frontal cortex as well as the temporal lobes. On H&E staining, microvacuolation is visible in the outer cortical layers of affected regions, becoming severe with increasing neuronal loss (Fig. 9). Diagnosis and sub-typing of disease are mainly dependent on immunohistochemical assessment, based on staged pathological examination.

- The commonest form is characterised by the presence of ubiquitin-immunoreactive inclusions in cortical and hippocampal neurons, together with ubiquitin-immunoreactive neurites, most evident in areas of microvacuolation. This type of disease appears pathologically very similar to cases of dementia associated with motor neuron disease [12, 19, 30, 31, 36, 37, 40, 45, 52, 58, 62, 64].
- Other cases are characterised by accumulation of tau protein in neurons and glia. In many instances the pathology is identical to that in the movement disorder termed corticobasal degeneration. Increasingly recognised are inherited forms of frontotemporal degeneration linked to mutations in the gene for tau protein on chromosome 17 (frontotemporal degeneration and parkinsonism linked to chromosome 17 or FTDP17). As indicated by this designation, clinical parkinsonism is a common feature in many cases [7, 18, 60, 63, 66].
- Classical Pick's disease is characterised by the presence of rounded Pick bodies and swollen Pick cells in the cortex. These may be detected with silver stains or antibodies to tau protein.

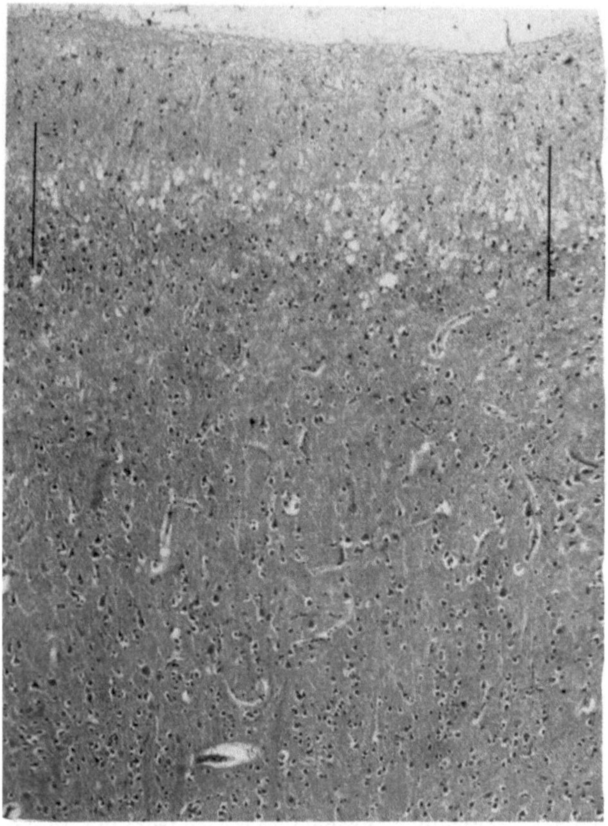

**Fig. 9.** Lower power view of frontal cortex showing microvacuolation in layer 2 (*between lines*). This is a common feature of frontotemporal dementias and should prompt application of a panel of immunohistochemical stains to characterise the disease

- In some cases, no inclusions or accumulations of tau protein can be seen. At present such cases are classified simply as frontotemporal dementia. It is anticipated that future insights will be able to relate such cases to a defined protein or genetic abnormality.

### 3.3.3 Problems in the Pathological Diagnosis of Frontotemporal Dementia

- Some elderly patients with frontotemporal dementia have a clinical diagnosis of alcoholic dementia. This is because a clinical feature of this type of dementia is disinhibition, leading to secondary alcoholism, termed symptomatic alcoholism.
- Self-neglect in the elderly is an indication to look for frontotemporal dementia syndrome.

- Microvacuolation seen in the cerebral cortex in cases of frontotemporal dementia can lead to a mistaken diagnosis of prion disease. Confirmation by immunohistochemistry for PrP and exclusion of defined causes of frontotemporal dementia by performing appropriate immunohistochemistry will avoid this confusion.
- Patients with the clinical syndrome of primary progressive aphasia show a range of pathologies which are the same as those encountered in frontotemporal dementia.

## 3.4 Vascular Dementia

### 3.4.1 Incidence and Classification

Vascular dementia, also termed multi-infarct dementia, describes cognitive decline caused by cumulative effects of multiple episodes of cerebral ischaemia. This definition excludes cases of diffuse cerebral cortical damage caused by a single episode of severe hypoxia or global cerebral hypoperfusion. While at one time this was thought to be the second commonest cause of dementia, recent clinicopathological studies have suggested that the incidence of pure vascular dementia may be lower than previously suspected.

### 3.4.2 Clinical Features of Vascular Dementia

Clinically, vascular dementia presents with early gait difficulties, strokes, urinary incontinence, parkinsonian features, pseudobulbar signs and cognitive impairment. Clinicians diagnose multi-infarct dementia on the basis of focal neurology consistent with the presence of strokes, a stepwise deterioration in condition suggestive of discrete insults to the brain and day-to-day fluctuation in cognitive performance. These are embodied in a clinical rating scale called the Hachinski score, which is frequently employed to assess whether a patient has multi-infarct dementia. Imaging studies are also used to support a diagnosis of vascular dementia, particularly the finding of white matter abnormality termed leuko-araiosis. Pathological studies have shown that the underlying abnormalities are non-specific and can be seen in normal elderly persons as well as in association with vascular risk factors and dementia. Because of difficulty with precise clinical and pathological diagnosis, an operational approach is recommended to establishing the diagnosis of a vascular dementia. Focal neurobehavioural syndromes caused by individual strokes are to be distinguished from vascular dementia. The diagnosis should only be used when memory impairment is associated with deficits in two other cognitive domains, including orientation, language skills, visuo-spatial skills, praxis, abstraction and judgement, sufficient to cause impairment in function and daily living [57]. Different operational criteria have different specificities for this diagnosis [9].

### 3.4.3 Neuropathological Features of Vascular Dementia

Vascular disease can cause dementia in several main ways [15, 43]:

- The commonest pathology is related to arteriolosclerosis, causing small vessel disease that affects deep white matter and subcortical grey matter regions. The dominant pathology is the presence of multiple lacunar infarcts and ischaemic white matter degeneration (Fig. 10). Ischaemic white matter degeneration can be recognised as pallor on myelin staining associated with varying degrees of astrocytic gliosis (Fig. 11). The term 'Binswanger's disease' is sometimes used in relation to dementia caused by ischaemic white matter degeneration.
- Small vessel disease may, less commonly, produce military areas of cortical microinfarction, macroscopically visible as so-called granular cortical atrophy (Fig. 12).

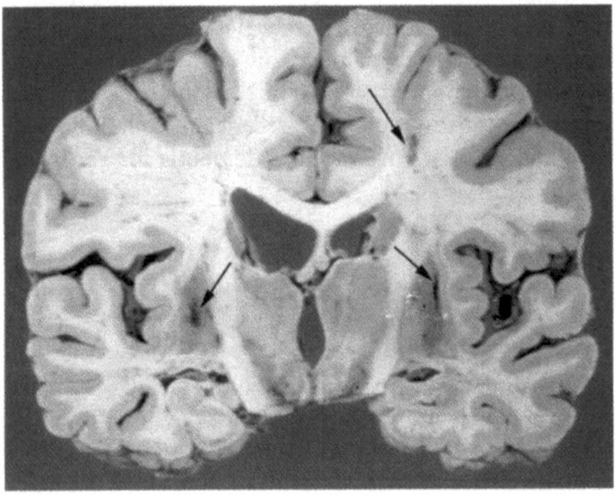

**Fig. 10.** Lacunar infarcts in basal ganglia and white matter

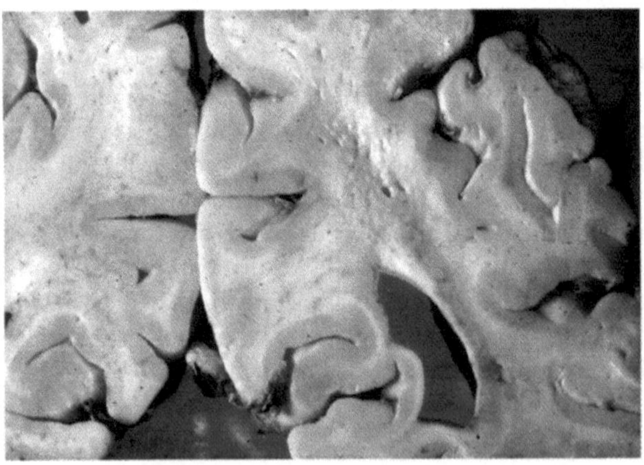

**Fig. 11.** Softening and granularity of white matter due to ischaemic degeneration

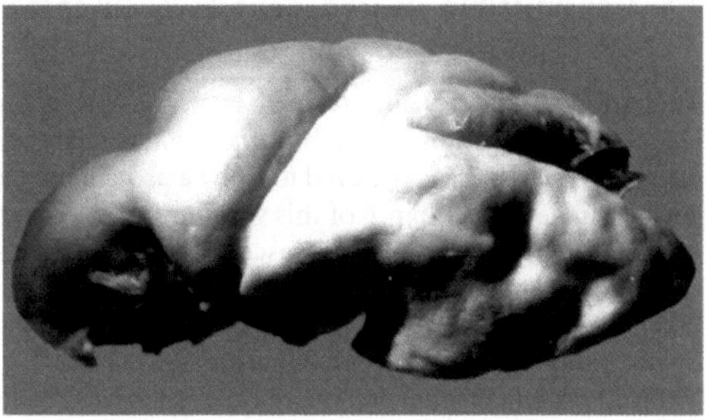

**Fig. 12.** Granular cortical atrophy in the tip of the temporal lobe

- Large regional infarcts may be associated with isolated neurobehavioural deficits related to dysfunction of the affected regions. The summation of deficits from multiple large infarcts may satisfy an operational diagnosis of vascular dementia.
- A small number of critically-sited infarcts may be responsible for a clinical diagnosis of dementia. Bilateral ischaemic damage to the hippocampal regions (hippocampal sclerosis) can cause a severe amnesic syndrome. Bilateral involvement of medial thalamic regions may also be associated with severe cognitive impairment.

Histological validation of cases of vascular dementia should always be performed. In many cases, associated features of AD or DLB are found, in which case a diagnosis of mixed dementia is appropriate. While arteriolosclerosis is the commonest reason for vascular dementia, other angiopathies may be encountered. Amyloid angiopathies, some being hereditary, are well described in a minority of cases of vascular dementia [55]. Increasingly, cases of CADASIL are being recognised as the cause of vascular dementia, with important genetic implications. This can be diagnosed by conventional histology, which reveals deposition of granular material within the walls of small vessels [14].

In many cases of suspected vascular dementia, histological examination reveals changes of Alzheimer's disease, warranting a diagnosis of mixed dementia.

### 3.4.4 Problems in Diagnosis of Vascular Dementia

- In clinico-pathological studies it has been found that the Hachinski score is not a very specific tool, and that the clinical diagnosis of multi-infarct dementia is not substantiated by autopsy in about one fifth of cases [17].
- Very often patients have changes of Alzheimer's disease plus strokes (mixed dementia); in other cases pure Lewy body dementia or Alzheimer's disease mimics the clinical features of vascular dementia.
- A patient with a single neurobehavioural deficit caused by a large cerebral infarct should not be diagnosed as having dementia.

## 3.5 Transmissible Neurodegenerative Disease

The prion disorders, also termed transmissible spongiform encephalopathies, represent a group of biologically unique conditions where transmission of a neurodegenerative disease is believed to be by a protein only agent. These conditions are covered in detail in Chap. 6 of this volume and are covered only briefly here. There has been great interest in the ascertainment of cases of human transmissible spongiform encephalopathy since the discovery of cases of variant Creutzfeldt-Jakob disease (vCJD) in the UK and its association with exposure to cattle infected by bovine spongiform encephalopathy (BSE) [11].

Prion protein is a normal membrane-associated cellular protein, with sequence and conformation conserved between species. It is believed that an abnormal conformation of protein develops which is responsible for the development of disease. In broad terms, the abnormal protein accumulates in neuronal cells eventually causing their death. It is believed that protein with an abnormal conformation brings about conversion of normal cellular prion protein to the abnormal form. Disease can be transmitted through administration of the abnormal protein either by inoculation or orally [10].

Clinical features which might suggest one of these diseases should be ascertained from case notes prior to undertaking an autopsy on a dementia case so that appropriate Health and Safety precautions can be taken if there is clinical suspicion of transmissible disease [3]. All pathologists involved in postmortem practice should be familiar with clinical features indicating a potential prion disease. Precautions should also be implemented for patients with a history of exposure to a known potential source of transmitted disease.

The transmissible agent is classed as a category III pathogen and must be handled according to appropriate Health and Safety requirements. In the UK, referral to the National CJD Surveillance Team in Edinburgh is encouraged of cases suspected of having CJD and those falling into high-risk categories. Similar national referral schemes exist in many other countries, reflecting increasing concern about the possibility of an epidemic of disease following population exposure to the agent in cattle with BSE. Separate protocols for autopsy and tissue handling in these cases have been produced and should be implemented in all laboratories handling such cases [3, 6, 28, 29, 56].

### 3.5.1 Classification and Incidence of Prion Diseases

Transmissible spongiform encephalopathies have been found in all populations studied with an incidence of around one per million population per year. Three types of disease are recognised:

- Genetic disease caused by mutation in the prion gene. These disorders are familial; however, tissue from such cases can cause disease by transmission. Familial Creutzfeldt-Jakob disease, Gerstmann-Straüssler-Scheinker syndrome, fatal familial insomnia and certain types of hereditary spastic paraparesis are the best-recognised forms of hereditary prion disease.

- Sporadic disease: believed to be caused by spontaneous conversion of normal prion protein to prion protein of abnormal configuration. Most cases conform to the clinical syndrome of Creutzfeldt-Jakob disease typified by a rapidly progressive dementia (causing death in under 2 years) associated with early myoclonus and characteristic EEG changes.
- Transmitted disease: caused by exposure to the agent from the environment. This applies to cases transmitted through neurosurgical procedures (dura mater grafts), cadaver-derived human hormone therapy or diet (acquisition of vCJD by eating products of cattle with BSE).

Higher incidence rates have been recorded in some regions or populations (such as amongst Libyan Jews, in areas of central Slovakia and Hungary). These high local rates are accounted for by large families with mutations in the prion gene. Approximately equal numbers of men and women are affected. About 10% of all prion diseases cases are familial. For sporadic disease, the age of onset is usually between 55 and 75 years with a peak incidence in the 60s. Young patients are characteristically encountered in cases of transmitted disease.

### 3.5.2 Pathological Features of Prion Disease

Postmortem and histological examination must be performed according to appropriate Health and Safety guidelines, bearing in mind that conventional fixation and histological processing does not inactivate the infective agent. Pathological confirmation of cases is possible by conventional histology, prion gene analysis (to exclude genetic causes of prion disease) and immunohistochemistry for PrP [29]. Protocols for performing such high-risk procedures have been published [3, 28].

Macroscopically, brain may appear atrophic but is often of normal size. The main histological features in prion disease are:

- Neuronal loss and astrocytic gliosis.
- Synaptic loss.
- Microvacuolation, termed spongiform change (Fig. 13).
- Accumulation of prion protein as amyloid plaques is seen in a small proportion of cases. This is a dominant pathological feature in cases of vCJD (Fig. 14).
- Paucity of lymphocytic inflammation.

Histological examination is usually performed after decontamination of tissue blocks by means of formic acid pre-treatment, a procedure which has been shown to reduce infective titres dramatically. Immunohistochemical demonstration of prion protein is possible by immunohistochemistry after section pre-treatment protocols for destruction of normal prion protein and antigen unmasking of pathological prion protein [2]. The morphological manifestations of the disease are affected by whether or not the disease is sporadic, familial or iatrogenic, the nature of the PrP gene defect (if familial) and the codon 129 PrP genotype, and the duration of the illness.

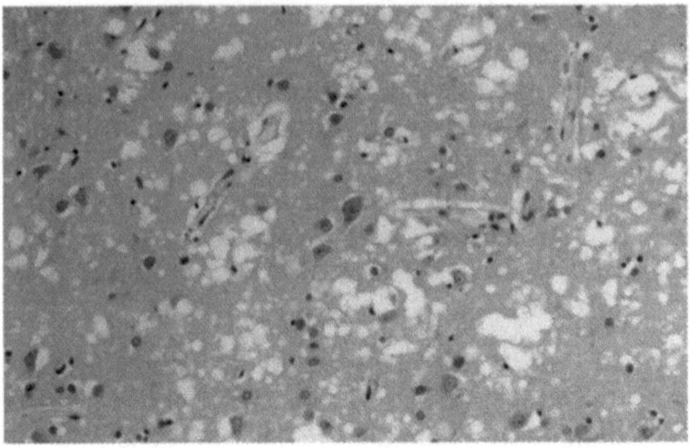

**Fig. 13.** Spongiform change in CJD

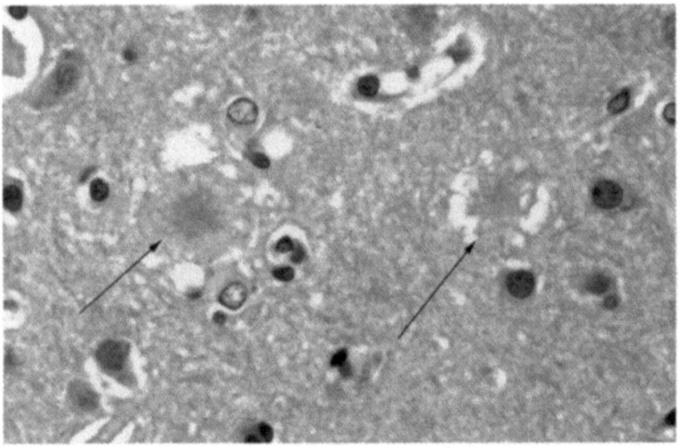

**Fig. 14.** Amyloid plaques in the cerebral cortex in vCJD

### 3.5.3 Problems in the Diagnosis of Prion Disease

- Rapidly progressive dementias may not just be caused by prion disease. Infective, metabolic, toxic and inflammatory conditions may all cause this picture.
- Rapidly progressive dementia associated with early myoclonus and characteristic EEG changes is often caused by dementia with Lewy bodies. Some cases of dementia with Lewy bodies have transcortical microvacuolation that mimics the spongiform change of prion disease. In DLB this is restricted to the mesial temporal lobe regions.
- Transcortical microvacuolation, neuronal loss and astrocytic gliosis are features of some of the pathological variants of frontotemporal dementia.
- There is a small subgroup of elderly patients with CJD who have a more protracted clinical course than is typical for classical CJD – so-called subacute CJD.

### 3.6 Unusual Dementia Syndromes

After the common causes of dementia have been excluded, one may be left with a situation in which dementia has been diagnosed but no firm pathological diagnosis is established.

- The most likely reason is that the clinical diagnosis of dementia is uncertain. Diagnosis by non-specialist clinicians may label confusional states as dementia. Depression in the elderly may have many of the clinical features of a specific dementia syndrome. In these instances the situation is often resolved by careful reading of the case notes to ascertain how the diagnosis of dementia was made and with what certainty.
- In addition to the main conditions of Alzheimer's disease, dementia with Lewy bodies, frontotemporal dementias and vascular dementia, there are many uncommon forms of dementia. These are usually given descriptive terms related to neuropathological features seen on special staining, for example argyrophilic grain dementia. Descriptions of the neuropathology of these rarer diseases is to be found in specialised textbooks and is outside the scope of this general review. In the diagnosis of unusual cases of dementia, referral to a specialist centre is advisable.
- Rarely, a confident clinical diagnosis of dementia is not accompanied by morphological changes in the brain.

## 4 Pathological Investigation of Dementia

The majority of postmortem examinations of patients who had a clinical dementia syndrome are performed by general histopathologists outside specialist clinical neuroscience centres. If a diagnosis of the cause of a dementia syndrome is required then it is usual for the complete brain to be retained and referred for examination by a specialist neuropathologist after fixation in formalin. In clinical neuroscience centres, postmortem procedures are usually performed by a specialist neuropathologist and brains are handled fresh, with samples preserved for more sophisticated examination in addition to routine diagnosis. This pattern of working may have to evolve in response to emerging pressures. It is apparent in many countries that retention of a whole brain following postmortem examination cannot be assumed to be part of a routine postmortem procedure, but may be performed only with specific informed consent from relatives of the deceased. Protocols that allow strategic sampling of the brain for histology, without retaining the whole brain (see "Appendix", pp 267) may be more acceptable to families but will require new ways of working to be developed in the laboratory. It is probable that public concerns related to CJD may drive up the demand for pathological verification of the precise nature of neurodegenerative diseases.

## 4.1 Aims of Neuropathological Assessment in Dementia

There are several possible objectives in performing a postmortem examination in a patient with a dementia syndrome:

- Establish a diagnosis of the cause of dementia based on clinical, macroscopic and histological assessment.
- Provide a clinicopathological correlation, including an opinion as to whether the disease made a direct contribution to the patient's death.
- Provide a written report to clinicians and pathologists or legal authorities involved in the case.
- Maintain a diagnostic index of cases to facilitate future review of cases for the purposes of genetic counselling of surviving relatives, teaching, audit and research.
- Archive material for audit teaching and research.
- Preserve material to facilitate genetic analysis.

Broadly speaking, there are two levels of sophistication of pathological assessment in dealing with a case of dementia syndrome:

- The diagnostic protocol can be limited to sampling and histological examination of key brain areas to establish a pathological diagnosis of disease.
- The protocol can be suited to detailed clinico-pathological correlation, in which sampling of many brain areas is performed, not merely to establish the diagnosis but also to stage the disease and relate the pathological findings to imaging and clinical abnormalities in life. This approach, largely restricted to cases seen in specialist clinical neuroscience centres, serves the purposes of diagnosis, audit, teaching and clinical research.

## 4.2 Postmortem Examination in Dementia

In the postmortem investigation of clinical dementia, the following, including documentation of relevant negative findings, should be a minimum routine standard. In cases where consent is limited to removal of only limited samples of brain tissue, some of these recommendations will not be possible.

- Autopsy procedures should be carried out in an appropriate facility in accordance with Health and Safety recommendations for autopsy practice.
- Adequate clinical data should be available to assess the potential risk of a transmissible neurodegenerative disease.
- A full postmortem examination should be performed with histology of all major organs. In the UK this is advised to be according to recommendations of the Royal College of Pathologists (2000).
- Careful examination for cerebrovascular disease is important (see also Chap. 2, this volume) and should include seeking potential sources of emboli from the heart and great vessels, opening the carotid vessels from their origin to the base of the skull, opening the vertebral arteries throughout their length.
- Examination of the venous sinuses with samples preserved for histology if appropriate.

- Consent should be obtained to retain the whole brain for fixation and later histological assessment. If dysphagia or motor weakness has been present in the latter stages of disease then the spinal cord, skeletal muscle and peripheral nerve should also be preserved (see also Chap. 7, this volume). If the postmortem examination is being performed for a legal authority, the authority should be advised that establishing the pathological cause of dementia frequently has a direct bearing on the cause of death.
- If consent to retain the whole brain cannot be obtained then tissue samples should be retained from key brain areas, sufficient to diagnose the common neurodegenerative disorders. The regions for suggested sampling are discussed later. An approach to obtaining tissue suitable for sampling is shown in the Appendix to this book.
- If facilities are available, CSF and portions of brain should be archived after freezing in liquid nitrogen and preserved at –70 °C. This will facilitate genetic analysis and microbiological or biochemical studies.
- The brain and spinal cord should be preserved in 8–10 times their volume of 10% formalin, changed weekly, for 3–4 weeks. The fixed brain is then sliced after 3–4 weeks. Brain tissue fixing in formalin waiting for examination should be stored in a dedicated, ventilated storage area. A ventilated area should be available that is suitable for regular changing of formalin during fixation process. Brains should be cut up in a dedicated ventilated cut-up area for dissection of fixed brains. The cut up area should be capable of decontamination according to protocols for handling of tissues containing the infective agent of Creutzfeldt-Jakob disease, as it is inevitable that these will be handled inadvertently at some time, despite precautions. In view of this potential risk of inadvertently handling tissue containing the agent transmitting Creutzfeldt-Jakob disease, brain-cutting knives should be disposable and should not be re-sharpened. Tools and areas used for brain cutting should be routinely decontaminated by a method which inactivates the agent [3].
- Histological sampling of brain and spinal cord should be performed in all cases. If it is not possible to retain a whole brain to ascertain the cause of a dementia, it is possible to preserve a restricted set of samples for histological diagnosis. If the pathologist is not certain of detailed neuroanatomy, preservation of large brain regions may be appropriate. For dementia, this would be large, thick slices of brain including the following regions (see "Appendix", pp 267):
  - Temporal lobe with hippocampus
  - Frontal lobe
  - Basal ganglia
  - Midbrain, pons and medulla
  - A slice of cerebellum

If the pathologist feels confident about neuroanatomy then it is possible to retain small specific tissue samples of a size that can be trimmed to fit into tissue processing cassettes. The areas most important for a routine screening for dementia would be:

- Hippocampus with parahippocampal gyrus
- Midbrain including substantia nigra
- Pons including locus coeruleus

- Medulla at the level of the hypoglossal nucleus
- Cerebellar cortex and dentate nucleus
- Globus pallidus and putamen
- Middle frontal gyrus
- Middle temporal gyrus
- Areas of macroscopic cortical atrophy not sampled in those above
- Areas of white matter abnormality not sampled above

Disadvantages of adopting a sampling strategy for diagnosis rather than retaining the whole brain are the risk of introducing artefact and compromising histology, the risk of missing focal pathologies and the fact that it will not be possible to perform correlative clinicopathological studies.

## 4.3 Histological Techniques for Dementia

For optimal histology, brain tissue requires longer processing schedules for embedding in paraffin wax than those used in general pathological practice. In the past, diagnostic neuropathologists relied greatly on the ability to process, embed

**Table 1.** Proteins detectable by immunohistochemistry and used in the diagnosis of dementia

| Protein | Summary |
|---|---|
| Ubiquitin | A highly conserved protein which is covalently attached to other proteins and flags them for degradation by the proteosome system. Labels a subset of neurofibrillary tangles, classical and cortical Lewy bodies, Lewy body neurites, intranuclear inclusions in triplet-repeat expansion diseases, inclusions and neurites in ALS and related dementia, inclusions of multiple system atrophy |
| Alpha synuclein | Originally identified as a non-amyloid component of plaques in AD now found in all Lewy bodies and Lewy-related neurites |
| Tau | In normal cells a microtubule-associated protein. Seen as a major component of neurofibrillary tangles in Alzheimer's disease. Also seen in tangles in other disorders. Found in glial cells as a distinctive feature of several degenerative diseases. Several different molecular forms associated with different diseases processes |
| Alpha B-crystallin | A chaperone protein related to one of the small heat-shock proteins. Normally found in glial cells. A marker of swollen neurons (formerly called Pick cells). Seen in a proportion of cortical Lewy bodies. Seen in inclusions of multiple system atrophy |
| A$\beta$ protein ($\beta$APP) | Derived from the amyloid precursor protein, this is a cleaved fragment that is the basis of the amyloid that accumulates in plaques in Alzheimer's disease and dementia with Lewy bodies. This is also the main protein found in vascular amyloid |
| PrP | Prion protein. A normal membrane-associated protein. What is widely believed to be a conformationally abnormal form accumulates in prion diseases such as Creutzfeldt-Jakob disease and bovine spongiform encephalopathy |

and cut whole lobes of brain to facilitate anatomical localisation of pathological changes. This is not required for establishing a diagnosis for dementia in the vast majority of cases; small samples that fit into routine tissue processing cassettes are perfectly adequate.

Laboratories should have well-established staining protocols for detection of pathological changes in neurodegenerative disease. A specialist neuropathology laboratory should have well-established techniques as follows:

- Haematoxylin and eosin
- Tinctorial stain for amyloid
- Myelin stain
- Nissl stain
- Stain sensitive for the detection of neurofibrillary tangles
- Stain sensitive for the detection of all forms of amyloid senile plaque
- Stain for the detection of astrocytic gliosis
- Immunostaining techniques should be routinely available in all neuropathology laboratories, and it is recommended that laboratories diagnosing neurodegenerative diseases have established methods for detection of $A\beta$ protein, tau protein, alpha-synuclein, ubiquitin, phosphorylated neurofilament protein, $\alpha$B crystallin, prion protein and glial fibrillary acidic protein (Table 1).

## 4.4 Histological Sampling and Staged Histological Examination

Establishing a diagnosis of the pathological cause of a dementia requires the staged examination of a case, often necessitating repeated histological sampling of several brain areas, and performing additional special histological stains. It is impractical and inefficient to perform a totally inclusive battery of histological samples and stains in all cases.

The initial choice of blocks is weighted to making a diagnosis of Alzheimer's disease, vascular dementia or dementia with Lewy bodies. The suggested blocks and stains are those required for a minimal diagnostic assessment for sampling a fresh brain (see above). Detailed clinicopathological study correlating function, imaging or unusual clinical features will require additional tissue sampling and additional special staining techniques.

Blocks are processed to paraffin wax and sections are cut from all areas sampled and stained for H&E and myelin. The temporal lobe and hippocampal blocks are stained by techniques sensitive to the presence of amyloid plaques and tangles. The initial screening of these preparations will enable diagnosis of the main types of dementia.

- Assessment made for Alzheimer's disease. Rare cases of dementia pugilistica and tangle-only dementias will also be revealed on analysis of sections stained to detect plaques and tangles.
- Assessment made for Lewy bodies in brain stem and, if present, in the cortex, to establish a diagnosis of dementia with Lewy bodies.
- Assessment made for vascular dementia and hippocampal sclerosis.

- Assessment made for tangles in the substantia nigra or for microvacuolation in outer cortex of frontal and temporal lobes. If present, additional immunostaining is performed to determine the sub-type of disease:
  - Tau immunostaining is performed to define specific types of disease as characterised by regional patterns of abnormal tau deposition, including senile dementia with tangles, progressive supranuclear palsy, Pick's disease, corticobasal degeneration, chromosome 17-linked neurodegeneration, argyrophilic grain dementia and multiple system atrophy.
  - Ubiquitin immunostaining defines diseases with inclusions related to motor neuron disease as well as dementia characterised by distinctive neurites.
  - Cases which show no inclusions, with variable numbers of swollen neurons, in the presence of cortical microvacuolation, can be considered as having dementia of frontal type or progressive subcortical gliosis.

Careful examination of the thalamus is indicated to define cases of thalamic dementia with inflammatory, vascular, neoplastic and degenerative aetiologies. Rare multi-system atrophies involving neuronal loss and astrocytic gliosis of subcortical nuclei can usually be related to one of the above disease groups using this staged examination strategy.

After excluding the above common causes of dementia, there remain many uncommon causes. Some of these are neurodegenerative disorders which are more usually seen in childhood. A detailed protocol for staged examination has been published and is suited for routine laboratory practice [44].

## References

1. Anderton BH (1997) Changes in the ageing brain in health and disease. Philos Trans R Soc Lond B Biol Sci 352 (1363):1781–1792
2. Bell JE, Gentleman SM, Ironside JW, McCardle L, Lantos PL, Doey L et al. (1997) Prion protein immunocytochemistry – UK five centre consensus report. Neuropathol Appl Neurobiol 23(1):26–35
3. Bell JE, Ironside JW (1993) How to tackle a possible Creutzfeldt-Jakob disease necropsy. J Clin Pathol 46(3):193–197
4. Bird TD (1998) Genotypes, Phenotypes, and Frontotemporal Dementia – Take Your Pick. Neurology 50(6):1526–1527
5. Bowler JV, Munoz DG, Merskey H, Hachinski V (1998) Fallacies in the Pathological Confirmation of the Diagnosis of Alzheimers-Disease. J Neurol Neurosurg Psychiatry 64(1): 18–24
6. Budka H, Aguzzi A, Brown P, Brucher JM, Bugiani O, Gullotta F et al. (1995) Neuropathological diagnostic criteria for Creutzfeldt-Jakob disease (CJD) and other human spongiform encephalopathies (prion diseases). Brain Pathol 5(4):459–466
7. Bugiani O, Murrell JR, Giaccone G, Hasegawa M, Ghigo G, Tabaton M et al. (1999) Frontotemporal dementia and corticobasal degeneration in a family with a P301S mutation in tau. J Neuropathol Exp Neurol 58(6):667–677
8. Chu CT, Caruso JL, Cummings TJ, Ervin J, Rosenberg C, Hulette CM (2000) Ubiquitin immunochemistry as a diagnostic aid for community pathologists evaluating patients who have dementia. Mod Pathol 13(4):420–426
9. Chui HC, Mack W, Jackson JE, Mungas D, Reed BR, Tinklenberg J et al. (2000) Clinical criteria for the diagnosis of vascular dementia: a multicenter study of comparability and interrater reliability. Arch Neurol 57(2):191–196
10. Collinge J (1997) Human prion diseases and bovine spongiform encephalopathy (BSE). Hum Mol Genet 6(10):1699–1705

11. Collinge J (1999) Variant Creutzfeldt-Jakob disease. Lancet 354(9175):317–323
12. Cooper PN, Jackson M, Lennox G, Lowe J, Mann DM (1995) Tau, ubiquitin, and alpha B-crystallin immunohistochemistry define the principal causes of degenerative frontotemporal dementia. Arch Neurol 52(10):1011–1015
13. Davis DG, Schmitt FA, Wekstein DR, Markesbery WR (1999) Alzheimer neuropathologic alterations in aged cognitively normal subjects. J Neuropathol Exp Neurol 58(4):376–388
14. Davous P (1998) CADASIL – A review with proposed diagnostic criteria. Eur J Neurol 5(3):219–233
15. Esiri MM (2000) Which vascular lesions are of importance in vascular dementia? Ann NY Acad Sci 903:239–243
16. Feany MB, Dickson DW (1996) Neurodegenerative disorders with extensive tau pathology: A comparative study and review. Ann Neurol 40(2):139–148
17. Fischer P, Jellinger K, Gatterer G, Danielczyk W (1991) Prospective neuropathological validation of Hachinski's Ischaemic Score in dementias. J Neurol Neurosurg Psychiatry 54(7):580–583
18. Goedert M, Spillantini MG (2000) Tau mutations in frontotemporal dementia FTDP-17 and their relevance for Alzheimer's disease. Biochim Biophys Acta 1502(1):110–121
19. Grimes DA, Bergeron CB, Lang AE (1999) Motor neuron disease-inclusion dementia presenting as cortical-basal ganglionic degeneration. Mov Disord 14(4):674–680
20. Grundman M, Thal LJ (2000) Treatment of Alzheimer's Disease: Rationale and Strategies. Neurol Clin 18(4):807–828
21. Gustafson L, Brun A, Passant U (1992) Frontal lobe degeneration of non-Alzheimer type. Baillieres Clin Neurol 1(3):559–582
22. Haltia M (2000) Human prion diseases. Ann Med 32(7):493–500
23. Hansen LA, Masliah E, Galasko D, Terry RD (1993) Plaque-only Alzheimer disease is usually the Lewy body variant, and vice versa. J Neuropathol Exp Neurol 52(6):648–654
24. Heyman A, Fillenbaum GG, Welshbohmer KA, Gearing M, Mirra SS, Mohs RC et al. (1998) Cerebral infarcts in patients with autopsy-proven alzheimer's-disease – CERAD, Part Xviii. Neurology 51(1):159–162
25. Holmes C, Cairns N, Lantos P, Mann A (1999) Validity of current clinical criteria for Alzheimer's disease, vascular dementia and dementia with Lewy bodies. Br J Psychiatry 174:45–50
26. Holmes C, Cairns N, Lantos P, Mann A (1999) Validity of current clinical criteria for Alzheimer's disease, vascular dementia and dementia with Lewy bodies. Br J Psychiatry 174:45–50
27. Hulette CM, Welsh-Bohmer KA, Murray MG, Saunders AM, Mash DC, McIntyre LM (1998) Neuropathological and neuropsychological changes in 'normal' aging: evidence for preclinical Alzheimer disease in cognitively normal individuals. J Neuropathol Exp Neurol 57(12):1168–1174
28. Ironside JW, Bell JE (1996) The 'high-risk' neuropathological autopsy in AIDS and Creutzfeldt-Jakob disease: principles and practice. Neuropathol Appl Neurobiol 22(5):388–393
29. Ironside JW, Head MW, Bell JE, McCardle L, Will RG (2000) Laboratory diagnosis of variant Creutzfeldt-Jakob disease. Histopathology 37(1):1–9
30. Jackson M, Lennox G, Lowe J (1996) Motor neurone disease-inclusion dementia. Neurodegeneration 5(4):339–350
31. Jackson M, Lowe J (1996) The new neuropathology of degenerative frontotemporal dementias. Acta Neuropathologica 91(2):127–134
32. Jellinger KA, Bancher C (1998) Neuropathology of Alzheimer's disease: a critical update. J Neural Transm Suppl (54):77–95
33. Jellinger KA, Bancher C (1998) Senile dementia with tangles (tangle predominant form of senile dementia). Brain Pathol 8(2):367–376
34. Jellinger KA, Bancher C (1998) Senile dementia with tangles (tangle predominant form of senile dementia). Brain Pathology 8(2):367–376
35. Jobst KA, Barnetson LP, Shepstone BJ (1997) Accurate prediction of histologically confirmed Alzheimer's disease and the differential diagnosis of dementia: the use of NINCDS-ADRDA and DSM-III-R criteria, SPECT, X-ray CT, and APO E4 medial temporal lobe dementias. The Oxford Project to Investigate Memory and Aging. Int Psychoger 9 (Suppl 1): 191–222; discussion 247–252

36. Kertesz A, Kawarai T, Rogaeva E, St (2000) George-Hyslop P, Poorkaj P, Bird TD et al. Familial frontotemporal dementia with ubiquitin-positive, tau-negative inclusions. Neurology 54(4):818–827
37. Kinoshita A, Tomimoto H, Suenaga T, Akiguchi I, Kimura J (1997) Ubiquitin-related cytoskeletal abnormality in frontotemporal dementia: immunohistochemical and immunoelectron microscope studies. Acta Neuropathol (Berl) 94(1):67–72
38. Knight R (1999) The relationship between new variant Creutzfeldt-Jakob disease and bovine spongiform encephalopathy. Vox Sang 76(4):203–208
39. Kosaka K, Iseki E (2000) Clinicopathological studies on diffuse Lewy body disease. Neuropathology 20(1):1–7
40. Kovari E, Leuba G, Savioz A, Saini K, Anastasiu R, Miklossy J et al. (2000) Familial frontotemporal dementia with ubiquitin inclusion bodies and without motor neuron disease. Acta Neuropathol (Berl) 100(4):421–426
41. Lebert F, Pasquier F, Souliez L, Petit H (1998) Frontotemporal behavioral scale. Alzheimer Dis Assoc Disorder 12(4):335–339
42. Lennox G, Lowe JS, Godwin-Austen RB, Landon M, Mayer RJ (1989) Diffuse Lewy body disease: an important differential diagnosis in dementia with extrapyramidal features. Prog Clin Biol Res 317:121–130
43. Leys D, Erkinjuntti T, Desmond DW, Schmidt R, Englund E, Pasquier F et al. (1999) Vascular dementia: the role of cerebral infarcts. Alzheimer Dis Assoc Disord 13 Suppl 3:S38–S48
44. Lowe J (1998) Establishing a pathological diagnosis in degenerative dementias. Brain Pathol 8(2):403–406
45. Mann DM (1998) Dementia of frontal type and dementias with subcortical gliosis. Brain Pathol 8(2):325–338
46. McKeith I, O'Brien J (1999) Dementia with Lewy bodies. Aust N Z J Psychiatry 33(6): 800–808
47. McKeith IG, Ballard CG, Perry RH, Ince PG, O'Brien JT, Neill D et al. (2000) Prospective validation of consensus criteria for the diagnosis of dementia with Lewy bodies. Neurology 54(5):1050–1058
48. McKeith IG, Galasko D, Kosaka K, Perry EK, Dickson DW, Hansen LA et al. (1996) Consensus guidelines for the clinical and pathologic diagnosis of dementia with Lewy bodies (DLB): report of the consortium on DLB international workshop. Neurology 47(5):1113–1124
49. Mirra SS, Hart MN, Terry RD (1993) Making the diagnosis of Alzheimer's disease. A primer for practicing pathologists. Arch Pathol Lab Med 117(2):132–144
50. Mirra SS, Heyman A, McKeel D, Sumi SM, Crain BJ, Brownlee LM et al. (1991) The Consortium to Establish a Registry for Alzheimer's Disease (CERAD). Part II. Standardization of the neuropathologic assessment of Alzheimer's disease. Neurology 41(4):479–486
51. Morris HR, Lees AJ, Wood NW (1999) Neurofibrillary tangle parkinsonian disorders–tau pathology and tau genetics. Mov Disord 14(5):731–736
52. Nakano I (2000) Frontotemporal dementia with motor neuron disease (amyotrophic lateral sclerosis with dementia). Neuropathology 20(1):68–75
53. Newell KL, Hyman BT, Growdon JH, Hedley-Whyte ET (1999) Application of the National Institute on Aging (NIA)-Reagan Institute criteria for the neuropathological diagnosis of Alzheimer disease. J Neuropathol Exp Neurol 58(11):1147–1155
54. Patterson WJ, Painter MJ (1999) Bovine spongiform encephalopathy and new variant Creutzfeldt-Jakob disease: an overview. Commun Dis Public Health 2(1):5–13
55. Rafalowska J (1999) Genetically determined vascular diseases. Folia Neuropathol 37(4): 210–216
56. Richard M, Biacabe AG, Perret-Liaudet A, McCardle L, Ironside JW, Kopp N (1999) Protection of personnel and environment against Creutzfeldt-Jakob disease in pathology laboratories. Clin Exp Pathol 47(3–4):192–200
57. Roman GC, Tatemichi TK, Erkinjuntti T, Cummings JL, Masdeu JC, Garcia JH et al. (1993) Vascular dementia: diagnostic criteria for research studies. Report of the NINDS-AIREN International Workshop. Neurology 43(2):250–260
58. Rossor MN, Revesz T, Lantos PL, Warrington EK (2000) Semantic dementia with ubiquitin-positive tau-negative inclusion bodies. Brain 123(Pt 2):267–276

59. Selkoe DJ (2000) The Genetics and Molecular Pathology of Alzheimer's Disease: Roles of Amyloid and the Presenilins. Neurol Clin 18(4):903–922
60. Spillantini MG, Van Swieten JC, Goedert M (2000) Tau gene mutations in frontotemporal dementia and parkinsonism linked to chromosome 17 (FTDP-17) Neurogenetics 2(4): 193–205
61. Tandon A, Rogaeva E, Mullan M, St George-Hyslop PH (2000) Molecular genetics of Alzheimer's disease: the role of beta-amyloid and the presenilins. Curr Opin Neurol 13(4):377–384
62. Tolnay M, Probst A (1995) Frontal lobe degeneration: novel ubiquitin-immunoreactive neurites within frontotemporal cortex. Neuropathol Appl Neurobiol 21(6):492–497
63. Tolnay M, Probst A (1999) REVIEW: tau protein pathology in Alzheimer's disease and related disorders. Neuropathol Appl Neurobiol 25(3):171–187
64. Tsuchiya K, Ozawa E, Fukushima J, Yasui H, Kondo H, Nakano I et al. (2000) Rapidly progressive aphasia and motor neuron disease: a clinical, radiological, and pathological study of an autopsy case with circumscribed lobar atrophy. Acta Neuropathol (Berl) 99(1):81–87
65. Weihl CC, Roos RP (1999) Creutzfeldt-Jakob disease, new variant Creutzfeldt-Jakob disease, and bovine spongiform encephalopathy. Neurol Clin 17(4):835–859
66. Wilhelmsen KC, Clark LN, Miller BL, Geschwind DH (1999) Tau mutations in frontotemporal dementia. Dement Geriatr Cogn Disord 10 (Suppl 1): 88–92
67. Will RG (1999) The transmission of prions to humans. Acta Paediatr Suppl 88(433):28–32

# Investigation of Prion Diseases

J. W. Ironside, D. Seilhean, M. W. Head, J.-J. Hauw



## 1 The Spectrum of Human Prion Diseases

The prion diseases, or transmissible spongiform encephalopathies, are a group of fatal neurodegenerative disorders which occur in animals and man [4]. The first of these to be identified was the disease in sheep known as scrapie, which is endemic in many parts of the world including Europe and the USA. Scrapie has been extensively studied in experimental models to investigate the nature of the unique transmissible agents responsible for this group of disorders. Early studies revealed that the scrapie agent had a unique spectrum of physical and chemical properties,

Current Topics in Pathology, Vol. 95
S. Love (Ed.): Neuropathology

**Table 1.** Human prion diseases

| Category | Disease | First reported |
|---|---|---|
| Idiopathic | Sporadic CJD | 1920–1921 |
| | Sporadic fatal insomnia | 1999 |
| Inherited | Familial CJD | 1924 |
| | Gerstmann-Straüssler-Scheinker syndrome | 1928–1936 |
| | Fatal familial insomnia | 1986 |
| Acquired | Kuru | 1957 |
| | Iatrogenic CJD | 1974 |
| | Variant CJD | 1996 |

with a marked resistance to conventional forms of microbial inactivation. In 1982, Prusiner published the prion hypothesis [62], which states that the transmissible agent responsible for this group of disorders is composed of a modified host protein, prion protein, which in humans is encoded by a gene on chromosome 20. Accumulation of the abnormal isoform of the prion protein ($PrP^{res}$) in the brain is a characteristic feature of all prion diseases, and the detection of this abnormal protein is now of major importance in their diagnosis [40, 58, 59].

The major groups of human prion diseases are listed in Table 1. The identification of human prion diseases depended for many years on neuropathological diagnosis, usually made at autopsy. The neuropathological features of Creutzfeldt-Jakob disease (CJD) allow a diagnosis to be made in the majority of cases, although it has been recognised for many years that the pathological features are extremely variable in different brain regions within a single CJD case; there is also marked variability in the distribution and intensity of the lesions between cases [5, 39]. Recent investigations have identified both host (patient) and agent (strain) factors which influence this marked pathological variability. In particular, the naturally occurring polymorphism at codon 129 in the prion protein gene (PRNP) has been found to exert a major influence on both disease susceptibility and the clinical and pathological phenotype of human prion diseases [17, 31, 57, 58]. Furthermore (as in experimental animal models) agent factors also influence the clinical and pathological features of the disease. The best example of this is in variant CJD (vCJD), in which the bovine spongiform encephalopathy (BSE) agent in man produces a relatively uniform disease phenotype which is markedly distinct from other forms of CJD [40, 68].

Since human prion diseases present as progressive neurological disorders with a wide range of initial clinical features and a variable rate of progression, most patients are investigated in neurological centres. Clinical investigations which are of particular diagnostic value include magnetic resonance imaging (MRI), electroencephalography (EEG) and studies of the 14.3.3 protein in the cerebrospinal fluid (CSF). MRI studies reveal characteristic abnormalities in sporadic CJD and vCJD; in the latter condition, the characteristic hyperintense posterior thalamic signal in T2-weighted images is incorporated as part of the diagnostic criteria for this disorder [71]. In sporadic CJD, the EEG shows characteristic periodic triphasic complexes in around 65%–70% of cases [8]. When present, this finding is a very helpful diagnostic aid and is incorporated in the clinical diagnostic criteria for sporadic CJD. Likewise, the presence of 14.3.3 protein in the CSF has a high sensitivity and specificity for the diagnosis of sporadic CJD (and is also incorporated in the current diagnostic criteria for this disorder) [37]. Current diagnostic criteria for sporadic CJD and vCJD are listed in Tables 2 and 3.

In order to exclude the possibility of familial CJD, Gerstmann-Straüssler-Scheinker syndrome (GSS) and fatal familial insomnia (FFI; see Table 1), it is necessary to screen the human PRNP for pathogenic mutations and insertions [59]. This is usually performed by extracting DNA from peripheral blood leucocytes while the patient is still alive, but can also be performed postmortem on

**Table 2.** Clinical diagnostic criteria for sporadic CJD

| | |
|---|---|
| I | Rapidly progressive dementia |
| II | A. Myoclonus<br>B. Visual or cerebellar problems<br>C. Pyramidal or extrapyramidal features<br>D. Akinetic mutism |
| III | Typical EEG |
| Definite: | Neuropathological/immunocytochemically confirmed |
| Probable: | I + two of II + III<br>or<br>Possible and +ve 14.3.3 |
| Possible: | I + two of II and duration of <2 years |

**Table 3.** Clinical diagnostic criteria for variant CJD

| | |
|---|---|
| I | A. Progressive neuropsychiatric disorder<br>B. Duration of illness >6 months<br>C. Routine investigations do not suggest an alternative diagnosis<br>D. No history of potential iatrogenic exposure |
| II | A. Early psychiatric symptoms [a]<br>B. Persistent painful sensory symptoms [b]<br>C. Ataxia<br>D. Myoclonus or chorea or dystonia<br>E. Dementia |
| III | A. EEG does not show the typical appearance of sporadic CJD [c] (or no EEG performed)<br>B. Bilateral pulvinar high signal on MRI scan |
| IV | A. Positive tonsil biopsy |
| Definite: | IA (progressive neuropsychiatric disorder) and neuropathological confirmation of vCJD [d] |
| Probable: | I and 4/5 of II and III A and III B |
| Probable: | I and IVA |
| Possible: | I and 4/5 of II and IIIA |

[a] Depression, anxiety, apathy, withdrawal, delusions.
[b] This includes both frank pain and/or unpleasant dysaesthesia.
[c] Generalised triphasic periodic complexes at approximately one per second.
[d] Spongiform change and extensive PrP deposition with florid plaques, throughout the cerebrum and cerebellum.

Table 4. PRNP codon 129 polymorphisms in human prion diseases

| Codon 129 genotype | Normal population (%) | Sporadic CJD (%) | Variant CJD (%) |
|---|---|---|---|
| MM | 37 | 71 | 100 |
| MV | 51 | 15 | – |
| VV | 12 | 14 | – |

frozen tissues. Additional techniques to sub-classify sporadic CJD include identifying the naturally occurring polymorphism at codon 129 in the PRNP, the distribution of which varies markedly between sporadic CJD, vCJD and the general population (Table 4). In particular, all cases of vCJD have so far occurred within a single genetic subgroup (methionine homozygotes at codon 129) [69].

Over the past few decades, a widening spectrum of human prion diseases has been identified (see [59] for review). This diversity requires a correspondingly broad approach to the investigation and diagnosis of prion diseases; in many countries there are now dedicated centres which specialise in this field. However, all neuropathologists and histopathologists can expect to encounter cases of human prion disease in their professional practice and should therefore be able to carry out the necessary procedures to enable a diagnosis to be made.

## 2 When to Suspect a Human Prion Disease at Autopsy

The commonest human prion disease is the sporadic form of CJD [67], which is therefore the disorder that neuropathologists are most likely to encounter at autopsy. As discussed above, there are now internationally accepted clinical criteria for the diagnosis of sporadic CJD (Table 2) and reference should be made to these criteria when the clinical suspicion of a human prion disease is raised. In the past, prion diseases were often suspected in cases of rapidly progressive dementia (particularly in those with a disease duration of less than 1 year) accompanied by other neurological abnormalities including ataxia, myoclonus, visual abnormalities and pyramidal or extrapyramidal rigidity. However, recent studies of sporadic CJD have revealed that the clinical phenotype is variable and depends critically on the codon 129 genotype in the PRNP and the PrP isotype as identified by Western blotting (see Sect. 8 below) [21, 58]. Although in some cases it is possible that the PrP genotype will be known prior to autopsy, in most cases this information is not readily available, and so the neuropathologist should bear in mind that the subtypes of sporadic CJD can have different clinical manifestations, which are summarised in Table 2. Perhaps the most useful antemortem investigative result is the detection of the 14.3.3 in the CSF, as this is positive in most cases of sporadic CJD, including some of the rarer subtypes [37]. However, it should be recalled that this protein may be released into the CSF in other conditions where there is widespread and rapid death of the nerve cells in the central nervous system, e.g. in herpes simplex encephalitis and acute stroke. However, it is normally possible to distinguish these disorders clinically from human prion diseases during life.

Another important factor to consider in the clinical history is the possibility of iatrogenic exposure to human prion agents, the commonest categories of which are listed in Table 5 [10]. Since around 10% of all human prion diseases occur as familial disorders [50], it is important to ascertain whether there is a family history of neurological disease. Because of the variable clinical phenotype in inherited prion diseases, the family history cannot always be relied upon for a specific diagnosis, and several families exist where earlier diagnoses made on clinical terms have included other neurological diseases, e.g. Alzheimer's disease or Huntington's disease. Although the clinical phenotype of inherited human prion diseases is markedly variable even within individuals in one affected family [29], broadly speaking, they are divisible into three groups (see [59] for review), those with the clinical features which resemble sporadic CJD (see above), those with a GSS-type presentation and fatal familial insomnia (Table 6). For these reasons, it seems reasonable that any patient with a family history of a progressive spinocerebellar syndrome of adult onset with accompanying dementia (regardless of the stage in the illness at which dementia occurs), and in whom no alternative diagnosis has been made, should be suspected of having a familial human prion disease.

The two most recently identified human prion diseases, vCJD and the sporadic form of fatal insomnia, have markedly different phenotypes. The sporadic form of fatal insomnia closely resembles fatal familial insomnia in terms of its clinical features but occurs in the absence of a family history [60]. This is an extremely rare disorder and only a small number of cases have so far been reported in the literature, although it is conceivable that such cases in the past may have been diagnosed as cases of thalamic dementia. In variant CJD, the clinical phenotype is

**Table 5.** Routes of transmission of iatrogenic CJD

| Category | Mode | Approximate number of cases worldwide |
|---|---|---|
| Neurosurgery | Neurosurgical instruments | 5 |
| | Intracerebral EEG electrodes | 2 |
| Tissue grafts | Corneal grafts | 3 |
| | Dura mater grafts | 106 |
| Tissue extracts | Human pituitary growth hormone | 125 |
| | Human pituitary gonadotrophins | 5 |

**Table 6.** Main clinical subgroups of inherited prion diseases (modified from PARCHI et al. [59])

| Subgroup | Clinical features |
|---|---|
| CJD-like | Dementia, myoclonus, ataxia, visual disturbances, extrapyramidal and pyramidal signs |
| FFI-like | Reduction of sleep time, enacted dreams, autonomic abnormalities, myoclonus, ataxia, dementia |
| GSS-like | Progressive cerebellar syndrome, eventually with dementia, extrapyramidal and pyramidal signs |
| Heterogeneous | Variably progressive dementia, with cerebellar signs; occasional cases have myoclonus, parkinsonism, extrapyramidal or pyramidal signs |

distinctive (Table 3) [68, 69]. In contrast to sporadic CJD, none of the patients exhibits characteristic periodic triphasic complexes on EEG studies and investigations of 14.3.3 protein in the CSF have yielded equivocal results, with roughly an equal number of positive and negative cases. The underlying reason for this finding is at present uncertain.

Neuroradiology is extremely helpful in the investigation of patients with suspected vCJD in life as there is a characteristic MRI abnormality which consists of a bilateral symmetrical region of hyperintensity in the pulvinar, often extending into the dorsomedial nucleus of the thalamus. Although this finding on its own is not entirely specific for vCJD, in the appropriate clinical context it appears to have a sensitivity of 78% and a specificity of 100% [71]. Accordingly, this has been incorporated into the clinical criteria for the diagnosis of vCJD (Table 3) [69]. vCJD also differs from other human prion diseases in that prion protein can be detected in lymphoid tissues during the clinical phase of the illness [36]. Although the figures for the sensitivity and specificity of this investigation are still under study, data from autopsy investigations suggest that the presence of the abnormal isoform of PrP (with the characteristic predominance of diglycosylated protein in western blots) in lymphoid tissues is strongly indicative that the patient suffers from vCJD.

There is no substitute for adequate communication between neuropathologists and neurologists when investigating human prion diseases, and each case should be discussed in order to obtain the maximum relevant information. Only by this collaborative approach can the appropriate postmortem investigations be arranged and the necessary samples prepared during autopsy to facilitate full examination of each case in the laboratory.

## 3 Autopsy in Creutzfeldt-Jakob Disease

Since neuropathological examination of the central nervous system is required to confirm a clinical diagnosis of human prion disease, the autopsy has a major role to play in the investigation of this group of disorders. In addition to providing diagnostic information, the autopsy has other important roles in research, teaching, clinicopathological correlation and audit. The transmissible agents responsible for human prion diseases are classified as Hazard Group 3, but as far as hospital autopsy and laboratory facilities are concerned, derogation from full category 3 facilities is generally acceptable (subject to local risk assessment) [1, 70]. For this reason, autopsies on patients with suspected CJD or other prion disorders can be performed in a routine mortuary as a 'high-risk' procedure. Although prion agents are transmissible, they are not contagious. None of the cases of human–human transmission of CJD (Table 5) has been associated with autopsy or laboratory procedures; although CJD has been reported in laboratory technical staff, epidemiological studies have failed to reveal an excess incidence of any form of human prion disease in health-care workers [67]. The main precautions that are required for the autopsy investigation of prion diseases relate to the prevention of accidental inoculation with contaminated tissues and minimising contamination of the mortuary environment. Prion agents are notoriously resistant to most conventional forms of disinfection and sterilisation. However, specialised protocols for cleaning and decontamination have been devised which allow a substantial reduction in potential infectivity [1, 9, 12, 70]. The highest levels of infectivity in prion diseases are present in the central nervous system and eye [1]. In sporadic CJD, most other tissues contain low levels of infectivity, but in vCJD lymphoid tissues throughout the body have been found to contain $PrP^{res}$.

## 3.1 Autopsy Procedures

The procedures to follow in a 'high-risk' neuropathological autopsy have been fully described by a number of authors [3, 12, 38, 63, 70]. These can be summarised as follows:

- The autopsy should be performed by an experienced pathologist, preferably with two trained mortuary assistants, one of whom does not handle the cadaver, but remains 'clean' and assists with instruments, specimen jars, labels, etc.
- Entry to and exit from the autopsy suite should be avoided while the autopsy is being performed.
- Staff should wear face masks and protective glasses, a disposable water-impermeable gown or body suit, an over-apron and two or three pairs of gloves, including puncture-proof gloves.
- Contamination of the mortuary environment should be minimised, e.g. by performing the autopsy within a body bag with absorbent wadding.
- Blunt-ended and disposable instruments should be used whenever possible; it is ideal to have a set of instruments which is used only on CJD cases.
- The skull can be opened with either a manual or electrical saw; the electrical saw may be used within a large, transparent plastic bag covering the head of the cadaver, to help reduce contamination of the mortuary.
- All tissue samples, fixed or not, should be clearly labelled 'risk of infection'.
- A special 'high-risk' autopsy suite should be used when available, but this is not mandatory [38].

## 3.2 Decontamination

The following methods should be used for decontamination of the mortuary working surfaces and instruments [1, 3, 12, 38, 63, 70]:

1. Porous load steam autoclaving at 134 °C for 18 min or six cycles at 134 °C for 3 min.
2. Gravity displacement steam autoclaving at 134 °C for 1 h.
3. Fresh sodium hypochlorite solution containing 20,000 parts per million available chlorine (this is highly corrosive to metals).
4. 2M sodium hydroxide for 1 h with constant rewetting of surfaces.
5. Incineration.

## 4 Biopsy in Prion Diseases

Brain biopsy has been widely employed for the diagnosis of prion diseases [14]. It is now performed less frequently, and its practice is discouraged in some countries, such as the United Kingdom [53].

### How to Choose Between Biopsy or Autopsy?

The diagnosis of human prion diseases is of both clinical and public health importance. What are the arguments for and against brain biopsy?

**In Favour of Biopsy.** This is a simple and fast procedure, and consent is often easily obtained from the family.

**Against Biopsy.** There are ethical issues to consider, and in many countries it is considered that a biopsy 'injuring' the brain should not be performed unless informed consent is obtained from the patient. This is not possible in prion diseases and other dementias. Furthermore, a brain biopsy might be considered an acceptable procedure only in those cases for which a treatment is possible. Neither prion diseases nor the other dementing disorders they can be mistaken for (and which could be recognised by cerebral biopsy) are curable. A few exceptions, such as Whipple's disease or intravascular lymphoma, may be treated by drugs, the efficacy and toxicity of which have to be evaluated in comparison to the hazards of a cerebral biopsy.

There are also economic and safety considerations. Surgical procedures on patients carrying the diagnosis of prion disease should be minimised [3]. The recommended practice in some countries, including France and the United Kingdom, is that neurosurgical instruments used on a patient with a proven prion disease should be incinerated to prevent potential transmission to another patient [1, 70].

There are, above all, technical arguments. The uneven distribution of lesions, of PrP immunolocalisation and of western blot results in CJD, emphasised by many authors [5, 13, 32, 59], indicates that cerebral biopsy is not a reliable, sensitive technique for diagnosing CJD. In addition, it does not allow the full characterisation of prion disease variants that is needed for epidemiological studies.

**Other Potential Tissues for Biopsy.** In biopsied tonsil, the presence of disease-specific PrP has been demonstrated by immunohistochemistry and western blotting in vCJD. In contrast, PrP has never been detected in tonsil in sporadic cases [36]. However, in view of the relatively small number of cases in which this investigation has been performed, its sensitivity and specificity remain to be established; a positive tonsil biopsy is at present included in the clinical criteria for the diagnosis of 'probable' vCJD.

**In Favour of Autopsy.** This is an efficient, relatively cheap and technically very satisfactory method for diagnosis. It also provides many opportunities for research, audit and teaching in addition to diagnosis.

**Against Autopsy.** This provides a diagnosis only after the patient has died, and may be difficult to accept for religious and cultural reasons. In the United Kingdom, the procedures and requirements for obtaining consent for the retention of tissues at autopsy have been the subject of much recent debate, and new guidelines emphasize the need to obtain informed consent for the removal for diagnosis of specified organs, such as the brain. Consent for this may be difficult to obtain. It is still usually possible to obtain sufficient material for diagnosis by careful sampling of the unfixed brain at autopsy (see 'Appendix' to book) although this limited approach may hinder research and impair clinicopathological correlation and the recognition of disease variants. In most other countries, such as France, the consent procedure and documentation do not make a distinction between different types of tissue sampling at autopsy (i.e. whether the investigation entails removal of the entire brain or limited sampling of the unfixed brain).

## 5 Diagnostic Laboratory Techniques: Tissue Handling and Brain Dissection

The storage of tissues obtained from patients with clinically documented and neuropathological validated diseases of the CNS and from well-chosen control cases forms a valuable resource for present and future research needs. To maximise their usefulness, it is desirable to store tissues in different forms, including fixed and frozen samples. The handling of any unfixed human tissue needs special precautions, and in many countries it is recommended that staff are protected against hepatitis B and tuberculosis [7]. However, storage of human prion disease tissues poses particular problems (taking into account the risk to future users), since the infective agents may well survive fixation and long-term storage at −80 °C. In addition to appropriate guidelines for acquisition, storage and transport of high-risk samples, the accurate postmortem detection of infectious agents such as prions should reinforce the safety of all brain-banking procedures [6].

### 5.1 Sampling Procedures

When handling fresh tissue from cases of suspected prion disease, protective clothing should be worn with particular attention to hands and eyes: chain-mail gloves worn between two pairs of rubber gloves, glasses with lateral protections or full-face visors, disposable gowns, overshoes and aprons, surgical masks and caps. The tissues are best handled in an extraction hood, which helps reduce contamination of the surrounding laboratory space. The use of sharp instruments (needles, knives, scissors etc.) should be minimised wherever possible; when the use of sharp disposable material is required it should be disposed of by incineration in sealed plastic 'sharps' containers.

### 5.1.1 Freezing Procedure

Frozen material is required for western blot analysis, occasionally for experimental transmission and strain typing and for cryostat microtomy. Fragments of tissue may be frozen by different methods: direct freezing at –80 °C, snap-freezing between aluminium plates chilled continuously on a metal stage bathed in liquid nitrogen or immersion either in liquid nitrogen or in isopentane cooled with liquid nitrogen. The frozen material should then be wrapped in sealed polythene bags which bear a 'risk of infection' label, the specimen number and date of sampling. For cryostat sections, the same precautions should be taken by the microtomist as for fresh tissue sampling, particularly the wearing of safety gloves and protection glasses. A dedicated cryostat and freezer are recommended for prion diseases research, but frozen material can be safely stored in a general freezer provided that the material is adequately packaged and labelled prior to its dispatch to a reference laboratory.

### 5.1.2 Fixation Procedure

Fixed tissues are best handled on a dissection bench with a downflow ventilation system. The duration of formalin fixation should always be kept as short as is compatible with good tissue preservation and timely neuropathological diagnosis. These two objectives may be fulfilled by performing a short duration fixation (3 or 4 days) of small selected brain tissue samples taken from the same areas as frozen specimens, allowing a rapid confirmation of the diagnosis. The rest of the brain is fixed for a longer time (at least 21 days) to allow detailed neuropathological examination, including morphometry. After dissection, blocks of tissue can be immersed in 96% formic acid for 1 h, and then washed in water prior to processing to paraffin wax [9]. This step helps reduce infectivity in the paraffin blocks, but it does result in the tissue becoming slightly more brittle than usual on microtomy. Microtomy can be performed on a general-purpose microtome, using a disposable blade and disposing of the trimmings by incineration. The microtomist should use hand and eye protection; in prion disease reference centres, a dedicated microtome should be available.

## 5.2 Procedure for Tissue Storage

Snap-frozen samples are stored at –80 °C in freezers labelled 'risk of infection' and equipped with a back-up system and alarm. Fixed material should be stored under standard conditions in ventilated rooms. Even after formic acid pre-treatment, blocks and slides should be labelled and separately stored.

### 5.2.1 Documentation

Clinical information, specimen listing and neuropathological results should be recorded and preferably computerised. This documentation is regularly updated as material is added to and removed from the brain store; the database should comply with national data protection acts or regulations.

## 5.3 Decontamination Procedures

The procedures listed above for the decontamination of autopsy rooms and equipment are also applicable to laboratory work surfaces, glassware and equipment. Spillages of contaminated fluids should be adsorbed with suitable material (e.g. sawdust), treated with 2M sodium hydroxide and disposed of by incineration.

## 5.4 Protocol for Accidents

All injuries and penetrating wounds which may have come into contact with contaminated material should be thoroughly washed with soap and cleaned with running water. Sodium hypochlorite is the most efficient skin disinfectant against prion agents, but is an irritant in use. A detailed record of any workplace accidents should be maintained and notified to local safety officers.

## 5.5 Transport of High-Risk Samples

Arrangements for safe transport from the bank to the user remain the responsibility of the sender until the arrival of the specimen. Courier companies specialised in the transport of hazardous material provide dedicated transport containers, labelled "risk of infection". They are also able to maintain frozen samples at the appropriate temperature for 48 h. The outer packaging should carry a destination address and an emergency contact telephone number.

# 6 Pathological Findings

## 6.1 Macroscopic Examination

Microscopic examination of the brain is required for the diagnosis of a human prion disease. At autopsy, no pertinent changes have been described in other organs, with rare exceptions which are described below. The patients often die from bronchopneumonia, seldom from pulmonary embolism or other general disorders. In most cases however, especially in cachectic patients, the cause of death may not be identifiable at autopsy. Cerebral atrophy and related ventricular dilatation are usually moderate or absent, and significantly low brain weights (under 1,000 g) are rare. Severe atrophy of cerebral or cerebellar hemispheres, or both, is occasionally seen, especially in disease of long duration [39]. In most cases, the contrast between the severity of dementia and the scanty macroscopic abnormalities of the brain is in itself a strong argument favouring the diagnosis of CJD.

## 6.2 Microscopic Examination

Diagnosis of a definite case of CJD or a related prion disease relies on two approaches: classic neuropathology and detection of $PrP^{res}$ in the central nervous system, by immunohistochemistry or western blotting. To recognise a spongiform encephalopathy on histological examination is straightforward in most cases, provided that sampling is sufficient and the technical quality of the sections is satisfactory. Since the distribution of lesions is the brain is markedly variable form case to case, extensive sampling of the brain for histology is required for diagnosis. This should include as a minimum:

- Frontal, occipital and temporal cortex (with hippocampus)
- Basal ganglia (with lentiform nucleus)
- Thalamus
- Cerebellum
- Brain stem (midbrain, pons and medulla)

More extensive sampling may be required for the identification of rare entities, the study of clinicopathological correlations, the delineation of lesion profiles and for differential diagnosis.

The classical histological triad of spongiform change (also called spongiosis), neuronal loss and astrogliosis is usually diagnostic [51]. Amyloid plaques are infrequent but their presence is characteristic in certain forms of sporadic, inherited and acquired prion diseases [13, 32]. In some cases, however, the diagnosis may be difficult because some of the classical lesions are missing or cannot be recognised.

### 6.2.1 Spongiform Change

Spongiform change consists of small (5–50 μm) rounded vacuoles of varying diameter, sometimes confluent, mainly present in the neuropil of the grey matter, i.e. between the cell bodies [51] (Fig. 1). Electron microscopy shows non-membrane-bound vacuoles largely located in neuronal processes, but vacuolation can also occasionally occur in neuronal cell bodies. The extracellular space is normal, and the astrocyte cell bodies and processes are free of vacuoles. The mechanism of spongiform change is unknown. A disturbance of cell membrane glycoproteins has been suggested (since PrP is glycosylated) [20], leading to impaired membrane fluidity and altered permeability. Another suggestion is more

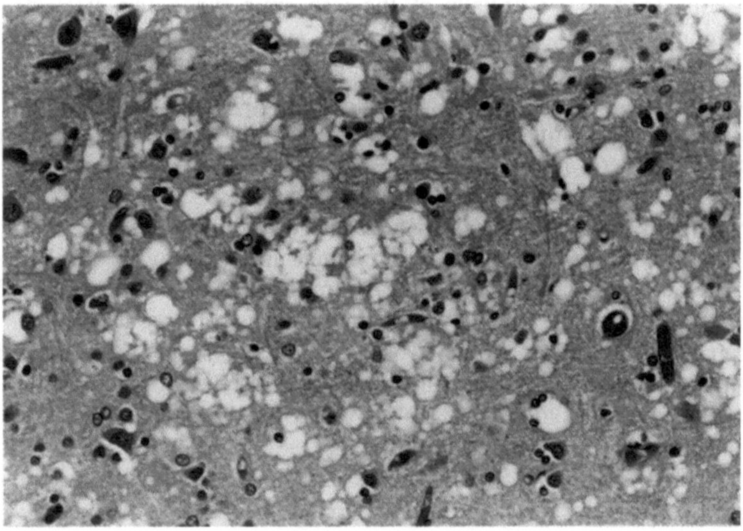

**Fig. 1.** Spongiform change in the cerebral cortex in sporadic CJD is characterised by numerous vacuoles in the neuropil. These can become confluent to produce larger cyst-like spaces. H&E, ×200

mechanistic: in CJD, astrogliosis is 'isomorphous', preserving tissue disorganisation by making a rigid frame which prevents cortical atrophy [46]; the cavities of spongiosis compensate for the loss of tissue volume due to nerve cell death. Vacuoles are found in most cases in a variable distribution in the cerebral cortex, where they occur either diffusely or in clusters ('morula-type') throughout the whole thickness of the cortical ribbon, or can predominate in the middle and deeper layers. Spongiosis can also be found in the basal ganglia, the thalamus, cranial nerve nuclei and the molecular layer of the cerebellar cortex. It is seldom found in other grey matter areas such as the spinal cord. The density of vacuoles varies greatly from case to case, from area to area and, in the same slide, from one microscopic field to another. Although it is the most characteristic lesion, in occasional cases, spongiform change may not be detectable even after extensive sampling [16].

A number of less-specific vacuolar changes have to be distinguished from the spongiform change associated with prion diseases. Vacuoles of various sizes (and which may be larger and less rounded than those in CJD) occur in the superficial layers of the cortex (I-II) in a variety of disorders of the central nervous system: frontal lobe degeneration lacking distinctive histology and other focal atrophies, Pick's disease, Alzheimer's disease, some alcoholic encephalopathies and AIDS [19, 32]. This may result from deafferentation of the superficial layers of the cortex due to degeneration of afferent nerve cell processes, as shown in the dentate gyrus in Alzheimer's disease [23]. In rare cases of encephalopathy associated with hepatic degeneration, microcavitation or coarser vacuoles are seen in the deep layers of the cortex and the adjacent white matter [64]. A very similar spongiosis to that of Creutzfeldt-Jakob disease can occur in the Alzheimer-type variant of dementia with Lewy bodies [30]. Spongiform change must also be distinguished from other lesions (oedema, especially of the ischaemic type) and artefacts. Differential diagnosis of spongiform change linked to prion diseases may thus be difficult. To be diagnostic, the vacuoles should be numerous and some of them should be found at a distance from small vessels and nerve cell bodies. In the cerebral cortex, they should be seen either throughout the whole thickness of the cortical ribbon or in the deep layers.

The 'status spongiosus' of German authors (tissue rarefaction displaying numerous cavities with massive neuronal loss and marked astrogliosis, often of the protoplasmic type, frequently distributed in large 'waves') can be seen in some cases of CJD, usually of long clinical duration [13]. It usually involves the isocortex and sometimes the head of the caudate nucleus, but is a non-specific feature, and can also be found in a number of degenerative diseases (especially Pick's disease and Alzheimer's disease) where the cortex is severely affected. In children and young adults, it is found in Canavan-van Bogaert-Bertrand disease, or spongiform leukodystrophy, where the lesions may extend from the white matter into the deeper layers of the cerebral cortex and the basal ganglia. It should be distinguished from the laminar necrosis seen in anoxic-ischaemic encephalopathies and boundary zone infarcts. This lesion, characterised by total neuronal loss, massive astrogliosis and vascular proliferation delineating very large cavities (up to 200 μm), predominantly affects the third and fifth cortical layers in the boundary zones between the main arterial territories of the brain, but may involve the full thickness of the cortical ribbon in a widespread distribution.

### 6.2.2 Astrocytic Gliosis and Macrophage-Microglial Activation

Astrocytic hypertrophy and proliferation (astrocytic gliosis) is usually present in human prion diseases. It can be recognised by the presence of densely packed or paired astrocytic nuclei seen in haematoxylin- and eosin-stained sections, but is best demonstrated by immunocytochemistry for glial fibrillary acidic protein. It usually involves areas of the grey matter severely affected by spongiform change and often extends to the adjacent white matter. It can be seen in the absence of either spongiform change or obvious neuronal loss. Marked astrocytic gliosis is a characteristic regional feature in certain conditions, particularly in the thalamus in fatal familial insomnia (anterior and medial nuclei) [49, 52] and in vCJD (pulvinar and periaqueductal grey matter) [40, 68]. In vCJD, astrocytic gliosis in the pulvinar occurs with severe neuronal loss and in the absence of marked spongiform change; this appears to be the pathological substrate of the high signal seen in the pulvinar in T2-weighted MRI scans, which are of diagnostic value in vCJD [71].

No 'classical' inflammatory changes (such as perivascular lymphocytic cuffing) are seen in human prion diseases [39], and no macrophage-microglial reaction is noticeable by conventional staining techniques, but immunohistochemistry for macrophage-microglial 'markers' (e.g. CD 68) demonstrates increased numbers of these cells, particularly in areas of neuronal loss. In CJD as in scrapie, there is evidence of functional activation of macrophage-microglial cells, which express the class II major histocompatibility complex [24]. These cells likely contribute to tissue damage by a cytokine-mediated mechanism, but whether they take part in

PrP processing is debated. Double-labelling with macrophage-microglial markers and anti-PrP antibodies showed that activated cells did not contain PrP-immunoreactivity, arguing against a primary role of these cells in PrP processing [55]. Macrophage-microglial activation, together with the absence of an inflammatory reaction as demonstrated by classical techniques, is associated with variable amounts of astrocytic gliosis and nerve cell loss in most, if not all, degenerative disorders of the central nervous system [22].

### 6.2.3 Neuronal Cell Death

In most cases of human prion disease, loss of nerve cells from the grey matter of the brain is difficult to ascertain, at least with conventional techniques, particularly if the neuronal loss is subtle and not associated with any other form of cellular reaction. In some cases, however, the cerebral or cerebellar cortex (particularly the granule cell layer) or the subcortical grey matter (such as the caudate or thalamic nuclei) is severely affected, leading either to status spongiosus or to obvious neuronal loss. This has led to the description of multiple variants of CJD (cerebellar, thalamic, occipital, etc.). These variable patterns of neuronal loss indicate 'targeting' of neuronal subpopulations by prion agents, possibly by interaction with particular forms of the normal prion protein ($PrP^c$) expressed in these subpopulations [20]. The mechanism of neuronal death in prion diseases is uncertain, but recent studies using an in situ end-labelling technique [27] suggest that neuronal death may be due to an apoptotic rather than a necrotic process.

### 6.2.4 Amyloid Plaques

The amyloid plaques which occur in the brain in prion diseases are formed from $PrP^{res}$ and are therefore very specific lesions. Although visible in haematoxylin- and eosin-stained sections and by silver impregnation, they are better demonstrated by Congo red (exhibiting the classic dichroism of amyloid substances) and especially by the periodic acid-Schiff technique. They are best shown by PrP immunohistochemistry; many morphological varieties may be distinguished, and they can schematically be described as follows [65]:

- The unicentric plaque is a single focal amyloid deposit with few or no adjacent dystrophic neurites.
- The kuru type plaque, 10–50 μm wide, has an unicentric amyloid core with radiating fibrils surrounded by a pale halo devoid of dystrophic neurites or reactive cells (Fig. 2). On electron microscopy, this plaque consists of 10-nm-wide radially arranged amyloid filaments. Their sharply delineated outline is demarcated by astrocytes, without any neuronal processes. A few exceptions have been reported in familial cases of CJD where dystrophic neurites can be seen. Microglial cells are infrequent.

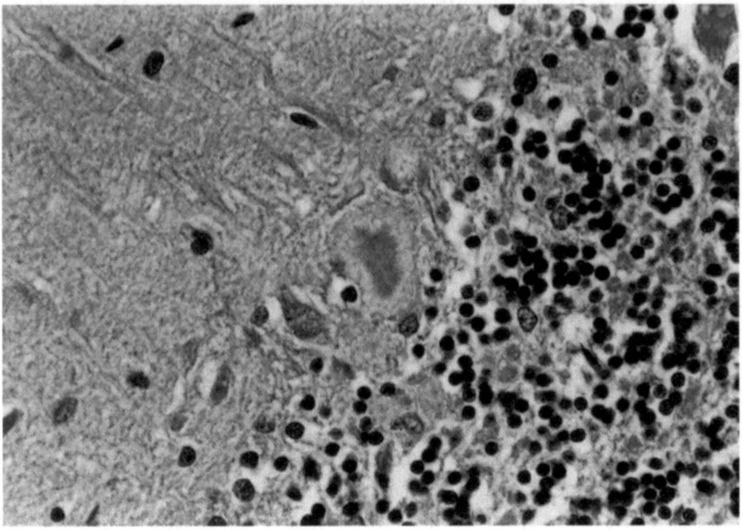

**Fig. 2.** A unicentric kuru-type plaque (*centre*) is present in the cerebellum in a patient with sporadic CJD who is heterozygous at codon 129 in the PRNP. The plaque has a dense eosinophilic core and pale radial peripheral fibrils. H&E, ×250

- The florid plaque is a kuru-type plaque surrounded by a zone of spongiform change in an otherwise intact neuropil [68] (Fig. 3). Electron microscopy shows loosely interwoven fibrils and some extracellular electron-dense bodies, pleomorphic vesicles and membrane debris, which react with anti-PrP antibodies. They are surrounded by degenerative and dystrophic neurites [25].
- The multicentric plaque is a composite structure, consisting of several focal amyloid deposits. By electron microscopy, it is made of foci of amyloid deposits lacking radial fibrils and associated with rods and amorphous deposits. Astrocytic processes are seen deep in the plaque and microglial cells in close proximity. No obvious abnormalities are found in the adjacent nervous tissue.

Plaques in CJD and other prion diseases differ from other types of plaque characteristic of Alzheimer's disease or ageing. These latter consist of deposits of another protein, A$\beta$ [19]: neuritic plaques contain a core of amyloid surrounded by a crown of various cell processes (neuronal, astroglial and microglial), some of which are dystrophic; diffuse deposits, seen only by immunohistochemistry, are less defined deposits lacking amyloid properties and dystrophic neurites. Interestingly, amyloid plaques, whatever the nature of the protein, are immunoreactive for sulphated glycosaminoglycans [28] and apolipoprotein E [56], which are believed to have chaperone properties, i.e. to participate in the conformational changes of proteins.

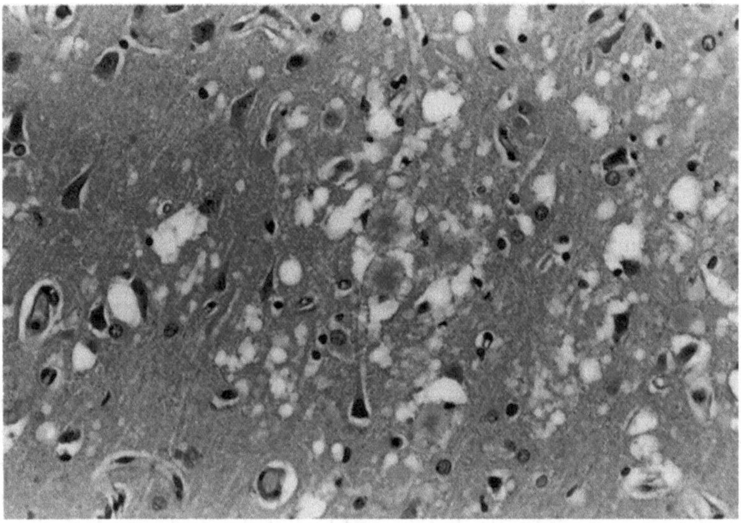

**Fig. 3.** Florid plaques in vCJD (*centre*) comprise a dense central core, pale radiating peripheral fibrils and a corona of spongiform change. H&E, ×180

### 6.2.5 Other Lesions

Vacuolation of neuronal cell bodies can be seen by light microscopy but is a rare finding in human prion diseases except kuru. This contrasts with natural and experimental prion diseases [15] and BSE [66]. Other non-specific lesions described in prion diseases include white matter changes: loss of myelinated fibres, axonal dystrophy, splitting and vacuolation of myelin with astrocytic gliosis and lipid-laden macrophages [48]. These usually occur in association with severe cortical involvement, particularly in cases with a long duration of illness. Extensive lesions of the white matter are seldom seen in Caucasians, but are more frequent in Japan, where they characterise the panencephalopathic variant of CJD [54]. Ballooned neurones similar to those in Pick's disease and other degenerative dementing processes are rare [42]. Amyloid angiopathy has, exceptionally, been associated with prion disease; with one exception [26], the amyloid deposited around the vessel walls was of the A$\beta$ type.

### 6.2.6 Electron Microscopy

Electron microscopy is of little diagnostic value in human prion diseases. No infectious agent has been regularly seen in conventional ultrathin brain sections; the tubulovesicular structures repeatedly found in human and animal prion diseases are not composed of PrP [47]. In contrast, the scrapie-associated fibres or rods seen by electron microscopy after negative staining of purified unfixed brain tissue are most likely to represent different varieties of PrP$^{res}$ aggregates.

## 7 Immunocytochemistry

The use of immunohistochemistry has greatly facilitated the neuropathological diagnosis of CJD and the other human and animal prion diseases. Identification of proteinase K-resistant PrP protein ($PrP^{res}$) in central nervous tissue by PrP immunohistochemistry, together with Western blotting, nowadays provides one of the most specific diagnostic tools. Unlike Western blot, PrP immunohistochemistry can be used on formalin-fixed tissues. $PrP^{c}$ (the normal cellular isoform of PrP) is proteinase K-sensitive and seems to be a very labile protein [19], whereas $PrP^{res}$ survives formalin fixation and paraffin processing. However, pre-treatments are required for the detection of $PrP^{res}$ by immunohistochemical techniques in sections of formalin-fixed and paraffin-embedded tissues. The molecular effects of these pretreatment are uncertain, but a combination of methods to remove any residual $PrP^{c}$ and enhance the immunoreactivity of $PrP^{res}$ appears to be most effective. Formic acid and enzymatic digestion with proteinase K or pepsin were first employed, followed by denaturation treatments using guanidine thiocyanate. Hydrolytic autoclaving or microwave irradiation and hydrated autoclaving techniques have been also developed. Various combinations of these methods were successfully tested (for review see [61]). Two multicentre prospective studies have assessed a variety of anti-

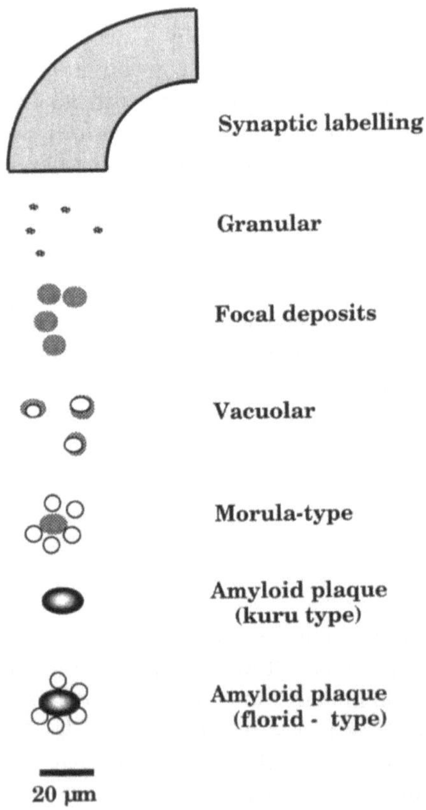


**Fig. 4.** Main varieties of PrP immunolabelled deposits in the brain. (Modified from Privat et al. [61])

bodies, including 3F4 [41], a commercially available widely used antibody (Senetek, USA; DAKO, UK) and numerous enhancement procedures [7, 35]. These have established a reliable consensus pre-treatment protocol for $PrP^{res}$ immunohistochemistry, regardless of the primary antibody used:

- Paraffin sections should be collected on coated slides (e.g. Vectabond) and baked overnight at 56 °C

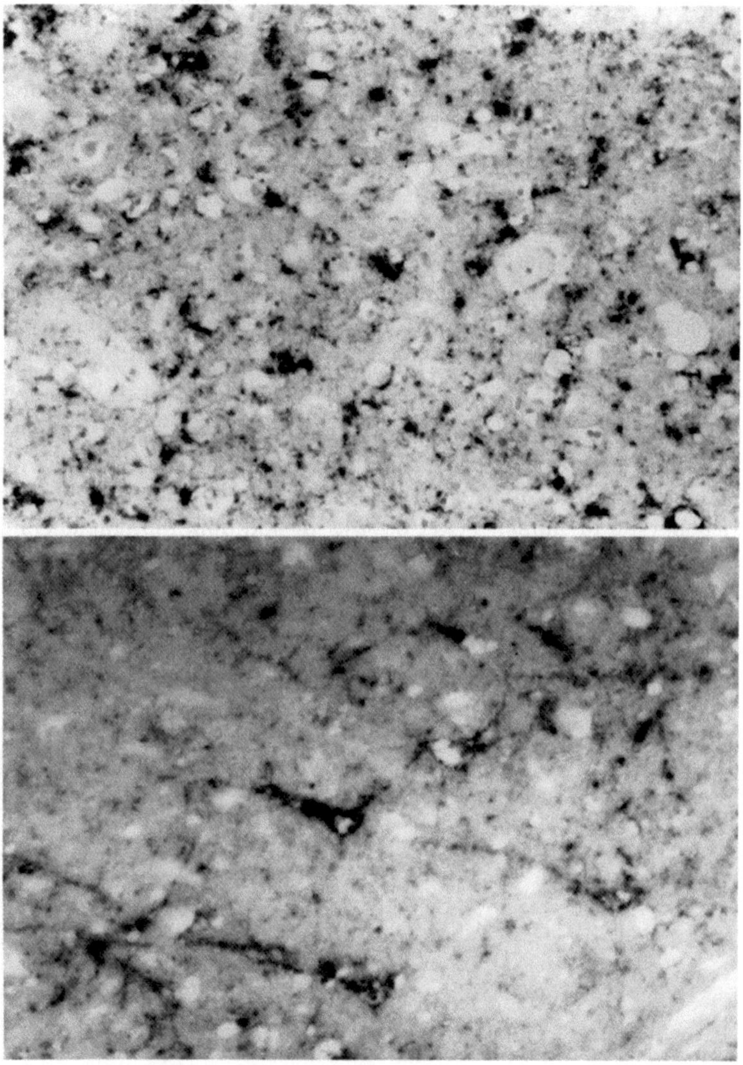

a

b

**Fig. 5a, b.** PrP deposition patterns in the cerebral cortex in sporadic CJD. **a** Granular and vacuolar deposits in a patient who is a methionine homozygote at codon 129 in the PRNP. **b** Strong perineuronal labelling of pyramidal cells in cortical layer V (with fainter synaptic labelling) in a patient who is a valine homozygote at codon 129 in the PRNP. 3F4 antibody, haematoxylin counterstain; **a** ×200, **b** ×180

- Hydrated autoclaving – 121 °C for 10 min
- Immersion in 96% formic acid for 5 min at room temperature
- Immersion in 4M guanidine thiocyanate at 4 °C for 2 h

A method that increases substantially the sensitivity of PrP immunohistochemistry, especially after prolonged formalin fixation, by the addition of enzymatic digestion by proteinase K has recently been developed [61]. Two commonly encountered pitfalls of PrP immunohistochemistry are low sensitivity, especially after long formalin fixation, and the difficulty in interpreting some apparently positive results. These difficulties can usually be resolved by adjusting the pre-treatment protocol (in cases which have undergone prolonged formalin fixation) and by extensive tissue sampling, always including the cerebellum and the regions which bear the brunt of pathology.

Various classifications of the patterns of immunolabelling with anti PrP antibodies have been proposed [7, 13, 31, 33, 43–45, 58, 61]. Six main varieties can be arbitrarily distinguished [31, 61] (Fig. 4):

- Synaptic labelling (diffuse staining, best seen at low magnification)
- Granular deposits (small, scattered, immunolabelled spots, less than 5 µm wide)
- Focal deposits (large, 5–50-µm-wide, non-amyloid, rounded, positive blots)
- Vacuolar deposits (surrounding vacuoles of spongiform change) (Fig. 5)
- Morula-type deposits (focal, non-amyloid deposits surrounded by vacuoles of spongiform change)
- Amyloid plaques (10- to 50-µm wide, usually of the kuru-type, immunolabel for PrP, but also identifiable in Congo red- and PAS-stained sections)

These patterns of immunolabelling may occur either in isolation or in a variety of combinations (Fig. 6) and do not in themselves imply any specificity for a particular type of human prion disease. In addition, immunolabelling of isolated

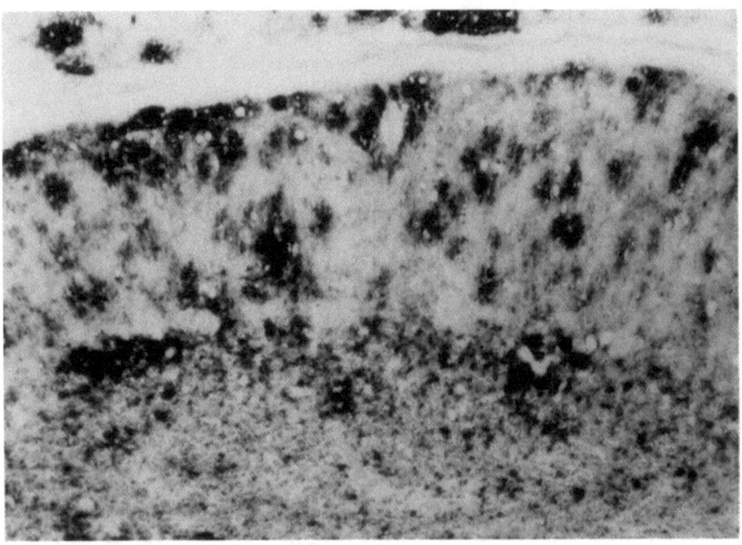

**Fig. 6.** In vCJD, the cerebellar cortex contains a mixture of florid plaques and widespread diffuse deposits in the molecular layer. 3F4 antibody, haematoxylin counterstain; ×180

neurones (cell body or processes) or astrocytes can occasionally be seen; its significance, especially when occurring in isolation, remains unclear.

## 8 Western Blotting

Western blotting techniques have assumed increasing importance in the investigation and diagnosis of human prion diseases [40, 58]. Western blotting requires unfixed tissue, which places a high priority on the retention of at least a portion of autopsy brain tissue to be frozen at –80 °C for future western blotting studies. As a minimum, samples should be taken from the non-dominant frontal lobe but for more advanced studies it may be preferable to dissect the brain unfixed and freeze alternate slices, or to freeze an entire cerebral hemisphere, cerebellar hemisphere and part of the brain stem [12, 13].

Since most of the anti-PrP antibodies that are currently available recognise both $PrP^c$ and $PrP^{res}$, the detection of the disease-associated isoform depends on digestion of the normal protein by proteinase K. A sample protocol for the western blotting technique is listed in the Appendix to this chapter. Proteinase K, under the conditions specified, will completely digest $PrP^c$ in the specimen, and will partially digest $PrP^{res}$ by cleavage at the N-terminus. Since PrP has two glycosylation sites, the protein can exist in di-, mono- or unglycosylated forms. This gives a characteristic three-band pattern in a western blot (Fig. 7); the size of the unglycosylated

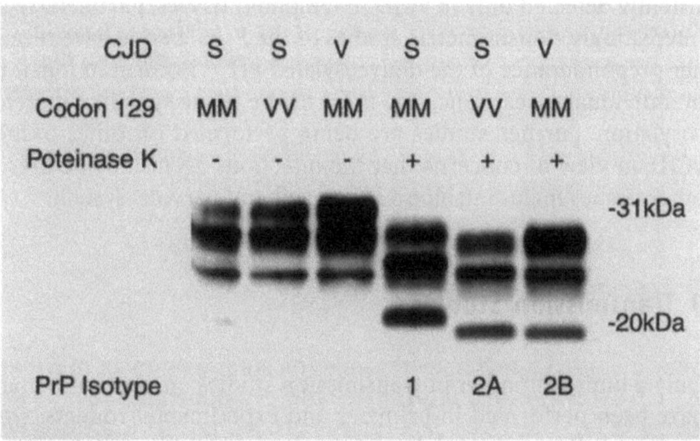


**Fig. 7.** Western blot analysis of PrP from the postmortem frontal cortex of patients with CJD of the sporadic (*S*) or variant (*V*) types. The PRNP codon 129 polymorphism is shown as *M* (methionine) or *V* (valine). Protein extracts were analysed with (+) or without (–) proteinase K treatment and the di-, mono- and non-glycosylated PrPs separated by SDS-PAGE (sodium dodecyl sulphate-polyacrylamide gel electrophoresis), transferred and detected with the monoclonal antibody 3F4. The molecular weights of standards are shown for reference. Prior to proteinase K digestion (–) PrPs from sCJD and vCJD have similar mobilities and glycoform ratios. Proteinase K digestion results in N-terminal cleavage, yielding PrP isotypes that differ in mobility of the non-glycosylated (*lowest*) band (type 1, ~21 kDa and type 2, ~19 kDa) and the proportion of the three glycoforms. vCJD is characterized by type 2 mobility and a preponderance of the diglycosylated (*top*) band (type 2B)

fragment is dependent on the extent of digestion by proteinase K and at least two major subtypes have been identified [58]. Most laboratories have identified bands that migrate at a mobility of around 21 kDa (Type 1) with the other major isotype having a mobility of around 19 kDa for the unglycosylated fragment. Samples for Western blot analysis can be further treated with enzymes that remove the sugar residues attached to $PrP^{res}$, thereby allowing more accurate visualisation of a single unglycosylated band. The differences in $PrP^{res}$ isotypes may be affected by the experimental conditions under which samples are prepared and western blotting is performed; a consensus study by the World Health Organisation is planned to attempt to identify standard procedures for this investigation and work towards a uniform nomenclature for $PrP^{res}$ isotypes.

All workers are agreed that there are differences between cases of sporadic CJD in terms of the major $PrP^{res}$ isotypes identified and that some of these, in conjunction with the codon 129 genotype, appear to influence the clinical and pathological phenotype of the disease [18, 40, 58]. All laboratories agree that in vCJD there is a distinct $PrP^{res}$ isotype with a predominance of the diglycosylated band, a pattern similar to that found in western blots of $PrP^{res}$ in BSE from cattle and in other BSE-related conditions in other species. This appearance has been considered as a molecular 'marker' of BSE infection in all species [18].

It is clear that additional investigative techniques such as 2D gel electrophoresis may allow further resolution of $PrP^{res}$ isotypes and may help to resolve some of the differences reported by various laboratories in terms of the identification and nature of the $PrP^{res}$ isotypes in human prion diseases. Western blotting can also be performed in non-neural tissues to detect $PrP^{res}$ and to date this has been consistently detected only in vCJD in lymphoid tissues, particularly in the tonsil [36]. Interestingly, densitometric studies of the $PrP^{res}$ bands have revealed an even higher preponderance of the diglycosylated $PrP^{res}$ isoform in tonsil than in the brain in individual cases, indicating there my be tissue specific differences in $PrP^{res}$ glycosylation. Further studies are being performed on other tissues from cases of vCJD, in view of concerns that the infectious agent may be present in a range of other tissues including blood and peripheral nervous system.

## 9 Transmission Studies

Only a limited number of transmission studies on cases of human prion diseases have been performed in primates and experimental rodents; work using a wide range of PrP-transgenic laboratory mice has greatly increased our understanding of the mechanism of spread of this agent and the pathogenesis of CNS infection. The evidence from studies of sporadic CJD is that there may well be several strains of the infectious agent [11] and there is a great deal of current interest in whether strains can be identified by their molecular properties in Western blots in addition to their characterisation by experimental transmission into rodents [18, 58].

Strain-typing studies in variant CJD have revealed transmission characteristics identical to those of the BSE agent both from cattle and from other species [11]. This has been the strongest evidence that variant CJD does indeed represent BSE infection in humans. Experimental transmissions are usually performed using brain tissue (a fact that underscores the need to retain some frozen brain tissue at autopsy) but the detection of $PrP^{res}$ in the lymphoreticular system in vCJD has led to further transmission studies involving panels of inbred and transgenic mice. The results of these studies are currently awaited.

Although transmission studies are unlikely ever to be a standard diagnostic procedure, they still represent the most sensitive method of identifying prion strains. Their use may help to answer questions concerning the aetiology of sporadic CJD, and such studies are needed to underpin investigation of molecular epidemiology and strain-specific epidemiology in human prion diseases.

## 10 Future Trends in Human Prion Diseases

The emergence of vCJD first in the United Kingdom and now in France and Ireland has emphasised the need for continuing surveillance of human prion diseases, particularly in countries which have reported cases of BSE or are at risk of BSE. In the United Kingdom, the CJD Surveillance project and its associated epidemiological studies have recently revealed a significant increase in the rate at which vCJD cases are occurring [2], but given the lengthy incubation period for this disorder, it is difficult to predict future numbers of cases. Other attempts to estimate population exposure to BSE (e.g. by studying large numbers of surgically removed lymphoid tissues for the presence of the abnormal prion protein) are limited by uncertainties as to the incubation period for the disease and the stage of the incubation period at which $PrP^{res}$ is detectable in these tissues. A better means of determining population exposure would be a blood-based diagnostic test which was able to detect low levels of $PrP^{res}$ in peripheral blood, but this has yet to be achieved for human prion diseases.

Although no screening tests are available for human prion disease, the possibility of a therapeutic approach to this disorder, or perhaps even a prophylactic approach, has not been overlooked. In animal models, there are several compounds that have been shown at least to delay substantially the onset of clinical disease and prolong the incubation period, and ever-increasing numbers of compounds show therapeutic potential without untoward toxic effects (see [34] for review). Additional studies are clearly required before any of these compounds can be tested in humans but the prospects for prophylaxis or treatment of human prion diseases are better at present than ever before, and it is anticipated that further advances will be made in the near future.

**Acknowledgements.** The CJD Surveillance Unit is funded by the Department of Health and the Scottish Executive. This work was supported by grants from the Medical Research Council (G9627376) and the European Commission (TSECFAC: BMH4-CT98-6015). The Raymond Escourolle Neuropathology Laboratory is funded by "Le Programme de Rechereche sur les EST et les Prions" and PHRC AOM 96117. We would like to thank Ms. A. Mackenzie for assistance in preparing the manuscript for publication. The support of neurologists and neuropathologists in France and the UK is gratefully acknowledged.

## Appendix: Protocol for Western Blot Detection of $PrP^{res}$ in CJD Brain [40]

1. Sample ~100 mg frozen cerebral cortical grey matter (usually frontal cortex).
2. Homogenise in 9 volumes (w/v) of non-denaturing detergent-containing buffer.
3. Clear homogenate by low speed centrifugation.
4. Digest supernatant with proteinase K (50 µg/ml, 1 h, 37 °C).
5. Separate 10 µl of SDS-denatured sample by mini-gel SDS-PAGE.
6. Semidry transfer to PVDF membrane.
7. Immuno-detection with monoclonal antibody 3F4 and an appropriate horseradish peroxidase-conjugated secondary antibody.
8. Enhanced chemiluminescent (ECL) detection.
9. Estimation of $PrP^{res}$ mobility by reference to (ECL) molecular weight markers or standard samples (Fig. 7).
10. Analysis of glycoform ratio by densitometry.

Note: Steps 1–8 should be carried out using appropriate personal protection in a category 3* laboratory with steps 1–4 being performed in a class 1 microbiological containment hood.

## References

1. Advisory Committee on Dangerous Pathogens (1999) Transmissible spongiform encephalopathy agents: Safe working and the prevention of infection. The Stationery Office, London
2. Andrews NJ, Farington CP, Cousens SN, Smith PG, Ward H, Knight RSG, Ironside JW, Will RG (2000) Incidence of variant Creutzfeldt-Jakob disease in the UK. Lancet 356:481–482
3. Baron H, Safar J, Groth D, De Armond S, Prusiner S (1999) Biosafety issues in prion diseases. In: Prusiner S (ed) Prion biology and diseases. Cold Spring Harbor Lab Press, New York, pp 743–777
4. Bastian FO (ed) (1991) Creutzfeldt-Jakob disease and other transmissible human spongiform encephalopathies. Mosby Year Book, St Louis
5. Bell JE, Ironside JW (1993) Neuropathology of spongiform encephalopathies in humans. Br Med Bull 49:738–777
6. Bell JE, Ironside JW (1997) Principles and practice of "high risk" brain banking. Neuropathol Appl Neurobiol 23:281–288
7. Bell JE, Gentleman SM, Ironside JW, McCardle L, Lantos PL, Doey L, Lowe J, Fergusson J, Luthert P, McQuaid S, Allen IV (1997) Prion protein immunocytochemistry – UK five centre consensus report. Neuropathol Appl Neurobiol 23:26–35
8. Bortone E, Bettoni L, Giorgi C, Terzano MG, Trabattoni GR, Mancia D (1994) Reliability of EEG in the diagnosis of Creutzfeldt-Jakob disease. Electroenceph Clin Neurophysiol 90:323–330
9. Brown P, Wolff A, Gajdusek DC (1990) A simple and effective method for inactivating virus infectivity in formalin-fixed tissue samples from patients with Creutzfeldt-Jakob disease. Neurology 40:887–890
10. Brown P, Preece MA, Will RG (1992) "Friendly fire" in medicine: hormones, homographs and Creutzfeldt-Jakob disease. Lancet 340:24–27
11. Bruce ME, Will RG, Ironside JW, McConnell I, Drummond D, Suttie A, McCardle L, Chree A, Hope J, Birkett C, Cousens SN, Fraser H, Bostock CJ (1997) Transmissions to mice indicate that "new variant" CJD is caused by the BSE agent. Nature 389:498–501
12. Budka H, Aguzzi A, Brown P, Brucher JM, Bugiani O, Collinge J, Diringer H, Gullotta F, Haltia M, Hauw J-J, Ironside JW, Kretzschmar HA, Lantos PL, Masullo C, Pocchiari M, Schlote W,

Tateishi J, Will RG (1995) Tissue handling in suspected Creutzfeldt-Jakob disease (CJD) and other human spongiform encephalopathies (Prion diseases). Brain Pathol 5:319-322
13. Budka H, Aguzzi A, Brown P, Brucher J-M, Bugiani O, Gullotta F, Haltia M, Hauw J-J, Ironside JW, Jellinger K, Kretzschmar HA, Lantos PL, Masullo C, Schlote W, Tateishi J, Weller RO (1995) Neuropathological diagnostic criteria for Creutzfeldt-Jakob (CJD) and other human spongiform encephalopathies (prion diseases). Brain Pathol 5:459-466
14. Castellani R, Parchi P, Stahl J, Capellari S, Cohen M, Gambetti P (1996) Early pathologic and biochemical changes in Creutzfeldt-Jakob disease: study of brain biopsies. Neurology 46:1690-1693
15. Cathala F, Court L, Hauw J-J, Escourolle R, Rohmer F, Castaigne P (1975). Clinical studies in primates inoculated with Kuru and Creutzfeldt-Jakob agents. In: Meldrum BS, Marsden CD (eds) Primate models of neurological disordeers. Raven Press Publishers, New York, pp 319-339 (Advances in Neurology, vol 10)
16. Collinge J, Owen F, Poulter M, Leach M, Crow TJ, Rossor MN, Hardy J, Mullan MJ, Janota I, Lantos PL (1990) Prion dementia without characteristic pathology. Lancet 336:7-9
17. Collinge J, Palmer MS, Dryden AJ (1991) Genetic predisposition to iatrogenic Creutzfeldt-Jakob disease. Lancet 337:1441-1442
18. Collinge J, Sidle CL, Meads J, Ironside JW, Hill AF (1996) Molecular analysis of prion strain variation and the aetiology of "new variant" CJD. Nature 383:685-690
19. DeArmond SJ, Dickson DW, DeArmond B (1997) Degenerative diseases of the central nervous system. In: Davis R, Robertson DM (eds) Textbook of neuropathology, 3rd edition. Williams & Wilkins, Baltimore, pp 1063-1178
20. DeArmond SJ, Qiu V, Sanchez H, Spilman PR, Ninchak-Casey A, Alonso D, Daggett V (1999) $PrP^c$ glycoform heterogeneity as a function of brain region: implications for selective targeting of neurons by prion strains. J Neuropathol Exp Neurol 58:1000-1009
21. de Silva R, Ironside JW, McCardle l, Esmonde TFG, Bell JE, Will RG (1994) Neuropathological phenotype and "prion protein" genotype correlation in sporadic Creutzfeldt-Jakob disease. Neurosci Lett 179:50-52
22. Dickson DW, Lee SC, Mattiace LA, Yen SC, Brosnan C (1993) Microglia and cytokines in neurological disease, with special reference to AIDS and Alzheimer's disease. Glia 7:75-83
23. Duyckaerts C, Colle MA, Seilhean D, Hauw J-J (1998) Laminar spongiosis of the dentate gyrus: a sign of disconnection, present in cases of Alzheimer disease. Acta Neuropathol 95:413-420
24. Eitzen U, Von, Egensperger R, Kösel S, Grasbon-Frodl E, Imai Y, Bise K, Kphsaka S, Mehraein P, Graeber M (1998) Microglia and the development of spongiform change in Creutzfeldt-Jakob disease. J Neuropathol Exp Neurol 57:246-256
25. Fournier J-G, Kopp N, Streichenberger N, Escaig-Haye F, Langeveld J, Brown P (2000) Electron microscopy of brain amyloid plaques from a patient with new variant Creutzfeldt-Jakob disease. Acta Neuropathol 99:637-642
26. Ghetti T, Piccardo P, Spillanti MG, Ichimiya Y, Porro M, Perini F, Kitamoto T, Tayeishi J, Seiler C, Giaccone G, Frangione B, Bugiani O, Giaccone G, Prelli F, Godert M, Dlouhy SR, Tagliavini F (1997) Vascular variant of prion protein cerebral amyloidosis with tau-positive neurofibrillary tangles: the phenotype of the stop codon 145 mutation in PRNP. Proc Natl Acad Sci USA 93:744-748
27. Gray F, Chretien F, Adle-Biassette H, Dorandeu A, Ereau T, Delisle MB, Kopp N, Ironside JW, Vital C (1999) Neuronal apoptosis in Creutzfeldt-Jakob disease. J Neuropathol Exp Neurol 58:321-328
28. Guiroy DC, Yanagihara R, Gajdusek DC (1991) Localization of amyloidogenic proteins and sulfatated glycosaminoglycans in non transmisible and transmissible cerebral amyloidoses. Acta Neuropathol 82:87-92
29. Hainfellner JA, Brantner-Inthaler S, Cercenakova L, Brown P, Kitamoto T, Tateishi J, Diringer H, Liberski PP, Regele H, Feucht M, Mayr N, Wessely P, Summer K, Seitelberger F, Budka H (1995) The original Gerstmann-Straussler-Scheinker family of Austria: divergent clinicopathological phenotypes but constant PrP genotype. Brain Pathol 5:201-211
30. Hansen LA, Masliah E, Terry RD, Mirra SS (1991) A neuropathological subset of Alzheimer's disease with concomitant Lewy body disease and spongiform changes. Acta Neuropathol 78:194-201

31. Hauw J-J, Sazdovitch V, Laplanche J, Peoc'h K, Kopp N, Kemeny J, Privat N, Delasnerie-Laupretre N, Brandel J, Deslys J, Dormont D, Alpérovitch A (2000) Neuropathologic variants of sporadic Creutzfeldt-Jakob disease and codon 129 of PrP gene. Neurology 54:1641–1646
32. Hauw J-J, Sazdovitch V, Seilhean D, Camilleri S, Lazarini F, Delasnerie-Lauprêtre N, Duyckaerts C (1996) The nosology and neuropathology of human conditions related to unconventional agents or prions. Eur J Neurol 3:487–499
33. Hayward PAR, Bell JE, Ironside JW (1994) Prion protein immunocytochemistry: reliable protocols for the investigation of Creutzfeldt-Jakob disease. Neuropathol Appl Neurobiol 20:375–383
34. Head MW, Ironside JW (2000) Inhibition of prion protein conversion: a therapeutic tool? Trends Microbiol 8:6–8
35. Hegyi I, Hainfellner J, Flicker H, Ironside J, Hauw J, Tateishi J, Haltia M, Bugiani O, Aguzzi A, Budka H (1997) Prion protein immunocytochemistry: reliable staining protocol, immunomorphology, and diagnostic pitfalls. Clin Neuropathol 16:262–263
36. Hill H, Butterworth R, Joiner S, Jackson G, Rossor N, Thomas D, Frosh A, Tolley N, Bell J, Spence M, King A, Al Sarraj S, Ironside J, Lantos P, Collinge J (1999) Investigation of variant Creutzfeldt-Jakob disease and other human prion diseases with tonsil biopsy samples. Lancet 353:183–189
37. Hsich G, Kenney K, Gibbs CJ Jnr, Lee KH, Harrington MG (1996) The 14.3.3 brain protein in cerebrospinal fluid as a marker for transmissible spongiform encephalopathies. New Eng J Med 335:924–930
38. Ironside JW, Bell JE (1996) The high risk neuropathological autopsy in AIDS and Creutzfeldt-Jakob disease: principles and practice. Neuropathol Appl Neurobiol 22:388–393
39. Ironside JW, Bell JE (1997). Pathology of prion diseases. In: Collinge J, Palmer M (eds) Prion diseases. Oxford University Press. Oxford, pp 57–88
40. Ironside JW, Head MW, Bell JE, McCardle L, Will RG (2000) Laboratory diagnosis of variant Creutzfeldt-Jakob disease. Histopathology 37:1–9
41. Kascsak RJ, Rubenstein R, Merz PA, Tonna-DeMasi M, Fersko R, Carp RI, Wisniewski HM, Diringer H (1997) Mouse polyclonal and monoclonal antibody to scrapie-associated fibril proteins. J Virol 61:3688–3693
42. Kato S, Hirano A, Umahara T, Llena J, Herz F, Ohama E (1992) Ultrastructural and immunohistological studies of ballooned cortical neurons in Creutzfeldt-Jakob disease: expression of $\alpha$B-crystallin, ubiquitin and stress-response protein 27. Acta Neuropathol 84:443–448
43. Kitamoto T, Doh-ura K, Muramoto T, Miyazono M, Tateishi J (1992) The primary structure of the prion protein influences the distribution of abnormal prion protein in the central nervous system. Am J Pathol 141:271–277
44. Kitamoto T, Ogomori K, Tateishi J, Prusiner SB (1987) Formic acid pretreatment enhances immunostaining of cerebral and systemic amyloids. Lab Invest 57:230–236
45. Kitamoto T, Shin RW, Doh-ura K, Tomokane N, Miyazono M, Muramoto T, Tateishi J (1992) Abnormal isoform of prion proteins accumulates in the synaptic structures of the central nervous system in patients with Creutzfeldt-Jakob disease. Am J Pathol 140:1285–1294
46. Lafarga M, Berciano MT, Suarez I, Viadero CF, Andres MA, Berciano J (1991) Cytology and organization of reactive astroglia in human cerebellar cortex with severe loss of granule cells: a study on the ataxic form of Creutzfeldt-Jakob disease. Neuroscience 40:337–352
47. Liberski P, Jeffrey M (2000) Tubulovesicular structures: what are they really? Microsc Res Technol 50:46–57
48. Liberski PP, Yanagihara R, Asher DR, Gibbs CJ Jr, Gajdusek DC (1990) Reevaluation of the ultrastructural pathology of experimental Creutzfeldt-Jakob disease. Brain 113:121–137
49. Lugaresi E, Medori R, Montagna P, Baruzzi A, Cortelli P, Lugaresi A, Tinuper P, Zucconi M, Gambetti P (1986) Fatal familial insomnia and dysautonomia with selective degeneration of thalamic nuclei. New Eng J Med 315:997–1003
50. Masters CL, Harris JO, Gajdusek DC, Gibbs CJ Jr, Bernoulli C, Asher DM (1979) Creutzfeldt-Jakob disease: patterns of worldwide occurrence and the significance of familial and sporadic clustering. Ann Neurol 5:177–188
51. Masters CL, Richardson EP (1978) Subacute spongiform encephalopathy (Creutzfeldt-Jakob disease). The nature and progression of spongiform changes. Brain 101:333–344

52. Medori R, Tritschler JH, LeBlanc A, Villare F, Manetto V, Ghen Hy, Xuf R, Leal S, Montagna P, Cortelli P, Tinuper P, Avoni P, Mochi M, Baruxxi A, Hauw JJ, Ott J, Lugarest E, Autilio-Gamettia L, Gambetti P (1992) Fatal familial insomnia, a prion disease with a mutation at codon 178 of the prion protein gene. New Eng J Med 7:444–449
53. Metters J (1992) Neuro and ophthalmic surgery procedures in patients with, or suspected to have, or at risk of developing CJD or GSS. (letter) Department of Health, London
54. Mizutani Y, Okumura A, Oda M, Shiraki H (1981) Panencephalopathic type of Creutzfeldt-Jakob disease. J Neurol Neurosurg Psych 44:103–115
55. Mühleisen H, Gehrmann J, Meyermann R (1995) Reactive microglia in Creutzfeldt-Jakob disease. Neuropathol Appl Neurobiol 21:505–517
56. Namba Y, Tomonoga M, Kawasaki H, Otomo E, Ikeda K (1991) Apolipoprotein E immunoreactivity in cerebral amyloid deposits and neurofibrillary tangles in Alzheimer's disease and kuru plaque amyloid in Creutzfeldt-Jakob disease. Brain Res 541:163–166
57. Palmer MS, Dryden AJ, Hughes JT, Collinge J (1991) Homozygous prion protein genotype predisposes to sporadic Creutzfeldt-Jakob disease. Nature 352:340–342
58. Parchi AU, Castellani R, Capellari S, Ghetti B, Young K, Chen SG, Farlow M, Dickson DW, Sima AA, Trojanowski JQ, Petersen RB, Gambetti P (1996) Molecular basis of phenotypic variability in sporadic Creutzfeldt-Jakob disease. Ann Neurol 39:767–778
59. Parchi P, Gambetti P, Piccardo P, Ghetti B (1998) Human prion diseases. In: Kirkham N, Lemoine NR (eds) Progress in Pathology (vol 4) Edinburgh, Churchill-Livingstone, pp 39–77
60. Parchi P, Capellari S, Chin S, Schwarz HB, Schecter NP, Butts JD, Judkins P, Burns DK, Powers JM, Gambetti P (1999) A subtype of sporadic prion disease mimicking fatal familial insomnia. Neurology 52:1757–1763
61. Privat N, Sazdovitch V, Seilhean D, Laplanche J-L, Hauw J-J (2000) Immunohistochemistry for human PrP: a new protocol. Microsc Res Technol 50:26–31
62. Prusiner SB (1982) Novel proteinaceous infectious particles cause scrapie. Science 216: 136–144
63. Richard M, Biacabe AG, Perret-Liaudet A, McCardle L, Ironside JW, Kopp N (1999) Protection of personnel and environment against Creutzfeldt-Jakob disease in pathology laboratories. Clin Exp Pathol 47:192–200
64. Victor M, Adams R, Cole M (1965) The acquired (non-Wilsonian) type of chronic hepatocerebral degeneration. Medicine 44:343–396
65. Watanabe R, Duchen LW (1993) Cerebral amyloid in human prion disease. Neuropathol Appl Neurobiol 19:253–260
66. Wells GAH, Scott AC, Johnson CT, Gunning RF, Hancock RD, Jeffrey M, Dawson M, Bradley R (1987) A novel progressive spongiform encephalopathy in cattle. Vet Rec 121:419–420
67. Will RG (1993) Epidemiology of Creutzfeldt-Jakob disease. Brit Med Bull 49:960–970
68. Will RG, Ironside JW, Zeidler M, Cousens SN, Estibeiro K, Alpérovitch A, Poser S, Pocciari M, Hofman A, Smith PG (1996) A new variant of Creutzfeldt-Jakob disease in the UK. Lancet 347:921–925
69. Will RG, Zeidler M, Stewart GE, Macleod MA, Ironside JW, Cousens SN, Mackenzie J, Estibeiro K, Green AJ, Knight RS (2000) Diagnosis of new variant Creutzfeldt-Jakob disease. Ann Neurol 47:575–582
70. World Health Organisation (2000) Infection control guidelines for transmissible spongiform encephalopathies. World Health Organisation, Geneva
71. Zeidler M, Sellar RJ, Collie DA, Knight R, Stewart G, Macleod MA, Ironside JW, Cousens SN, Colchester AF, Hadley DM, Will RG (2000) The pulvinar sign on magnetic resonance imaging in variant Creutzfeldt-Jakob disease. Lancet 355:1412–1418

# Autopsy Investigation of Disorders of Skeletal Muscle and Peripheral Nerves

D. A. Hilton, R. O. Weller



## 1 Introduction

Postmortem examination of peripheral nerve and skeletal muscle will often provide useful information for understanding clinical conditions in which neuromuscular features are present. A common misconception is that postmortem sampling of nerves, and particularly muscle, is of limited value because of autolytic change and loss of enzyme activity. Many of the histochemical techniques used for the analysis of muscle biopsies, however, can be used even if there is a postmortem delay of several days. Simple morphology may also be informative, even in muscle samples taken from a 3,200-year-old mummy, which allowed the diagnosis of trichinella

Current Topics in Pathology, Vol. 95
S. Love (Ed.): Neuropathology

infection (de Boni et al. 1977). A neuromuscular disorder may be either the primary disease which has led to the death of the individual or a complication of a systemic disorder, e.g. paraneoplastic diseases or critical illness myoneuropathy. Many skeletal muscle disorders also affect cardiac muscle, e.g. muscular dystrophies and mitochondrial myopathies, which can lead to conduction defects, cardiomyopathy and sudden cardiac death. Involvement of respiratory muscles may result in respiratory failure. Involvement of bulbar muscles predisposes to choking; this occurs in neurogenic disorders, such as motor neuron disease and in myopathic disorders, including the muscular dystrophies. As in all autopsies, a clear understanding of the underlying pathology is of great educational value to clinicians and helps in explaining the cause of death to family members. Autopsy allows more extensive sampling of different muscles and nerves than is possible during life and, therefore, provides a better understanding of the full extent and severity of the disease process. The underlying diagnosis may also have other implications for relatives, as many neuromuscular disorders have a hereditary basis.

The most important role of the pathologist is to ensure that the correct samples are retained at autopsy and that they are properly handled to allow the maximum amount of information to be obtained from their examination. This chapter is intended as general advice for histopathologists, rather than a comprehensive guide to neuromuscular disorders. Consultation with the local neuropathology centre is recommended in most cases. Interpretation of muscle and nerve disease at autopsy is greatly aided by adequate clinical information, which would usually include the findings of a neurological examination, electrophysiological results, family history and results of blood tests. Occasionally magnetic resonance imaging (MRI) or computed tomography (CT) imaging may be available to aid in the sampling of limb muscles.

## 2 Skeletal Muscle

### 2.1 Sampling of Muscles at Autopsy

The sampling of muscle groups should include those muscles which are clinically involved, but should not concentrate upon those with severe wasting, as histology may just show end-stage disease. In most primary muscle diseases, the proximal muscle groups such as serratus anterior, deltoid, biceps brachii and quadriceps femoris are predominantly involved; however, certain muscular dystrophies have a much more selective distribution, e.g. scapulo-peroneal-humeral muscular dystrophy. Limb muscles are generally more useful than axial muscles, such as psoas, because preservation tends to be better, due to more rapid postmortem cooling; furthermore, there are more data available on the normal appearances of limb muscles. It is best to avoid sites of tendon and fascial insertion, as muscle in these areas may be difficult to interpret because of increased numbers of central nuclei and fibre splitting, which resemble changes seen in myopathic disorders. A muscle should be sampled so that it can be easily orientated, by taking a strip along the long axis of the muscle approximately 1.5 cm in length and 0.5 cm in diameter.

## 2.2 Preparation of Tissue

Perhaps the most critical step in tissue preparation is the correct freezing of muscle to avoid ice-crystal artefact. Muscle should be snap-frozen in isopentane that has been cooled in liquid nitrogen until it has a syrup-like texture. Alternatively, if isopentane is not available, the muscle may be coated in talc (glove powder) and snap-frozen in liquid nitrogen (the talc helps prevent the insulating layer of bubbles forming on the tissue surface that slows freezing and leads to ice-crystal formation). If ice-crystal formation does occur, it is recognised as clear holes in histological sections of muscle fibres. When sectioning the muscle for histology, the fibres should be orientated in the transverse plane so that an assessment of fibre size and shape can be made. A small amount of muscle, approximately 1 $cm^3$, should be frozen for possible genetic or biochemical analysis. It is also worthwhile taking additional muscle for paraffin wax histology. Although of more limited value, paraffin wax histology allows for more extensive sampling, which is particularly useful in the assessment of inflammation, fibrosis and vasculitis, and is often adequate for the diagnosis of polymyositis and other inflammatory disorders and for detecting denervation. A small amount of muscle may be fixed in glutaraldehyde for electron microscopy, if required. Postmortem autolysis will probably preclude the detailed assessment of many ultrastructural features, such as mitochondria, but more robust structures such as filamentous and rod bodies, may be adequately preserved to allow their recognition.

## 2.3 Histological Techniques

A number of stains and histochemical preparations are performed on cryostat sections of skeletal muscle as part of routine assessment. Histochemical preparations do not always work in autopsy tissue; however, if the body has been refrigerated soon after death, most are of value for several days (see Table 1).

Immunocytochemistry is also often of value in the diagnosis of muscular dystrophies. Perhaps the best-known antibodies are to dystrophin, which show loss of membrane immunoreactivity in Duchenne and Becker muscular dystrophies. Other antibodies commonly used include those directed against sarcoglycans and dysferlin (deficient in many autosomal recessive forms of limb-girdle muscular dystrophy), merosin (deficient in some forms of congenital muscular dystrophy) and emerin (deficient in Emery-Dreifuss muscular dystrophy).

Immunocytochemistry may also be of value in other situations. For example, class I MHC antigen expression is increased in muscle fibres in cases of myositis, even in areas distant from inflammation; antibodies to slow and fast myosin allow fibre typing in paraffin sections; desmin immunoreactivity is increased in desmin storage disorders and critical illness neuromyopathy. Lymphocyte markers are also often helpful in characterising the nature and full extent of any inflammatory cell infiltrate.

**Table 1.** Tinctorial stains and histochemical preparations used in the assessment of muscle histology

| Tinctorial stain | Purpose | Postmortem delay during which the technique may still be of value |
|---|---|---|
| H&E[a] | General pathological reactions – fibre necrosis, regeneration, hypertrophy, atrophy, inflammation, vasculitis | > 10 days |
| PAS[a] | Demonstrates glycogen – accumulates in glycogen storage diseases, steroid myopathy, hypothyroid myopathy | Usually severely depleted in post-mortem muscle |
| ORO | Demonstrates neutral lipids – accumulate in lipid disorders, alcoholic myopathy, steroid myopathy | > 10 days |
| VG[a] | Demonstrates collagen – increases in most chronic muscle disorders, especially the dystrophies | > 10 days |
| Reticulin[a] | Demonstrates basement membrane – useful in fibre size estimation | > 10 days |
| GT | Muscle fibres appear green, mitochondria and some cytoplasmic bodies e.g. nemaline rods, appear red. 'Ragged-red' fibres are seen in mitochondrial myopathies. Also useful to demonstrate a red border of 'rimmed' vacuoles, seen in disorders such as inclusion body myositis | > 10 days |
| Histochemical preparations | | |
| ATPases | Demonstrate fibre types by varying the pH – type I fibres react strongly at acid pH, type II fibres at alkaline pH. In certain disorders only one muscle fibre type may be affected. Fibre-type grouping indicates denervation with subsequent reinnervation | > 10 days |
| NADH | Oxidative enzyme present on the sarcoplasmic reticulum and in mitochondria. Useful as a general marker of internal fibre architecture. Denervated fibres stain darkly and may form 'target fibres' | > 10 days |
| SDH | Oxidative enzyme, specific to mitochondria. Used as an indicator of the number of mitochondria, which often accumulate in mitochondrial myopathies | > 10 days |
| COX | Oxidative enzyme in mitochondria. In mitochondrial myopathies there are often fibres with segments deficient in COX. | > 10 days |
| Myophosphorylase | Deficient in McArdle's disease | 12 h |
| Myoadenylate deaminase | Deficient in myoadenylate deaminase deficiency | > 10 days |

ATPases, myosin adenosine triphosphatase; COX, cytochrome oxidase; GT, Gomori trichrome; H&E, haematoxylin and eosin; NADH, nicotine adenine dinucleotide dehydrogenase tetrazolium reductase; ORO, oil red O; PAS, periodic acid Schiff; SDH, succinic dehydrogenase; VG, van Gieson.

[a] Also of value in paraffin sections.

## 2.4 Histology of Normal Muscle

Muscle fibres may be several centimetres in length; they are syncytia formed by fusion of fetal myoblasts. They have peripherally situated nuclei and a hexagonal outline in transverse sections. There are usually 4–6 subsarcolemmal nuclei in each section, and approximately 30 nuclei/mm muscle. Muscle fibre diameters (defined as the shortest transverse distance) range from 40–80 μm in adult males and 30–70 μm in adult females. They can be divided into two major fibre types: type I fibres contract relatively slowly, are more important for postural activity and are rich in oxidative enzymes, lipids and myoglobin; type II are fast-twitch fibres, relying more on glycolysis for energy for contraction and containing relatively more glycogen and fewer mitochondria. Type II fibres can be further subdivided on the basis of their reactions with adenosine triphosphatases (ATPases) at different pHs, into IIa, IIb and in infants, IIc. The fibre type is determined by the innervation that the fibre receives. Each motor neuron innervates variable numbers of fibres, forming a motor unit, ranging from about ten fibres in external ocular muscles to several hundred in limb muscles. The fibres from each motor unit are randomly distributed throughout the muscle fascicle, producing a 'chequerboard' pattern with ATPase preparations (Fig. 1). The fibre-type distribution of different muscles may vary considerably, depending upon function. There are also individual variations and differences between superficial and deep parts of a muscle (Johnson et al. 1973), so any interpretation of abnormalities in fibre-type distribution should be based on knowledge of the normal range. In superficial parts of deltoid and quadriceps femoris there are approximately equal numbers of type I, IIa and IIb fibres.

Skeletal muscle fibres (extrafusal fibres) are surrounded by a thin layer of connective tissue, the endomysium, and grouped into fascicles which are surround-

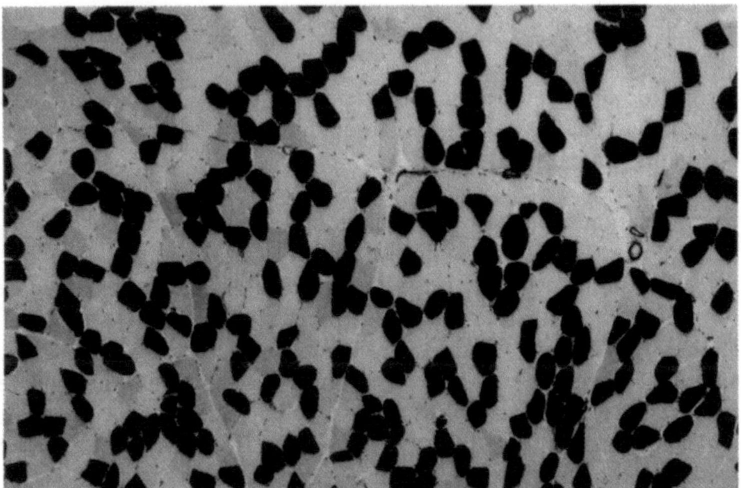

**Fig 1.** Section of autopsy muscle following a histochemical reaction for ATPase at pH 9.4. Type I fibres (*pale*) and type II fibres (*dark*) are randomly mixed producing a 'chequerboard' pattern

ed by a thicker connective tissue layer, the perimysium. Muscle spindles and neurovascular bundles are found between fascicles. Spindles consist of 3–14 specialised (intrafusal) muscle fibres within a fibrous capsule that measure muscle fibre tension and length.

## 2.5 Clinical Features of Muscle Disease

Muscle diseases can be broadly divided into primary muscle disorders (myopathies), muscle disease secondary to denervation or disorders of the neuromuscular junction.

In myopathic disorders symptoms of muscle weakness are usual, although myalgia and cramps may be present in inflammatory and metabolic diseases. Neurogenic weakness is often accompanied by loss of reflexes, although in motor neuron disease involvement of upper motor neurons may lead to increased muscle tone (spasticity) and brisk reflexes. Rapidly progressive denervating conditions, such as motor neuron disease, may produce spontaneous muscle twitching (fasciculations). Sensation may be abnormal in peripheral neuropathies, but is normal in disorders affecting anterior horn cells and neuromuscular junctions. The results of electromyography and nerve conduction studies usually allow distinction between neurogenic and myopathic disease, and may help in deciding which muscles (and nerves) to sample. Electromyography is particularly valuable in defining disorders of the neuromuscular junction, such as myasthenia gravis.

## 2.6 Pathology of Skeletal Muscle

### 2.6.1 General Pathological Reactions

Myopathic and neurogenic disorders produce well-characterised and distinct pathological changes in muscle, although in some conditions both neurogenic and myopathic changes may occur.

Myopathies are characterised by changes in individual muscle fibres, ranging from variation in fibre size to muscle fibre destruction, phagocytosis and regeneration. Fibrosis and severe fibre atrophy ensue when muscle destruction is widespread. In some myopathies, specific inclusions or defects in enzyme staining may be typical of the disorder.

Neurogenic muscle disease, for the most part, is typified by atrophy of small or sometimes large groups of muscle fibres that have lost their nerve supply. Reinnervation of denervated muscle fibres can be detected in ATPase stains as they all adopt the same muscle fibre type (I, IIa or IIb) and the normal chequerboard pattern of the muscle is disrupted.

### 2.6.2 Neurogenic Disorders

Following denervation, muscle fibres undergo atrophy; however, unlike myopathic atrophy, the fibres have an angular outline, appearing to be indented by the surrounding fibres which may be of normal size or undergo compensatory hypertrophy. In denervation, both fibre types are affected, which is helpful in distinguishing selective type II fibre atrophy, which is a non-specific myopathic change, and the atrophic fibres often occur in groups (Fig. 2). Eventually, if reinnervation does not occur, the fibre will appear as a clump of pyknotic nuclei with little remaining cytoplasm. Denervated fibres may appear dark on nicotinamide adenine dinucleotide reductase (NADH) preparations, and fibres may have a 'target' appearance. Target fibres have a central area lacking NADH activity, with a surrounding dark intermediate zone and outer normal area; they are characteristic of denervation and seen most often in peripheral neuropathies. Denervated fibres may be scattered throughout a muscle fascicle or in small groups (disseminated neurogenic atrophy). Reinnervation occurs by collateral sprouting of surviving intramuscular nerves, resulting in adjacent muscle fibres being supplied by the same neuron, and therefore becoming the same fibre type. Fibre-type grouping is highly characteristic of reinnervation, and may be defined as either two fibres of one fibre-type being completely surrounded by fibres of the same type or a group of 12 adjacent fibres of the same type. However, care should be taken in diagnosing fibre-type grouping if there is an overall predominance of one fibre type, as groups of the predominant fibre type may occur by chance. Groups of reinnervated fibres may undergo grouped atrophy if the nerve supplying them becomes affected by the denervating process. Necrotic fibres may occasionally be seen in denervated muscles.

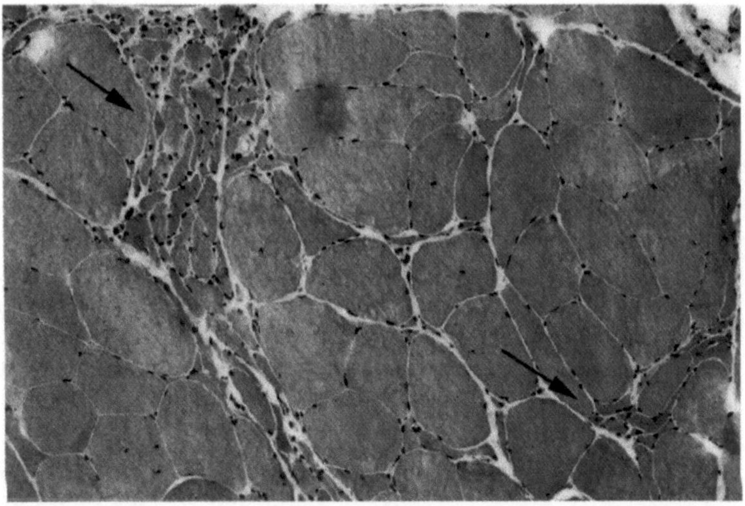

**Fig. 2.** Denervation showing scattered atrophic fibres, some of which are in characteristic groups (*arrows*)

In chronic denervating conditions, secondary myopathic changes can occur which may be quite prominent and may result in an appearance resembling a muscular dystrophy; however, enzyme histochemistry will usually reveal fibre-type grouping in such cases.

Disorders affecting anterior horn cells, peripheral motor nerves, including the nerve roots or the neuromuscular junction may result in neurogenic muscular atrophy. Therefore, if a neurogenic process were suspected clinically, it is important to sample peripheral nerves and the spinal cord as well as skeletal muscle. In some cases, examination of the brain may also be useful; for example, patients with motor neuron disease and paraneoplastic disorders may develop dementia associated with characteristic histological changes in the brain.

---

Neurogenic disorders

Anterior horn cell diseases: motor neuron disease, spinal muscular atrophies, enterovirus infection (e.g. polio), primary spinal cord disorders (e.g. syringomyelia)

Nerve root disease: Guillain-Barré syndrome, chronic inflammatory demyelinating neuropathy

Peripheral neuropathies

Neuromuscular junction: Myasthenia gravis, Eaton-Lambert disease

---

#### *2.6.2.1 Anterior Horn Cell Disorders*

Motor neuron disease usually presents between the ages of 50 and 70 years with progressive upper and lower motor neuron signs. There is relative sparing of ocular movements and patients are continent; death from respiratory failure is usual within 5 years. The aetiology of most cases is unknown, although about 10% of cases are familial, of which a minority are due to mutations in the superoxide dismutase gene. Skeletal muscle shows widespread denervation atrophy, which is particularly severe in respiratory muscles. Reinnervation may be present, particularly in limb muscles. Occasional necrotic fibres may also be seen. Although sensory signs are not a feature, abnormalities have been reported in the sural nerve of long survivors (Heads et al. 1991). The spinal cord may show pallor of the corticospinal tracts due to degeneration of axons, and some of the remaining anterior horn cells usually contain filamentous inclusions that show ubiquitin immunoreactivity. Neuron loss may also be seen in the lower cranial nerve nuclei and motor cortex. In 10%–20% of cases there is also a frontal lobe dementia in which there is spongiosis of the superficial frontotemporal cortex with neuronal loss and ubiqitinated neuronal inclusions.

**Spinal Muscular Atrophies.** These are usually inherited in an autosomal recessive manner, with most cases having deletions in the survival motor neuron (SMN) gene on chromosome 5, resulting in lower motor neuron loss with progressive weakness and muscle wasting. The early onset form, type I (Werdnig-Hoffmann disease), usually presents in early life as a 'floppy baby'. Survival is usually less than 2 years. Skeletal muscle shows numerous rounded atrophic fibres (unlike most neurogenic disorders) with a few normal sized or hypertrophic fibres. Muscle spindles are unaffected. In type II, spinal muscular atrophy (SMA) onset is usually after 6 months of age and prognosis much more variable. The muscle shows less severe changes and fibre-type grouping may be present. Type III SMA (Kugelberg-Welander disease) presents in later childhood and type IV in adulthood; both are only slowly progressive and do not produce a reduction in life expectancy. In these latter forms, fibre-type grouping and secondary myopathic change are prominent features in the muscle. In SMA there is neuronal loss from the spinal cord, brain stem and, in some cases, from the thalamus and dorsal root ganglia.

In active enterovirus infections, inflammatory infiltrates may be present in the cord and leptomeninges, initially neutrophil polymorphs, followed by lymphocytes and by active neuronophagia. Coxsackie viruses produce an acute 'poliomyelitis', and should be considered in young adults with an unexplained rapid onset anterior horn cell disease. Other organs, including the brain, heart and pancreas may also show inflammatory lesions. Although acute poliovirus infection is now extremely rare in the UK, individuals who have suffered poliomyelitis in the past may develop post-polio syndrome in later life, with progressive weakness of the affected muscles. The muscle may show myopathic change, fibre-type grouping and scattered denervated fibres.

Primary spinal cord lesions such as syringomyelia and tumours and compression from degenerative disease of the spine may also cause a combination of upper and lower motor neuron signs, that can be confused clinically with motor neuron disease. Many other conditions including toxic and metabolic disorders may lead to anterior horn cell loss (see Washington University Neuromuscular Disease Index web page).

Disorders affecting the peripheral nerves and roots are discussed below. Neurogenic changes in the muscle in these disorders will depend on the severity and duration of the disease.

#### 2.6.2.2 *Disorders of Neuromuscular Junctions*

Myasthenia gravis presents with progressive weakness on effort and is caused by autoantibodies directed against acetyl choline receptors on the post-synaptic neuromuscular junction (NMJ) membrane. The muscle may only show type II fibre atrophy, although denervation and aggregates of lymphocytes can occasionally be seen. In approximately 70% of cases the thymus is hyperplastic and in 10% a thymoma is present.

Eaton-Lambert syndrome is a rare disorder causing weakness, which may improve with exercise, and is caused by autoantibodies directed against calcium channels on the presynaptic NMJ, reducing release of acetyl choline. The muscle does not show specific abnormalities, but an underlying malignancy, particularly small-cell carcinoma of the lung, should be carefully looked for at autopsy.

## 2.6.3 Myopathies

An increase in variation in fibre size is seen in most myopathies (Table 2), with both hypertrophic and atrophic fibres (as a general rule the diameter of the largest fibres should not exceed more than twice that of the smallest in normal muscle). Prominent fibre hypertrophy is most frequently seen in dystrophies and is often associated with fibre splitting and an increase in the number of fibres with internal nuclei (usually no more than 3% fibres have internal nuclei; Fig. 3). In many myopathic disorders, and also atrophy resulting from disuse, the atrophic fibres are predominantly type II; however, in a few disorders type I atrophy may occur, e.g. myotonic dystrophy and fibre-type disproportion. Type I fibre predominance is common in chronic, particularly childhood-onset, myopathic disorders. Necrotic fibres have amorphous eosinophilic cytoplasm and lack nuclei. Later macrophage infiltration is seen, and regenerating fibres, characterised by basophilic cytoplasm, enlarged nuclei and prominent nucleoli, follow a few days after muscle damage. Necrotic and regenerating fibres are prominent in toxic and inflammatory myopathies and in some dystrophies. Disturbances in internal fibre architecture, seen easily on NADH preparations, are common and may produce a 'moth-eaten', 'whorled', or 'lobulated' appearance. 'Ring' fibres, which have peripheral spirally arranged myofibrils, may be prominent in myotonic dystrophy. Increased endomysial collagen and adipose tissue is seen in chronic myopathies.

**Table 2.** Myopathic disorders

| | |
|---|---|
| Inflammatory muscle disease | Metabolic myopathies |
| Idiopathic | Glycogen storage diseases |
| Polymyositis | Disorders of lipid metabolism |
| Dermatomyositis | Mitochondrial cytopathies |
| Inclusion body myositis | Myoadenylate deaminase deficiency |
| Sarcoid | |
| Localised myositis | Congenital myopathies |
| Giant cell myositis | Nemaline myopathy |
| Eosinophilic myositis | Central core disease |
| | Centronuclear myopathy |
| Infective | |
| Viruses | Periodic paralyses |
| Bacteria | |
| Protozoa | Toxic and drug-induced myopathies |
| Metazoa | Alcoholic |
| | Drug-induced |
| Dystrophies | Critical illness neuromyopathy |
| Duchenne | |
| Becker | |
| Fascioscapulohumeral | |
| Limb-girdle | |
| Myotonic | |
| Congenital | |

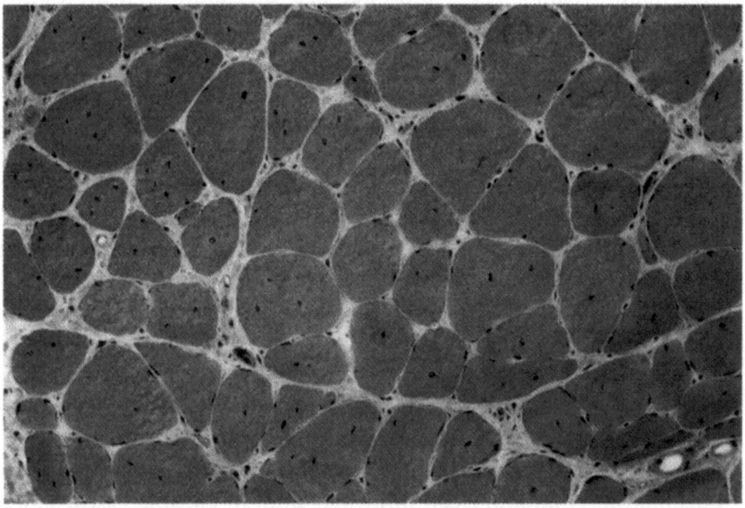

**Fig. 3.** Myopathic change characterised by hypertrophic fibres, rounded atrophic fibres, increased numbers of fibres with central nuclei and an increase in endomysial collagen

### 2.6.3.1 *Inflammatory Muscle Diseases*

Polymyositis is an uncommon condition that most often presents in mid to late life over a period of weeks or months, with a painful proximal myopathy. Some cases have an acute presentation with severe weakness, rhabdomyolysis and subcutaneous oedema. Rarely there may be a nodular presentation, with multiple painful muscle swellings. In more chronic cases, sparing of facial and ocular muscles can be helpful in distinguishing polymyositis from dystrophies. Some cases occur as a pure muscle disorder, but other features such as Raynaud's phenomenon, arthralgia and lung fibrosis may also occur. Polymyositis may be associated with autoimmune and connective tissue diseases and malignancy. In the majority of cases, serum creatine phosphokinase is elevated, reflecting muscle fibre necrosis, and electromyography characteristically shows short polyphasic motor-unit potentials, spontaneous activity and high-frequency repetitive discharges. A number of muscle autoantibodies have been found in patients with polymyositis, although most are not specific (Plotz et al. 1989). Histology of skeletal muscle shows focal changes with fibre necrosis, regeneration and inflammatory infiltrates. The infiltrates are often seen in relation to necrotic fibres and consist largely of T lymphocytes with variable numbers of plasma cells, macrophages and eosinophils. Muscle fibres show increased sarcolemmal and sarcoplasmic expression of class I major histocompatibility antigen, which can be helpful if inflammatory cells are not prominent. Chronic cases show replacement of muscle by fibroadipose tissue, increased central nucleation and variation in fibre size, although fibre hypertrophy is not usually prominent. Although symptomatic cardiac disease is uncommon in these patients, about 40% have either coronary vessel abnormalities or myocarditis at autopsy (Haupt and Hutchins 1982).

Dermatomyositis has a bimodal age distribution with juvenile and adult presentations. In addition to muscle involvement, patients have an erythematous rash, which typically has a butterfly distribution over the face and a lilac colour around the eyes. Dusky red, scaly, elevated patches occur over the elbows, knuckles (Gottron's sign – which spares the phalanges in contrast to the rash of systemic lupus erythematosus) and, to a lesser extent, over the knees and medial malleoli. Although extremely rare in juvenile cases, about 20% of adult cases are associated with underlying malignancy. Like polymyositis, inflammation, fibre necrosis and regeneration are seen in skeletal muscle. Inflammatory infiltrates are predominantly perivascular with a larger proportion of B lymphocytes than in polymyositis. Areas of muscle infarction and vascular thrombosis may be present, particularly in association with underlying malignancy (Basset-Seguin et al. 1990). Perifascicular atrophy (Fig. 4) is a characteristic feature seen in 90% of juvenile cases and 50% adult cases, associated with loss of capillaries at the periphery of fascicles. In juvenile cases, vascular lesions may occur in other organs, including the gastrointestinal tract. Skin shows epidermal atrophy, basal degeneration and occasional inflammatory cell infiltrates and, in chronic cases, subcutaneous calcification may be seen.

Inclusion body myositis presents in the elderly with progressive, painless weakness, that may involve distal as well as proximal muscles. Most cases are sporadic with a male predominance, although it may rarely be inherited, most often in an autosomal dominant manner. Creatine phosphokinase levels are only mildly elevated. Skeletal muscle shows a necrotising, inflammatory myopathy with cytoplasmic vacuoles that have a basophilic rim and eosinophilic inclusions that are present both in the cytoplasm and nuclei. These inclusions have been shown to contain a number of proteins including amyloid, tau, ubiquitin and prion protein (Askanas et al. 1993). By electron microscopy, the inclusions consist of a mixture

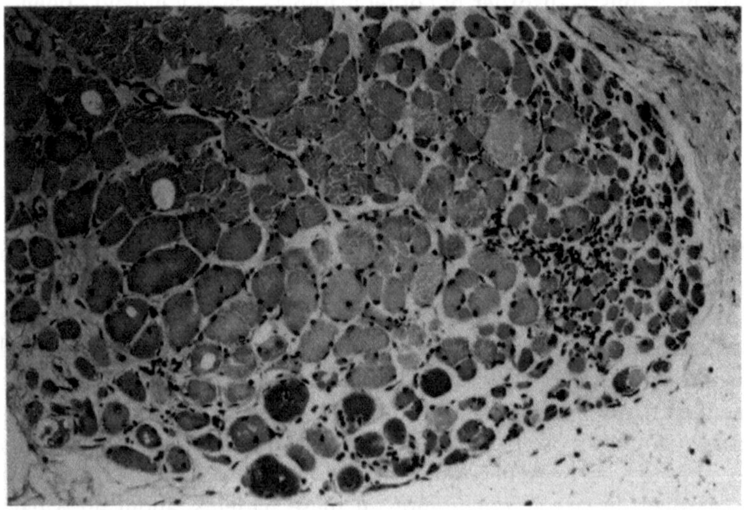

**Fig. 4.** Juvenile dermatomyositis with scattered collections of perivascular lymphocytes and perifascicular atrophy

of 15-nm tubulofilaments, 8-nm fine filaments and amorphous granular material. The inflammatory infiltrates consist predominantly of T lymphocytes, which often surround and infiltrate non-necrotic fibres. Other features include the frequent occurrence of muscle fibres showing mitochondrial abnormalities and clusters of atrophic fibres, resembling those seen in denervation. In view of the intriguing nature of the inclusions and the presence of features resembling denervation it would be of great interest to know whether there is pathological involvement of the central or peripheral nervous system, but unfortunately autopsy findings have not been reported.

Sarcoid granulomata may involve muscle, but extensive destruction of muscle is not a feature. A giant cell myositis may occur in association with thymoma. Localised myositis presents as a focal mass, usually in the thigh or calf. Eosinophilic myositis may occur as part of a systemic hypereosinophilia syndrome.

A number of viruses have been associated with acute myositis, most commonly influenza A. Presentation may be with fever, myalgia, rapid onset weakness, and myoglobinuria. Renal impairment may lead to death, but most cases make a good recovery. Muscle shows necrotic and regenerating fibres, but inflammation is variable. Human immunodeficiency virus (HIV) may cause a myopathy resembling polymyositis. Generalised bacterial and fungal infections of muscle are rare. Cysticercosis and *Trichinella spiralis* may cause muscle infestation from ingestion of undercooked meat.

#### *2.6.3.2 Dystrophies*

Muscular dystrophies are a group of inherited, often destructive, progressive myopathies that are usually diagnosed during childhood or early adult life. They may present with proximal limb muscle weakness or have a restricted pattern of muscle involvement. Many are now known to be caused by mutations in genes encoding dystrophin and dystrophin-associated proteins (Fig. 5); some of these proteins can be demonstrated by immunocytochemistry. In many of the muscular dystrophies, cardiac involvement may lead to sudden death or a dilated cardiomyopathy (Moriuchi et al. 1993). In some dystrophies, such as myotonic dystrophy, other tissues, including the central nervous system, may be involved.

**Dystrophin-Deficient Muscular Dystrophies.** Duchenne and Becker muscular dystrophies are X-linked recessive disorders caused by mutations in the dystrophin gene. Mutations that result in severe gene disruption, such as frame-shift mutations, produce the more severe Duchenne phenotype, whereas in-frame deletions which may allow the formation of a truncated form of the protein result in Becker phenotype. Duchenne muscular dystrophy (DMD) presents at 4–6 years of age with a waddling gait, difficulty in getting up (they may 'climb up their legs' when getting up from the floor – Gower's sign) and lumbar lordosis. The calves may undergo hypertrophy, and creatine phosphokinase levels are markedly elevated to over 1,000 IU. Most become wheelchair bound by their early teens, and death from respiratory or cardiac failure before the age of 30 is usual. Becker muscular dystrophy (BMD) has a later onset and slower progression than DMD, and affected in-

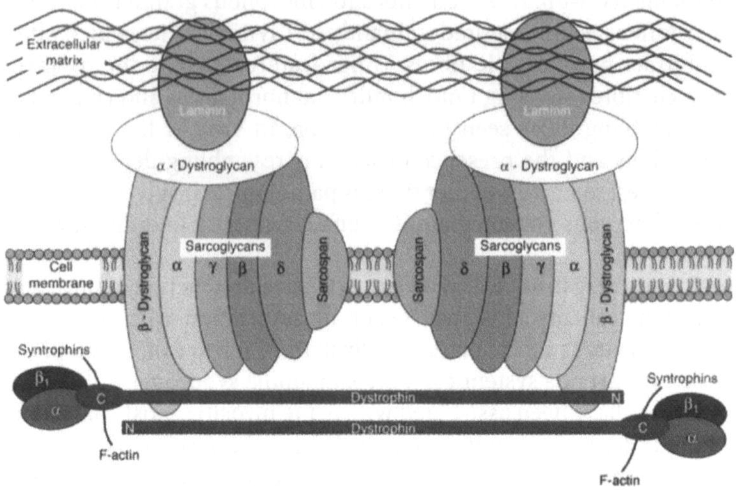


**Fig. 5.** Diagram of dystrophin complex illustrating the proteins which are defective in some of the muscular dystrophies: dystrophin – Duchenne and Becker dystrophies; sarcoglycans – autosomal recessive limb-girdle dystrophies; $\alpha$2-laminin (merosin) – congenital muscular dystrophy

dividuals may be able to walk independently until late adulthood. Dystrophin is expressed in cardiac muscle, so there may also be a cardiomyopathy, and in some cases cardiac involvement may predominate. Central nervous system involvement may result in a reduced IQ or psychiatric features. Female carriers may have mild symptoms and elevation of creatine phosphokinase.

Muscle changes depend upon the stage of disease; early in the disease there is muscle fibre necrosis and regeneration with characteristic hypercontracted 'hyaline' fibres. Later there is fibre hypertrophy and splitting, increased central nucleation and eventually extensive fibrosis and fatty replacement. Fibre-type differentiation may be poor in ATPase preparations. Dystrophin immunocytochemistry shows loss of normal membrane immunoreactivity; in DMD there may be a complete absence of fibre staining apart from occasional positive fibres which have undergone somatic 'corrective' mutations (revertant fibres). In BMD a variety of immunocytochemical patterns may occur, including generalised reduced intensity of staining, discontinuous membrane immunoreactivity and variable immunoreactivity between fibres. It is important to use antibodies to different regions of the dystrophin molecule (rod domain, amino and carboxyl termini) otherwise some cases will be missed; use of a control antibody to spectrin is essential to confirm integrity of the sarcolemma. Also, it is important to note that a secondary reduction in dystrophin immunoreactivity may be seen in sarcoglycan-deficient limb-girdle muscular dystrophy. Antibodies to the rod and carboxyl domains also work in paraffin-embedded tissue following microwave antigen-retrieval. Myocardial fibrosis occurs in both BMD and DMD (Moriuchi et al. 1993) and Purkinje cell loss from the cerebellum may occur in DMD (Jagadha and Becker 1988).

**Fascioscapulohumeral Muscular Dystrophy.** A rare dominantly inherited dystrophy with onset in childhood or early adult life due to deletions on a gene localised to chromosomal region 4q35 whose product has not been characterised. Clinical presentation is with slowly progressive weakness, predominantly affecting facial, shoulder girdle and upper arm muscles. In addition there may be retinal microvascular abnormalities and mild sensorineural hearing loss. Involved muscle usually shows mild myopathic abnormalities, although endomysial inflammation is often a prominent feature.

**Limb-Girdle Muscular Dystrophy.** There are a number of different forms of limb-girdle muscular dystrophy (Bushby 1999), with onset varying from childhood to adulthood. Inheritance is usually autosomal recessive, but may be autosomal dominant. Progression is usually slow and creatine phosphokinase only mildly elevated. Muscle shows chronic myopathic changes. In some, usually the more severe childhood-onset cases with hypertrophic calf muscles, there may be loss of membrane sarcoglycan immunoreactivity. A minimum of two antibodies (to $\alpha$ and $\gamma$ sarcoglycans) should be used to exclude sarcoglycan deficiency. If a firm diagnosis has not been made in life, it is important to exclude spinal muscular atrophy, which may present with a similar clinical syndrome, by demonstrating the absence of fibre-type grouping on ATPase preparations (or by immunocytochemistry with antibodies to slow and fast myosin) and the absence of anterior horn cell loss in the spinal cord.

**Myotonic Dystrophy.** This dystrophy is a dominantly inherited condition, and one of a growing number of diseases associated with expansions of normally occurring trinucleotide repeat sequences, in this case in a gene encoding a protein kinase on chromosome 19. Patients have weakness, particularly in distal muscles, an inability to relax muscles after contraction (myotonia), frontal balding, cataracts, facial and sternomastoid wasting, ptosis, gonadal atrophy, diabetes, dysphagia and cardiac conduction defects, which may result in sudden death. Many have mild mental subnormality. Like most other trinucleotide disorders, the disease shows anticipation in succeeding generations (earlier onset and more severe), due to increase in length of the repeat sequence. A severe form which presents in infancy, with hypotonia and respiratory difficulties, is usually maternally inherited. Skeletal muscle shows mild chronic myopathic change, usually with a striking increase in numbers of internal nuclei (which form 'chains' in longitudinal sections), atrophy of type I fibres, ring fibres and increased numbers of fibres within muscle spindles, due to fibre splitting. Myocardial fibrosis also occurs. The brain shows abnormalities including tau-positive neurofibrillary tangles in the temporal lobe and olfactory bulbs (Kiuchi et al. 1991).

**Congenital Muscular Dystrophy.** This condition presents with neonatal hypotonia and developmental delay. Most cases have a good prognosis and muscle shows myopathic features with fibroadipose replacement. Occasional necrotic muscle fibres may be seen. There are, however, a number of different forms, some of which are associated with abnormalities of the central and peripheral nervous system. Cases in which merosin ($\alpha$-2-laminin) is absent from the sarcolemma have more severe features and white matter abnormalities in the brain.

There are many other muscular dystrophies including the distal muscular dystrophies, Emery-Dreifuss dystrophy (X-linked deficiency of the muscle protein emerin, resulting in a dystrophy associated with contractures and cardiac conduction defects), scapuloperoneal muscular dystrophy, oculopharyngeal muscular dystrophy and ocular muscular dystrophy.

### *2.6.3.3 Metabolic Myopathies*

Although, like muscular dystrophies, these disorders have an underlying genetic basis, they result in enzyme deficiencies or mitochondrial dysfunction, rather than loss of structural proteins and muscle fibre destruction. As a result, symptoms such as muscle fatigue, myalgia and cramps are the usual presenting features, instead of weakness. Some, for example myophosphorylase and carnitine palmitoyltransferase deficiency, may also be associated with episodes of acute rhabdomyolysis.

**Glycogen Storage Diseases.** These are rare defects of the glycolytic pathway, some of which result in the accumulation of glycogen in muscle, and are due to mutations in the genes encoding glycolytic enzymes. As both glycogen and glycolytic enzyme activity are not well preserved at autopsy, it is important to obtain muscle samples as soon as possible after death when investigating these disorders. The first described and best known is myophosphorylase deficiency (McArdle's disease), which usually presents in young adults with myalgia, premature fatigue and cramps on exercise and mild rhabdomyolysis with myoglobinuria. The muscle fibres show subsarcolemmal accumulation of glycogen with absent myophosphorylase activity. A number of mutations in the myophosphorylase gene have been described. Several other glycogen-associated enzyme deficiencies may result in similar features; however, in some of these disorders muscle weakness may be the predominant symptom, such as in acid maltase deficiency. In adults, acid maltase deficiency presents with a progressive proximal weakness, often with prominent respiratory muscle involvement. In infants, a more severe form occurs (Pompe's disease) with hypotonia, weakness, cardiomegaly, hepatomegaly, respiratory difficulties and an enlarged tongue; death usually occurs by the age of 2 years. In both forms, glycogen accumulates in vacuoles in muscle, much within lysosomes, but the changes are much more marked in the infantile form. Glycogen accumulation is also seen in cardiac and skeletal muscle. The spinal cord should be assessed at autopsy because of the suggestion of anterior horn cell involvement (Karpati et al. 1997).

**Disorders of Lipid Metabolism.** Long-chain fatty acids are utilised as a muscle energy source during prolonged exercise and fasting. Carnitine palmitoyltransferase deficiency leads to myalgia, weakness and rhabdomyolysis following prolonged exercise or fasting. This disorder usually presents in young men and skeletal muscle may appear normal or show a slight increase in neutral lipid. Carnitine deficiency on the other hand produces a myopathy with a striking increase in muscle lipid. It should be noted that lipid accumulation may also occur in a number of other disorders including steroid myopathy, alcoholic myopathy and the mitochondrial cytopathies.

**Mitochondrial Cytopathies.** Mitochondria are an important site of oxidative metabolism, producing ATP for muscle contraction. Mitochondria have their own DNA, which encodes for a number of mitochondrial proteins (the remainder being encoded by nuclear genes). Abnormalities of mitochondrial DNA result in a number of different clinical disorders which predominantly involve non-dividing cells including neurons and cardiac and skeletal muscle. Muscle symptoms include weakness, myalgia, cramps, ophthalmoplegia and ptosis. In the Kearns-Sayre syndrome in which deletions of mitochondrial DNA occur, there may be cerebellar ataxia, cardiac conduction defects, dementia, deafness, hypoparathyroidism, diabetes mellitus and short stature, in addition to muscle symptoms. Other syndromes include myoclonic epilepsy with ragged red fibres (MERRF), mitochondrial encephalopathy with lactic acidosis and stroke-like episodes (MELAS), neuropathy, ataxia and retinitis pigmentosa (NARP), due to different point mutations in the mitochondrial genome.

At autopsy it is important to sample the central and peripheral nervous system, cardiac and smooth muscle, endocrine organs, in addition to skeletal muscle, in order to properly assess the extent and pattern of the disease. Skeletal muscle shows mild myopathic changes, fibres with increased numbers of mitochondria, predominantly in a subsarcolemmal distribution ('ragged-red fibres') (Fig. 6) and cytochrome oxidase deficient fibres. Mitochondria show ultrastructural abnormalities which include pleomorphic forms, abnormal cristae, electron-dense bodies and paracrystalline inclusions; however, ultrastructural preservation of mitochondria is poor in postmortem tissue. Oxidative enzymes are usually well preserved even if autopsy has been delayed for several days after death. It should be remembered that mitochondrial changes in muscle are not diagnostic of mitochondrial disorders as they also occur in normal ageing, although not normally affecting

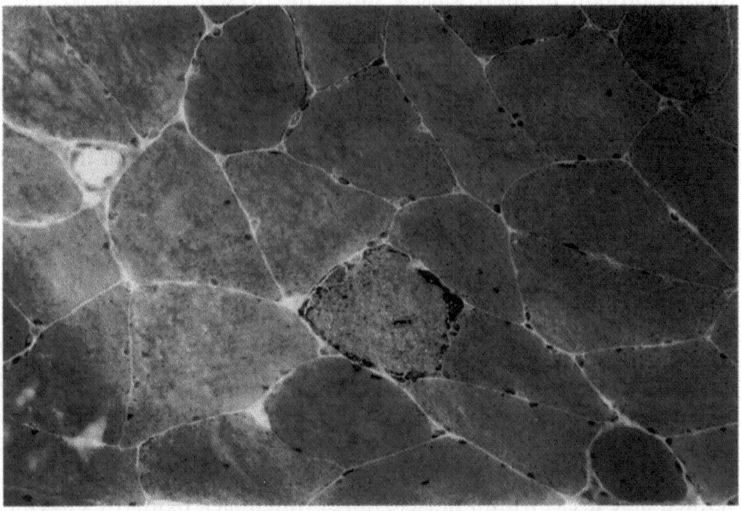

**Fig. 6.** Gomori trichrome preparation, which stains mitochondria red, showing a fibre with increased numbers of mitochondria. These 'ragged-red' fibres are numerous in mitochondrial myopathies, but may also be occasionally seen in other myopathies and normal muscle

more than 0.1% fibres. The brain may show infarct-like lesions in MELAS and myelin vacuolation in Kearns-Sayre syndrome.

**Myoadenylate Deaminase Deficiency.** This has been associated with muscle fatigue and rhabdomyolysis, but may occur in the absence of symptoms. The muscle shows a marked reduction in myoadenylate deaminase activity, but appears otherwise normal.

### *2.6.3.4 Congenital Myopathies*

Congenital myopathies are a group of either non-progressive or very slowly progressive myopathies which have characteristic histological or histochemical changes in skeletal muscle. They usually present in infancy with hypotonia, the 'floppy baby syndrome' or, later in childhood, with mild weakness. Rarely they may present in adulthood. Most have an underlying genetic basis.

**Nemaline Myopathy.** This usually presents in childhood with weakness, reduced muscle bulk and dysmorphic features including a long thin face and high arched palate. Cases sometimes present in adults, but there may be a history of weakness dating back to childhood. Some cases are progressive and a cardiomyopathy may occur. In adult-onset cases, an underlying immunodeficiency, including HIV infection, should be excluded. A severe form, presenting with hypotonia at birth, respiratory and swallowing difficulties, has a poor prognosis. Most cases have an autosomal dominant pattern of inheritance and are due to mutations in the gene encoding the muscle protein tropomyosin. Some cases, especially the severe infantile form, are autosomal recessive and due to mutations in the gene encoding another protein, nebulin. Muscle shows the presence of rod-like inclusions, which are most numerous in subsarcolemmal regions, and usually a type I fibre predominance. The inclusions are best seen with a Gomori trichrome preparation, where they appear as aggregates of small red structures, and are easy to identify in autopsy muscle. The rods are negative with histochemical preparations. Ultrastructural examination reveals rectangular structures with the characteristics of Z-discs. Consistent abnormalities of the peripheral or central nervous system have not been found at autopsy.

**Central Core Disease.** This is a dominantly inherited condition which presents with mildly delayed motor milestones in early childhood and may be associated with dislocation of the hip. The heart is unaffected in the majority of cases. In a minority of cases there is a susceptibility to malignant hyperthermia during anaesthesia. Central core disease (and some cases of malignant hyperthermia) is due to mutations in ryanodine receptor gene, which has roles during muscle maturation and in the release of sarcoplasmic calcium during contraction. Cores are sharply defined pale areas within muscle fibres which lack oxidative enzyme activity and are either central or subsarcolemmal. They run the length of the fibre and at ultrastructural examination either consist of intact myofibrils with focal Z-line streaming ('structured cores') or show extensive myofibrillar disarray and advanced

Z-line streaming ('unstructured cores'), although these ultrastructural features may be difficult to recognise in autopsy tissue. Central core disease should not be confused with another congenital myopathy, minicore disease, in which there are multiple short cores in each fibre, and cardiac conduction defects and cardiomyopathy may occur.

**Centronuclear Myopathy.** This condition is also known as myotubular myopathy because of the resemblance of fibres to foetal myotubules. The severe neonatal form is X-linked and due to mutations in the gene for the nuclear protein myotubularin. Infants may be dysmorphic with large heads, narrow faces and long digits; and polyhydramnios is common. There is generalised hypotonia, respiratory muscle weakness, ophthalmoplegia and ptosis. These cases have a poor prognosis and death usually occurs in the first year from respiratory muscle weakness. Less severe forms, that may be either recessively or dominantly inherited, present in later childhood or in adulthood with ophthalmoplegia and proximal limb- and facial-muscle weakness. Skeletal muscle shows type I fibre predominance, large numbers of central nuclei and reduced numbers of peripheral nuclei. There may be reduced ATPase and NADH activity in the central part of the muscle fibres, and type I fibre atrophy may be a prominent feature.

There are a large number of other congenital myopathies including congenital fibre-type disproportion and myopathies with distinctive structures at ultrastructural examination (e.g. 'finger-print' myopathy, 'zebra-body' myopathy, tubular aggregate myopathy), although diagnosis of these latter disorders may be difficult if there has been a long postmortem delay before sampling of the muscle.

Investigation of infants dying with the 'floppy-baby' syndrome should not be restricted to examination of skeletal muscle as a number of conditions affecting the central and peripheral nervous system may produce infantile hypotonia (Table 3).

**Table 3.** Causes of infantile hypotonia

| | |
|---|---|
| Central nervous system | Peripheral nerves |
| Cerebral palsy | Congenital hypomyelinating neuropathies |
| Cerebellar disease | Muscle |
| Spinal cord injury | Congenital myopathies |
| Spinal muscular atrophy | Congenital dystrophies |
| Polio | Metabolic myopathies |
| Tumours | Endocrine |
| | Hypothyroidism |
| Neuromuscular junction | |
| Neonatal myasthenia gravis | Benign congenital hypotonia |

### *2.6.3.5 Periodic Paralyses*

Periodic paralyses comprise a group of disorders characterised by episodes of flaccid paralysis which are usually associated with disturbances of serum potassium levels. There are two main forms: hypokalaemic, in which episodes may last for up to 3 days, and hyperkalaemic, in which episodes last less than 3 h. Both forms are inherited in a dominant manner and are due to mutations in calcium-channel and sodium-channel genes respectively. Occasional cardiac deaths have been reported in hyperkalaemic periodic paralysis. In both types, particularly during attacks, muscle fibres contain clear vacuoles that may contain faintly PAS-positive material. Episodes of weakness with muscle vacuolation may also be seen in hypokalaemia due to other causes and in association with thyrotoxicosis, especially in Japanese patients.

#### *2.6.3.6 Toxic and Drug-Induced Myopathies*

A number of drugs and toxins may cause extensive muscle necrosis (rhabdomyolysis) resulting in muscle pain, flaccid paralysis, elevated creatine phosphokinase, myoglobinuria and acute renal failure. Muscle shows fibre necrosis and regeneration, with little inflammation. A number of other acute muscle disorders may also lead to extensive fibre necrosis (see Table 4). Steroid use may result in progressive weakness associated with type IIb fibre atrophy. Penicillamine can result in an inflammatory myopathy or syndrome resembling myasthenia gravis and chloroquine can cause a vacuolar myopathy. Azidothymidine can cause a mitochondrial myopathy with 'ragged-red' fibres and paracrystalline mitochondrial inclusions, which usually improves on drug withdrawal.

Malignant hyperthermia may occur during or following general anaesthesia with halothane and suxamethonium in susceptibility individuals, and unless rapidly treated has a high mortality. Susceptibility to malignant hyperthermia is dominantly inherited, in some families due to mutations in the same gene that causes central core disease, the ryanodine receptor gene. Patients develop widespread muscle necrosis, and about half have an underlying myopathy with increased numbers of central nuclei, 'short' cores and 'moth-eaten' fibres. Central core disease is present only in a minority of cases.

Neuroleptic malignant syndrome is a rare and sometimes fatal complication of dopaminergic drugs such as chlorpromazine which results in hyperthermia, autonomic disturbance, muscle rigidity, dystonia and abnormal movements. Muscle shows extensive necrosis and regeneration. Purkinje cell loss has been reported in the cerebellum (LEE et al. 1989). This disorder may be associated with Lewy body dementia.

Critical illness neuromyopathy is a cause of severe weakness and poor recovery of patients in intensive care units. The aetiology is unknown, although non-depolarising neuromuscular blockers, steroids and sepsis have all been implicated. A variety of muscle changes have been described including widespread fibre atrophy with increased desmin immunoreactivity in atrophic fibres, loss of thick filaments at ultrastructural examination and fibre necrosis (HELLIWELL et al. 1998). There may also be an associated axonal polyneuropathy.

#### *2.6.3.7 Rhabdomyolysis*

Table 4 shows a variety of disorders that are associated with widespread necrosis of muscle fibres resulting in the release of enzymes, such as creatine kinase, and other relatively low molecular weight proteins such as myoglobin. This results in high creatine kinase levels in the serum and myoglobin escaping into the urine. Crystallisation of myoglobin within the kidney may result in acute renal failure.

**Table 4.** Causes of acute rhabdomyolysis

| |
|---|
| Drugs, e.g. clofibrate, lovastatin, emetine |
| Toxins, e.g. venoms, alcohol |
| Acute polymyositis |
| Viral myositis, e.g. influenza A, coxsackie virus |
| Crush injury, e.g. trauma, prolonged unconsciousness |
| High body temperature, e.g. heat stroke, malignant hyperpyrexia |
| Metabolic myopathies, e.g. carnitine palmitoyltransferase (CPT) deficiency, myophosphorylase deficiency |
| Severe exercise |

# 3 Peripheral Nerves

## 3.1 Sampling of Peripheral Nerves at Autopsy

Autopsy sampling of peripheral nerves will depend on the clinical features, but in many situations will include sampling of both proximal and distal nerves, and occasionally examination of autonomic nerves and nerve plexuses may be required. In general the more distal nerves are better preserved at autopsy and in many neuropathies, distal fibres in the limbs are more severely affected. There is a large amount of data on the range of changes in the normal population for the sural nerve, which is the most commonly sampled nerve during life. The sural nerve is therefore one of the nerves that can be sampled at autopsy. It is easy to locate as it runs between the lateral malleolus and Achilles tendon, usually immediately deep to the short saphenous vein (Fig. 7). The sural nerve is a pure sensory nerve so is of limited value in the assessment of predominantly motor neuropathies. Other nerves that are relatively easy to sample at autopsy and include both motor and sensory fibres are the femoral nerve in the upper thigh and the median, ulnar and radial nerves in the forearm. If there is autonomic involvement clinically then sampling of the cervical sympathetic trunk (deep to the carotid sheath), vagus nerve (along side the lower oesophagus) and prevertebral ganglia (overlying the upper abdominal aorta) should be undertaken. Nerve roots and plexuses should be examined when proximal disease is suspected (e.g. inflammatory demyelinating neuropathies) or there is specific plexus involvement (e.g. plexus neuropathies,

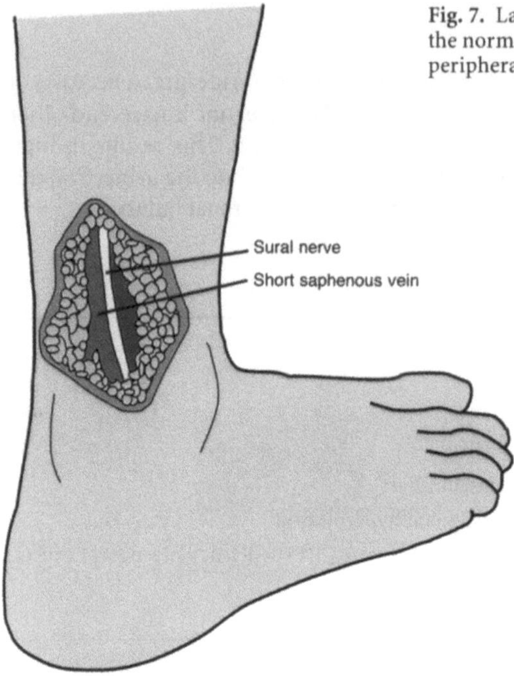


Fig. 7. Lateral aspect of the lower leg showing the normal site for sampling the sural nerve in peripheral neuropathies

traumatic damage). The spinal cord is often of value and if removed anteriorly by sawing through the anterior pedicles, also exposes the dorsal root ganglia. Examination of the spinal cord is required when there is prominent motor involvement to exclude anterior horn cell disease and also for the assessment of autonomic neurons in intermediolateral cell column. The dorsal root ganglia may show inflammation and neuronal loss especially in paraneoplastic neuropathies. Nerve conduction studies may indicate the best sites for sampling, particularly in asymmetric or multifocal neuropathies, and help in distinguishing axonal from demyelinating conditions.

## 3.2 Preparation of Tissue

When removing peripheral nerves it is very important to handle the samples very carefully prior to fixation because of their susceptibility to stretch and crush artefact which, if marked, may render the nerve useless for histology. At autopsy, several centimetres of nerve can be taken and roughly half fixed in glutaraldehyde, half in formalin and a small amount snap frozen in liquid nitrogen and stored frozen.

Peripheral nerves taken at autopsy can be prepared in a variety of ways, including embedding in epoxy resin or paraffin wax, frozen for cryostat sections or mounted as teased fibre preparations.

Epoxy resin embedding requires osmicated glutaraldehyde or formalin fixed pieces of nerve carefully prepared as blocks for transverse or longitudinal sections.

Teased fibre preparations can also be prepared from osmicated glutaraldehyde or formalin fixed material and then teased in liquid epoxy resin; permanent mounts can be prepared by hardening the resin. Alternatively, fibres can be teased in glycerine and either mounted wet or in glycerine jelly.

For autopsy nerves, embedding of nerve specimens in paraffin wax for transverse and longitudinal sections is probably the most rewarding. Care must be taken to always ensure that exact cross sections are cut, as the histology of peripheral nerves is difficult to evaluate in oblique sections. Cryostat sections can be obtained from snap frozen material or from formalin-fixed material that is subsequently frozen.

### 3.3 Histological Techniques

Although ideal for examination of nerve biopsies, 0.5-μm resin sections stained with toluidine blue may be difficult to evaluate in autopsy material due to the presence of postmortem artefact. Myelinated fibres become swollen and disrupted so that they obscure the fine details of the nerve. Nevertheless, much can be gained by examining exact cross-sections of resin-embedded material, particularly in estimating the degree of large myelinated fibre loss (Jacobs and Love 1985).

Osmicated teased fibre preparations are very valuable for detecting segmental demyelination in which short lengths of the fibre have lost myelin but retained the axon. Axonal degeneration with myelin ovoids and axonal regeneration with short internodes can be observed in teased preparations.

Perhaps the most useful general technique for postmortem nerves are transverse and longitudinal paraffin sections. Haematoxylin and eosin will reveal the general histological view of the nerve and is particularly useful for detecting inflammatory cells in the epineurium or perineurium, or for detecting abnormalities in vessels. Haematoxylin van Gieson will stain myelin black and Luxol fast blue, or the Klüver Barrera stain will identify the myelinated fibres as blue structures. Specific stains such as Congo red for amyloid and Ziehl-Neelsen for *Mycobacterium leprae* are ideally performed on paraffin sections. Immunocytochemistry for neurofilament protein is ideal for identifying and quantifying axons and S100 protein for locating Schwann cells. Myelin can be stained with antibodies against myelin basic protein and the perineurium expresses epithelial membrane antigen. Macrophages (CD68), lymphocyte subsets and immunoglobulins in myelin sheaths in paraproteinaemic neuropathies can also be identified by immunocytochemistry.

Frozen sections of peripheral nerve are particularly useful for detecting abnormalities of lipids in peripheral nerves and, in particular, lipid storage in metachromatic leukodystrophy by staining with cresyl violet.

### 3.4 Histology of Normal Peripheral Nerves

A normal nerve, such as the sural nerve, consists of several fascicles of nerve fibres, surrounded by perineurium and embedded in epineurial connective tissue and fat. Epineurial arteries receive segmental branches from adjacent arteries and several small veins are also seen in the epineurium. Within the perineurial sheath is the endoneurium, which contains myelinated nerve fibres, ranging in size from 2–17 μm in total diameter, with a peak of small myelinated fibres at 5 μm and of large myelinated fibres at 13 μm. There are large numbers of non-myelinated fibres in the endoneurium which are surrounded by Schwann cells but lack myelin sheaths; these are best seen in 0.5-μm resin-embedded sections and by electron microscopy, but they can be detected as very fine fibres by neurofilament protein immunocytochemistry. Surrounding each fibre is an S100-positive Schwann cell with a small number of fibroblasts present in the endoneurium. Between the myelinated and non-myelinated fibres, Schwann cells are longitudinally orientated bundles of collagen fibres embedded in a mucoprotein matrix. Fine capillaries are also seen within the endoneurium.

## 3.5 Clinical Features of Peripheral Nerve Diseases

Diseases of the peripheral nerve are characterised by muscle weakness and wasting, sensory disturbance or loss of sensation, especially distally in the limbs, and occasionally by autonomic disturbances.

Motor symptoms consist of weakness and muscle wasting and occasionally fasciculation in muscles close to the skin. Sensory symptoms, on the other hand, are characterised by loss of sensation such as light touch, pain, temperature and vibration. Light touch, proprioception and vibration are mediated by fast-conducting large myelinated fibres, whereas pain and temperature sensation involve small myelinated fibres and non-myelinated fibres. In addition to reduced sensation, paraesthesiae and pain may be present in peripheral neuropathies.

In addition to careful clinical examination for the identification of functional defects in peripheral nerves, electromyography is a valuable diagnostic tool, as it will detect denervation in muscle. Nerve-conduction studies are used to examine peripheral nerve function during life. Loss of axons in peripheral nerves may leave some of the fastest conducting fibres undamaged, so there may be little or no change in the recorded conduction velocities. In contrast, however, demyelination of fast conducting fibres reduces the conduction velocity of large myelinated fibres from 45–70 m/s to a velocity that is often below 20 m/s and may be unrecordable.

Particularly pertinent to the autopsy examination of peripheral nerves is the pattern of clinical involvement. Polyneuropathy is symmetrical with all limbs affected, whereas a mononeuritis may affect just one nerve or several nerves (mononeuritis multiplex). Sampling of peripheral nerves at autopsy should reflect the clinical distribution.

Autonomic neuropathies may be characterised by postural hypotension, tachycardia, impotence, incontinence or retention. Lack of sweating may also occur and wound healing in the skin may be delayed.

## 3.6 Pathology of Peripheral Nerves

### 3.6.1 General Pathological Reactions

Peripheral nerves show two major pathological reactions. These are axonal degeneration and segmental demyelination.

The majority of peripheral neuropathies (Table 5) are characterised by axonal degeneration in which the distal segment of the axon degenerates and the myelin forms ovoids that are eventually broken down by Schwann cells and macrophages. Soon after axonal transection, the distal end of the preserved proximal part of the nerve swells to form an axon balloon from which regenerating axons arise and grow along bands of Schwann cells left by the process of axonal degeneration. These 'bands of Büngner' may support several axons in a regenerating cluster that can be recognised histologically in cross sections of the peripheral nerve (Fig. 8). Axonal degeneration can be recognised in histological sections either by the absence of axons, a reduction in the number of myelinated nerve fibres, or by the presence of neutral lipid stainable by Sudan dyes or oil red O within the damaged nerve. Regeneration in peripheral nerves is very effective over short distances and as long as the integrity of the nerve bundle is maintained. An axonal reaction (chromatolysis) occurs in neuron cell bodies 8–10 days after axonal degeneration

**Table 5.** Peripheral polyneuropathies

| |
|---|
| Inherited |
| Hereditary sensory neuropathy (HSN) |
| Hereditary sensorimotor neuropathy (HSMN) |
| Amyloid |
| leukodystrophy |
| Porphyria |
| Refsum's disease |
| Metabolic |
| Diabetes mellitus |
| Vitamin deficiency |
| Uraemia |
| Toxic |
| Drugs |
| Toxins |
| Inflammatory |
| Guillain-Barré syndrome |
| Chronic inflammatory demyelinating neuropathy (CIDP) |
| Infective |
| Leprosy |
| HIV |
| CMV |
| Lyme disease |
| Diptheria |
| Vascular disease |
| Paraneoplastic |

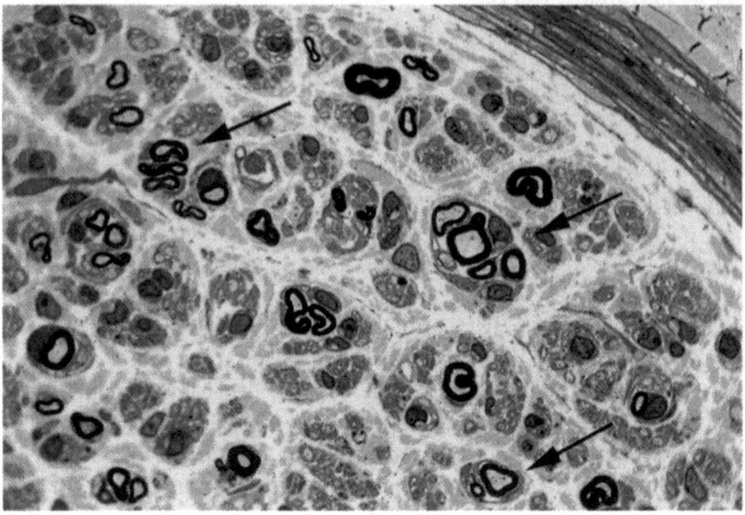

**Fig. 8.** Toluidine blue-stained resin section from an axonal neuropathy showing regeneration clusters (*arrows*)

commences; it is characterised by a loss of Nissl substance and an increase in polyribosomal RNA and by peripheral displacement of the nucleus and hypertrophy of the nucleolus. Segmental demyelination is a minor component of many neuropathies but is a major pathological feature of some hereditary motor and sensory neuropathies, chronic inflammatory demyelinating polyradiculopathy and diphtheritic neuropathy. In segmental demyelination, the axon remains intact but

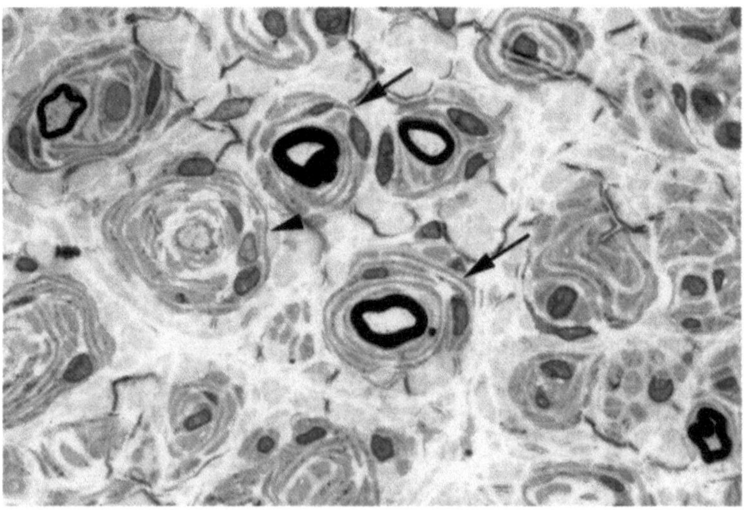

**Fig. 9.** Toluidine blue-stained resin section from a chronic demyelinating neuropathy (HMSN type I) showing concentric arrays of Schwann cells ('onion-bulb' formations) surrounding a demyelinated axon (*arrow head*) and remyelinated axons (*arrows*)

the myelin sheath is selectively damaged with loss of one or more segments myelinated by individual Schwann cells. Such pathology results in slowing of conduction across the demyelinated segment but remyelination begins within a few days and the myelin sheath may be quickly restored. In chronic demyelinating neuropathies, repeated episodes of segmental demyelination occur and result eventually in imbricated whorls of Schwann cells ('onion-bulb' formations) and enlargement of the nerves as hypertrophic neuropathy (Fig. 9). Segmental demyelination is best demonstrated in teased nerve fibres but histological sections and, in particular, 0.5-μm resin sections, often reveal large demyelinated axons. Remyelinating fibres can be identified as large axons with thin myelin sheaths.

### 3.6.2 Inherited Neuropathies

Hereditary sensory neuropathies present in infants and children with progressive distal sensory loss, sometimes with prominent autonomic disturbance. Nerves may show loss of small diameter sensory fibres and unmyelinated fibres. Inheritance can be dominant or recessive.

Hereditary motor and sensory neuropathies (HMSN) present in young adults with slowly progressive distal sensory loss and weakness. HMSN I (Charcot-Marie-Tooth disease/peroneal muscular atrophy) is dominantly inherited in most cases, due to duplication of the peripheral myelin protein (PMP-22) gene. Progression is slow leading to muscle wasting, pes cavus, scoliosis and thickened nerves. Nerves show widespread demyelination in childhood with hypertrophic changes becoming prominent during adolescence. An autopsy report described loss of anterior horn cells, dorsal root ganglia neurons and posterior column degeneration (Smith et al. 1980). HMSN II presents in a similar manner, although is less common than HMSN I, and nerves show a predominantly axonal changes. Hereditary neuropathy with liability to pressure palsies (HNPP) is a related disorder that presents with multiple nerve palsies at sites of pressure and in some a peripheral neuropathy. HNPP is dominantly inherited and due to a deletion of the PMP-22 gene. Nerves show variable demyelination and remyelination with numerous sausage-shaped enlargements of the myelin sheath (tomacula), which are best seen on teased fibre preparations. Severe, recessively inherited, forms of sensory and motor neuropathy which present in early childhood also occur.

Amyloid neuropathies may be either acquired, in association with light chain-associated systemic amyloidosis, or inherited due to mutations in the transthyretin gene. In both types, autonomic involvement may occur and there are multifocal amyloid deposits in nerve fascicles with axonal loss, particularly of non-myelinated and small myelinated fibres. Immunocytochemistry using antibodies to transthyretin and light chains may help in demonstrating the nature of the amyloid.

A number of rare inherited disorders including Fabry's disease, Krabbe's disease, metachromatic leucodystrophy, porphyria, Refsum's disease and Tangier disease also involve peripheral nerves.

### 3.6.3 Metabolic Neuropathies

Diabetes mellitus is commonly associated with a peripheral neuropathy, usually as a slowly progressive, symmetrical distal sensorimotor neuropathy. Autonomic involvement is common. Nerves show predominantly axonal changes and marked thickening of the basal lamina of perineurial cells and around small endoneurial blood vessels. Many other patterns can also occur (Thomas 1999) including a painful lower limb motor neuropathy and acute mononeuropathies, which are probably of vascular origin.

Vitamin deficiencies, particularly group B, in association with alcoholism may lead to distal axonal neuropathies. Vitamin $B_{12}$ deficiency causes a peripheral neuropathy, as well as subacute combined degeneration of the spinal cord. Vitamin E deficiency, for example in chronic liver disease, can also lead to both a peripheral neuropathy and tract degeneration in the spinal cord.

Uraemia leads to a distal symmetrical sensory and motor neuropathy. Cranial and autonomic nerves are usually spared. Distal nerves show predominantly axonal changes, proximal nerves are usually normal. Posterior column degeneration may be seen in the upper spinal cord.

### 3.6.4 Toxic Neuropathies

Numerous drugs and chemical toxins can cause peripheral nerve damage. Most cause a distal, predominantly axonal, neuropathy and examples include vincristine, izoniazid, metronidazole, acrylamide, organophosphates and the anti-HIV drugs, zalcitabine and stavudine. Lead toxicity may result in a mononeuropathy with wrist or foot drop and may have a demyelinating component.

### 3.6.5 Inflammatory Neuropathies

Guillain-Barré syndrome is an immune-mediated, acute ascending paralytic condition, usually progressing over days. Most cases follow an acute viral illness and more than 75% make a full recovery. Investigations usually reveal reduced nerve conduction velocity and increased protein in CSF. It is an immune-mediated post-infectious process which affects predominantly proximal peripheral nerves and nerve roots as a multifocal inflammatory demyelinating process. Autopsy examination should include brainstem and spinal cord for assessment of proximal nerve roots and, particularly if motor features are prominent, to exclude anterior horn cell disease.

Chronic inflammatory demyelinating polyradiculopathy (CIDP) evolves more slowly, over a period of several weeks, with a symmetric polyradiculopathy and polyneuropathy affecting both motor and sensory fibres. Recovery is slow and often incomplete. Postmortem cases of remitting CIDP show multifocal, predominantly proximal demyelinating disease affecting spinal roots, spinal nerves, major plexuses and elsewhere in the peripheral nervous system. Segmental demyelination, onion bulbs and some axonal loss are seen together with scattered lymphocytic infiltrates in the endoneurium and epineurium. Within the CNS there may be loss of myelin in the posterior columns and chromatolysis of the anterior horn and intermediolateral cell columns. More distal nerves such as the sural nerves, may also show demyelination.

### 3.6.6 Neuropathies Associated with Infectious Agents

Leprosy, although rare in the UK, is the most common cause of peripheral neuropathy world-wide. In tuberculoid leprosy there are well-defined areas of sensory loss with thickening of underlying nerves and an intense granulomatous inflammatory reaction in the skin and cutaneous nerves, with few organisms. Lepromatous leprosy results in larger areas of sensory loss and nerves show infiltration by foamy macrophages and numerous bacilli in Schwann cells and macrophages.

HIV infection can be associated with acute and chronic inflammatory demyelinating neuropathies, particularly early in the disease, vasculitic neuropathy and in late disease, a chronic axonal sensory neuropathy. An inflammatory neuropathy due to cytomegalovirus (CMV) also occurs in the late stages of acquired immunodeficiency syndrome (AIDS), in which CMV inclusions may be seen in Schwann cells and in vascular endothelium. CMV may also involve nerve roots and the lower spinal cord.

Lyme disease causes an inflammatory neuropathy but *Borrelia* spirochaetes cannot usually be identified in the nerves.

Diphtheria toxin causes a severe demyelinating, predominantly motor, neuropathy.

### 3.6.7 Vascular Disease

Peripheral neuropathy is common in the elderly and it is also seen in association with peripheral vascular disease. Accompanying muscle infarction in patients with intermittent claudication and pain in the calf muscles are the histological features of denervation, suggesting that vascular damage to limb nerves is as common as vascular damage to muscle (Clyne et al. 1982).

Vasculitis involves peripheral nerves in many cases, usually producing multiple nerve palsies (mononeuritis multiplex), but sometimes a symmetric polyneuropathy. Vasculitis may be part of a systemic disorder such as polyarteritis nodosa, rheumatoid arthritis and Wegener's granulomatosis, or occur as an isolated peripheral nerve vasculitis. In most cases there is involvement of epineurial arteries and florid acute Wallerian degeneration of nerve fibres. Extensive sampling of both peripheral nerves and other tissues including muscle should be undertaken at autopsy.

### 3.6.8 Paraneoplastic Neuropathy

Clinical neuropathy occurs in about 5% of patients with malignancy, although subclinical involvement is more common. Most common is sensorimotor neuropathy that may be either rapidly or slowly progressive. Nerves may show both axonal and demyelinating changes, occasionally with inflammatory cell infiltrates. A subacute sensory neuropathy which progresses over weeks with sensory ataxia, paraesthesia and limb pain may present before the tumour is apparent, particularly in association with small-cell carcinoma of the lung. There may be an associated paraneoplastic encephalopathy, particularly in association with a sensory neuropathy. Nerves may show extensive fibre loss and ongoing Wallerian degeneration. The spinal cord may show posterior column degeneration and there may be loss of dorsal root ganglionic cells with perivascular inflammatory cell infiltrates. Inflammation within the brain stem and cerebral hemispheres and Purkinje cell loss may be seen if there is CNS involvement. Rarely vasculitic neuropathies and acute Guillain-Barré syndrome have been described in patients with malignancies. Direct tumour infiltration of peripheral nerves and roots most often occurs in association with non-Hodgkin's lymphoma. Presentation is variable, but often pain is a feature.

### 3.6.9 Neuropathies Associated with Paraproteins

Some patients with paraproteinaemias, particularly of the IgM type, develop a sensorimotor neuropathy due to cross reactivity between the immunoglobulin and myelin proteins. Immunoglobulin is deposited in peripheral nerve myelin sheaths and there is a demyelinating and axonal neuropathy with characteristic separation of myelin lamellae at electron microscopy. Patients may have either a benign monoclonal gammopathy or malignant plasma cell proliferation.

## 4 Conclusions

The study of muscle and nerve disease at autopsy has many advantages over investigating these diseases during life. More adequate sampling can be obtained giving a clearer picture of the clinicopathological correlation. In the majority of muscle diseases, the proximal limb muscles are more affected than the distal muscles, whereas in peripheral nerve diseases, the distal nerves are more involved than the proximal. Different phases of the disease process, from mild to severe can be assessed by studying tissue samples from a variety of proximal and distal sites.

In addition to sampling clinically involved muscles and nerves, muscles or nerves that can be visualised by imaging, but are not available for biopsy during life, can be very fruitfully examined at autopsy. Finally, although the techniques of enzyme histochemistry, transmission electron microscopy, and some genetic studies may be somewhat limited in autopsy material, more adequate study of different nerves and muscle and different parts of the same nerve and muscle is only possible at autopsy. Changes in nerves and muscles can also be correlated with those in other organs.

## References

Askanas V, Bilak M, Engel WK, Alvarez RB, Tome F, Leclerc A (1993) Prion protein is abnormally accumulated in inclusion-body myositis. Neuro Report 5:25–28

Basset-Seguin N, Roujeau JC, Gherardi R, Guillaume JC, Reuz J, Touraine R (1990) Prognostic factors and predictive signs of malignancy in adult dermatomyosis. A study of 32 cases. Arch Dermatol 126:633–637

de Boni U, Lenczner MM, Scott JW et al. (1977) Autopsy of an Egyptian mummy (Nakht – Rom1). Can Med Assoc J 117:461–476

Bushby KM (1999) Making sense of the limb-girdle muscular dystrophies. Brain 122:1403–1420

Clyne CA, Weller RO, Bradley WG, Silber DI, O'Donnell TF, Callow AD (1982) Histochemical and capillary adaptation of gastrocnemius muscle to occlusive peripheral vascular disease. Surgery 92:434–440

Haupt HM, Hutchins GM (1982) The heart and cardiac conduction system in polymyositis-dermatomyositis: a clinicopathologic study of 16 autopsied patients. Am J Cardiol 50:998–1005

Heads T, Pollock M, Robertson A et al. (1991) Sensory nerve pathology in amyotrophic lateral sclerosis. Acta Neuropathol 82:316–320

Helliwell TR, Wilkinson A, Griffiths RD, McClelland P, Palmer TEA, Bone JM (1998) Muscle fibre atrophy in critically ill patients is associated with the loss of myosin filaments and the presence of lysosomal enzymes and ubiquitin. Neuropathol Appl Neurobiol 24:507–517

Jacobs JM, Love S (1985) Qualitative and quantitative morphology of human sural nerve at different ages. Brain 108:897–924

Jagadha V, Becker LE (1988) Brain morphology in Duchenne muscular dystrophy: a Golgi study. Pediatr Neurol 4(2):87–92

Johnson MA, Plogar J, Weightman D, Appleton D (1973) Data on the distribution of fibre types in thirty-six human muscles: An autopsy study. J Neurol Sci 18:111–129

Karpati G, Carpenter S, Eisen A, Aube M, DiMauro S (1977) The adult form of acid maltase deficiency. Ann Neurol 1:276–280

Kiuchi A, Otusuka N, Namba Y, Nakano I, Tomonaga M (1991) Presenile abundant Alzheimer neurofibrillary tangles without senile plaques in the brain in myotonic dystrophy. Acta Neuropathol 82:1–5

Lee S, Merriam A, Kim TS, Liebling M, Dickson DW, Moore GR (1989) Cerebellar degeneration in neuroleptic malignant syndrome: neuropathologic findings and review of the literature concerning heat-related nervous system injury. J Neurol Neurosurg Psychchiatry 52:387–391

Moriuchi T, Kagawa N, Mukoyama M, Hizawa K (1993) Autopsy analyses of the muscular dystrophies. Tokushima J Exp Med 40:83–93

Plotz PH, Dalakas M, Leff RL, Love LA, Miller FW, Cronin ME (1989) Current concepts in the idiopathic inflammatory myopathies: polymyositis, dermatomyositis and related disorders. Ann Int Med 111(2):143–157

Smith TW, Bhawan J, Keller RB, De Girolami U (1980) Carcot-Marie-Tooth disease associated with hyperytrophic neuropathy. A neuropathologic study of two cases. J Neuropathol Exp Neurol 39:420–440

Thomas PK (1999) Diabetic neuropathy: mechanisms and future treatment options. J Neurol Neurosurg Psychiatry 67:277–279

## Useful Textbooks

Thomas PK, Landon DN, King RHM (1997) Diseases of peripheral nerves. Weller RO, Cumming WJK, Mahon M. Diseases of muscle. In: Graham DI, Lantos PL (eds) Greenfield's neuropathology, 6th edn. Arnold
Midrioni G, Bilbao JM (1995) Biopsy diagnosis of peripheral neuropathy. Butterworth-Heinemann
Mastaglia FL, Walton JN (1992) Skeletal muscle pathology, 2nd edn. Churchill Livingstone
Swash M, Schwartz MS (1991) Biopsy pathology of muscle, 2nd edn. Chapman & Hall

## Useful Internet Sites

The National Center for Biotechnical Information has a well referenced and constantly updated summary of many inherited disorders at: http://www.ncbi.nlm.nih.gov/omin/

The Washington University Neuromuscular Disease Center has a very up to date synopsis of many neuromuscular disorders which includes clincal features, differential diagnoses, pathology, genetic and biochemical changes at: http://www.neuro.wustl/edu/neuromuscular/index.html

# Lymphoma and the Nervous System

D. W. Ellison, B. S. Wilkins



## 1 Introduction

This chapter considers the cellular pathologist's perspective of the patient whose nervous system is affected by malignant lymphoma. This perspective is mainly gained through the assessment of surgical biopsies or cytological preparations, which are obtained from sites within or outside the central nervous system (CNS). But it is also influenced by postmortem findings, notably histological examination of the fixed brain in disorders that pose a significant diagnostic challenge, such as intravascular large-cell lymphoma.

Lymphoma is most often encountered in the nervous system when it spreads there from another site, to be termed secondary CNS lymphoma (SCNSL). However, primary central nervous system lymphoma (PCNSL) does occur, despite an absence of lymphoid tissue in the CNS, and its variants form an important group among the extra-nodal non-Hodgkin's lymphomas (NHL). The classification and origins of PCNSL have aroused considerable scientific interest. In particular, re-

Current Topics in Pathology, Vol. 95
S. Love (Ed.): Neuropathology

search has attempted to address the ontogenetic relationship between PCNSL and other NHL [70, 80, 113, 126].

In addition to the detrimental mass effect of tumour located around or within the nervous system, lymphomas can produce paraneoplastic neurological syndromes, in which either CNS or peripheral nervous system may be affected. These syndromes have an immunogenic basis, and are unrelated to the presence of tumour within the nervous system. Aside from classifying the systemic lymphoma, the cellular pathologist's involvement in such cases is usually limited to postmortem examination of the brain, spinal cord or peripheral nerves.

Optimal evaluation of the patient with a neurological syndrome and known or suspected lymphoma requires a multidisciplinary approach. It is obvious that discussion of the patient's condition by clinician and pathologist facilitates the diagnostic process. Clinical assessment of symptoms and signs usually precedes a range of imaging techniques, and the cellular pathologist becomes involved when tissue is submitted for examination. Tissue is usually derived from a mass discovered clinically or during imaging studies. However, the evaluation of a neurological syndrome associated with lymphoma may involve sural nerve biopsy or cytological examination of the CSF or rarely the vitreous of the eye. Staff involved in obtaining samples must ensure that they reach the laboratory in a suitable condition for a range of analytic techniques.

The following sections cover classification and the processing of tissue for analysis, PCNSL, SCNSL and paraneoplastic syndromes.

## 2 Lymphoma Classification

Terminology used to describe lymphoid neoplasms continues to evolve as understanding of normal and neoplastic lymphoid cell behaviour increases. In 1994, a considerable advance in classification occurred with the publication of the Revised European-American Lymphoma (REAL) proposals [61]. This classification categorised lymphomas, as far as possible, into clinicopathologically relevant entities. The requirement for consideration of clinical features, immunophenotype and genetic analysis, in addition to descriptive morphological characteristics, was acknowledged for the first time by the REAL classification. With rapidly increasing knowledge of the molecular genetic basis of many lymphomas, the REAL classification has now been modified by a WHO working party of haematopathologists, assisted by a clinical advisory committee. The newly proposed WHO classification [60] encompasses the principles of the REAL system and provides flexibility to incorporate future developments, particularly in the field of molecular genetic analysis.

The REAL classification was the first to recognise the distinctive clinicopathological features of several types of extranodal lymphomas, and this recognition has been maintained within the WHO system. Extranodal marginal zone B-cell lymphomas of the gastro-intestinal tract, derived from mucosa-associated lymphoid tissue (MALT), are perhaps the best known of these extranodal lymphomas. It could be argued that diffuse large B-cell lymphomas (DLC-B) arising in the CNS, the most prevalent form of PCNSL, should be recognised as a distinct group of extranodal lymphomas, as should primary testicular DLC-B. However, all DLC-B in the REAL and WHO classifications are grouped together into a single category, regardless of nodal or extranodal origin. The WHO haematopathologists have acknowledged that this may require modification in future. However, at present, it is unclear on what basis biologically relevant subtypes of DLC-B can be defined.

A further refinement of lymphoma classification offered by the WHO is specific categorisation of lymphomas associated with human immunodeficiency virus (HIV) infection. A significant proportion of DLC-B presenting as PCNSL arise in the context of HIV infection or the acquired immunodeficiency syndrome (AIDS). Rarely, PCNSL may also arise in inherited immunodeficiency states or associated with acquired immunodeficiency unrelated to HIV infection (e.g. post-transplantation and in other patients receiving immunosuppressive therapy).

## 3 Processing Tissue from Suspected CNS Lymphomas for Analysis

Haematopathologists are often envious of the consistency with which most neuropathologists obtain CNS biopsy samples promptly and unfixed from their neurosurgical colleagues. This culture of handling fresh tissue is a great bonus for the diagnosis of lymphoma, whether suspected before the sample was collected or only recognised later, once initial tissue sections have been examined histologically. Prompt receipt of fresh tissue allows fixation to be arranged under optimal conditions in the pathology department. In most cases, a small portion of tissue is examined rapidly in frozen sections and/or smear preparations; if lymphoma is suspected at this stage, cells can be dispersed from a portion of the tissue for fluorescent immunocytochemistry by flow cytometry. This technique allows rapid demonstration of a wide range of antigens in lymphoid cells. Such cells can also be investigated by cytogenetic analysis. If sufficient tissue is available for cryostorage, DNA and RNA analyses are possible retrospectively.

Even if there is insufficient tissue for such investigations, rapid fixation of small biopsy samples generally preserves DNA well for molecular genetic analysis following polymerase chain reaction (PCR) amplification. Well-fixed small biopsy samples generally permit good-quality histology and are very satisfactory for immunohistochemical staining. Antigen retrieval techniques involving proteolysis or modifications of wet-heat exposure may be required for successful immunohistochemistry, depending on the antigens studied. However, these requirements are similar to those for other fixed tissues and there are no limitations specific to CNS tissue. The possibility of unexpected antibody cross-reactivity with neural or glial cells should always be borne in mind.

At postmortem examination, it has been usual for suspected CNS pathology to be examined after prolonged formalin fixation of the intact brain. This approach allows the macroscopic appearances of tumours such as lymphomas to be examined optimally and provides tissue for high quality histological sections [97]. However, prolonged fixation means that parameters for antigen retrieval prior to immunohistochemistry are altered. In generally, longer proteolysis or longer exposure to wet heat is required to achieve equivalent immunohistochemical results to those obtained with rapidly fixed tissues. Unfortunately, DNA and RNA are poorly preserved by the prolonged, slow fixation achieved by immersion of the intact brain in formalin. Perfusion fixation provides one means to increase the rate of formalin penetration, but no data exist to demonstrate whether this yields nucleic acids of satisfactory quality for molecular genetic studies.

A satisfactory compromise in cases of suspected CNS lymphoma may be to slice the brain while fresh and sample areas of tumour and standard reference areas. Although macroscopic information will be less accurate, fixation will be superior and investigations such as immunohistochemistry and molecular genetic analysis will be possible without additional technical modifications. This approach to the sampling of brain tissue in suspected lymphoma may also be more acceptable to the next-of-kin at a time of increasing public sensitivity about the retention of organs at postmortem examination.

Immunohistochemistry is needed in all cases of suspected involvement of the CNS by lymphoma. It is required to determine the lymphoid nature of neoplastic cells, to assign the lymphoma to its correct lineage (B cell, T cell or other) and to provide information of potential prognostic importance. At present, prognostic use of immunohistochemistry is much more advanced in node-based lymphomas than in PCNSL, but this area of knowledge is advancing rapidly. In the assessment of PCNSL, it is currently important to document the presence or absence of antigen-expression patterns known to be of prognostic importance in nodal NHL. Only by accumulating this information and correlating it with clinical outcome data in large series of patients will it be possible to determine whether it has similar value in predicting outcome in PCNSL as in non-CNS lymphomas. In addition, in the assessment of PCNSL from any patient suspected of having underlying immunodeficiency, it is important to establish whether or not neoplastic lymphoid cells harbour latent infection with Epstein-Barr virus (EBV). This can be done by immunohistochemistry for EBV latent membrane protein-1 (LMP-1) and Epstein-Barr virus nuclear antigen-2 (EBNA-2). In laboratories able to offer mRNA in situ hybridisation, demonstration of Epstein-Barr virus early RNA species (EBER) by this method is currently the most sensitive way of demonstrating the presence of EBV in fixed histological material. In fresh or frozen samples, EBV DNA can be studied by Southern blot analysis, and clonality of the viral infection can be demonstrated. There is ongoing controversy as to whether EBV latent infection is also associated with PCNSL in fully immunocompetent individuals. As a counsel of perfection, it would be desirable to investigate EBER expression in all large B-cell PCNSL until sufficient experience is accumulated to prove or disprove a role for EBV in this lymphoma in immunocompetent patients. There are also published claims that the Kaposi's sarcoma-associated virus, human herpesvirus 8 (HHV8), has been demonstrated in a proportion of PCNSL in HIV-positive and HIV-negative individuals [6, 31]. These data have technical limitations and are contradictory; it remains to be determined whether HHV8 has a role in the pathogenesis of PCNSL.

Table 1 contains details of useful antibodies for immunohistochemistry in suspected PCNSL.

Molecular genetic studies are of most value in small biopsies that allow only limited morphological and immunohistochemical interpretation. In general, PCR amplification of frozen or fixed tissue sections is practised to maximise the amount of DNA template available. The presence of a monoclonal lymphoid cell population

**Table 1.** Antibodies used in the assessment of CNS lymphomas

| Antigen | Antibody | Specificity | Comments |
|---|---|---|---|
| CD45 | PD7/26 | Cells of lymphoid and myeloid origin | |
| CD20 | L26 | Most B cells | Absent from some primitive B cells and down-regulated in plasma cells |
| CD79a | Mb1, HM47/A9 | Most B cells | Expressed by more primitive cells than CD20 and in plasma cells. Some neoplastic plasma cells are negative. |
| CD5 | 4C7 | Most T cells; subset of B cells | Expressed by neoplastic B cells of CLL and MCL, plus rare DLC-B |
| CD23 | 1B12 | Follicular dendritic cells and subset of B cells | Expressed by neoplastic B cells of CLL |
| CD10 | 56C6 | Subset of B cells | Expressed by germinal centre B cells, in Burkitt's lymphoma and in a proportion of DLC-B |
| Terminal deoxynucleotidyl transferase (TdT) | NPT26 | Primitive lymphoid cells | Expressed in most cases of B- or T-ALL and in occasional cases of AML |
| P63 (rough endoplasmic reticulum-associated protein) | VS38c | Plasma cells | Expressed in most cases of plasma cell neoplasia. Other cell types with high content of RER may be positive |
| CD138 | B-B4 | Plasma cells | Expressed in most plasma cell neoplasms; also in some DLC-B and non-lymphoid tumours. |
| Epithelial membrane antigen (EMA) | GP1.4 | Plasma cells | Many neoplastic plasma cells are negative |
| Kappa light chain | Polyclonal antisera | Plasma cells (cytoplasmic) | Some lymphomas without plasma cell differentiation may have detectable membrane expression |
| Lambda light chain<br>Mu heavy chain<br>Gamma heavy chain<br>Delta heavy chain<br>Alpha heavy chain<br>Cyclin D1 | DCS-6, P2D11F11 | B cells of mantle-cell lymphoma | Up to 20% of cases of MCL are negative; occasional other B cell NHL are +ve |
| BCL2 | 124, BCL2/100 | T cells, mantle B cells, neoplastic germinal centre lymphoid cells, and many cases of DLC-B | Expression in DLC-B may be of prognostic importance (see text) |
| BCL6 | P1F6, PG-B6p | Germinal centre cells and some cases of DLC-B | Expression in DLC-B may be of prognostic importance (see text) |

**Table 1** (continued)

| Antigen | Antibody | Specificity | Comments |
|---|---|---|---|
| CD3 | CD3–12 | Most T cells | |
| CD45RO | UCHL1, OPD4 | Antigen-experienced T cells | OPD4 has less reactivity with myelomonocytic cells such as reactive macrophages |
| CD43 | MT1, DFT1 | Most T cells; subset of B cells | Strong expression by myelomonocytic cells |
| CD4 | 1F6 | Helper T-cell subset | Cross-reactivity with macrophages |
| CD8 | 4B11 | Cytotoxic/suppressor T-cell subsets | |
| CD56 | 1B6 | Natural killer cells and some cytotoxic T cells | Cross-reactivity with neurones and neuro-ectodermal cells |
| CD57 | Leu7 | | |
| Anaplastic lymphoma-associated kinase (ALK) | ALK-1 | Cells of anaplastic large-cell lymphoma (nuclear and/or cytoplasmic location) | Most paediatric cases are positive; a higher proportion of adult cases are negative |
| Epithelial membrane antigen (EMA) | E29 | Cells of anaplastic large-cell lymphoma | Cross-reactive with cells of many carcinomas |
| CD30 | BerH2 | Cells of anaplastic large-cell lymphoma and Reed-Sternberg cells in Hodgkin's lymphoma | Cross-reactive with cells of some malignant germ cell tumours, particularly embryonal carcinomas |
| CD15 | LeuM1 | Reed-Sternberg cells of Hodgkin's lymphoma | Cross-reactive with myelomonocytic cells |
| Ki67 | MIB-1, MM1 | Proliferating cells (nuclear expression) | |
| p53 | DO-7 | Cells with mutant p53 genes or with excess expression of wild-type p53 | Expressed in many DLC-B, high grade T-cell lymphomas, some astrocytic tumours and some carcinomas |
| LMP-1 | CS1–4 | Cells with latent EBV infection (cytoplasmic and membrane expression) | Expressed in cases of lymphoma associated with EBV latency, especially in immunosuppressed patients |
| EBNA-2 | PE2 | Cells with latent EBV infection (nuclear expression) | |

can be inferred if clonal products are obtained using primer pairs specific for selected immunoglobulin heavy chain gene or T-cell receptor gene sequences. There is a theoretical risk of obtaining a false positive result if very few lymphoid cells are present in the starting material but, in practice, we have not encountered this problem with CNS biopsy material. A problem that does occur, however, is the detection of a monoclonal T-cell receptor gene rearrangement in a lymphoid infiltrate that appears to have a B-cell immunophenotype. Molecular genetic clonality analysis of the type described above does not assign neoplastic lymphoid cells accurately to T- or B-cell lineages; approximately 10% of B-cell lymphomas show T-cell receptor gene rearrangements and vice versa [132]. In some cases, monoclonal PCR products will be obtained with both T-cell receptor and immunoglobulin heavy chain gene primers in a single neoplasm. Molecular genetic analyses and the interpretation of their results should always be undertaken by fully trained, experienced technical staff in laboratories specialised to perform this work, and should be interpreted with expert assistance. Future use of molecular genetic analysis is certain to increase as the molecular processes underlying lymphoma development and progression are revealed. Detection of gene rearrangements, such as those involving BCL1, BCL2 and ALK genes, is becoming increasingly important in the assessment of systemic lymphomas. It may only be a short time before specific genetic abnormalities associated with PCNSL become known.

## 4 Primary CNS Lymphoma

Primary CNS lymphomas (PCNSLs) are extranodal lymphomas that present with neurological disease in the absence of tumour outside the brain, spinal cord, meninges or retina and vitreous of the eye [65, 68, 88, 101, 127].

### 4.1 Background

The distinction between PCNSLs and other primary CNS tumours of neuro-epithelial lineage was first made during early attempts at the histological classification of brain tumours in the first half of the twentieth century. At that time, PCNSL was labelled 'perithelial sarcoma' to reflect a striking relationship between the tumour cells and the perivascular spaces of the brain [20]. Derivation of these tumours from lymphoid cells was not considered because no lymphoid cells normally reside in the CNS. Later, following the use of silver stains on these tumours, attention was focused on a possible relationship between PCNSL and microglia [116]. Native microglia and a population of cells within PCNSL showed a similar staining pattern with silver impregnation. Derivation from microglia was inferred, leading to the label 'microglioma'. However, an alternative viewpoint regarded the silver-positive cells within PCNSL as a reactive population of microglia, and preferred the term 'reticulum cell sarcoma'. In time, and with the benefit of electron microscopy, the similarities between PCNSL and NHL outside the CNS became evident, this relationship being reinforced by the advent of immunohistochemistry.

## 4.2 Epidemiological Aspects

Rising steadily, the incidence of PCNSL has tripled over the last 20 years [3,32,82,118]. Several factors account for this, including increased recognition of the disease and the increased incidence of HIV infection, PCNSL being associated with immunocompromised states [33, 44, 53]. A tissue diagnosis is made more frequently because developments in surgical technique, particularly the introduction of stereotactic guidance for needle biopsy, have encouraged neurosurgeons to operate on an older population of patients with intracranial tumours. Also, PCNSL is increasingly recognised by histopathologists, helped by the use of a continuously expanding range of immunohistochemistry. The association between PCNSL and immunosuppression has contributed significantly to its increased incidence. The contribution from a burgeoning programme of transplant surgery [2, 59], with which PCNSL was traditionally associated, has been supplemented in the past 20 years by its occurrence in association with HIV infection and the acquired immunodeficiency syndrome (AIDS).

Current data indicate that PCNSL accounts for 2%–3% of primary intracranial tumours and approximately 1% of all NHL. PCNSL is a tumour of adults; very few examples have been documented in children. More males than females (3:2) are affected. The median age at presentation is different in the non-immunocompromised (59 years) and AIDS (38 years) groups. PCSNL occurs in 3%–12% of patients with AIDS. Presentation with PCNSL may precede the development of AIDS in HIV-infected individuals and, as mortality from opportunistic infections in Western patients with AIDS is falling, mortality due to PCNSL is rising. Several immunodeficiency states other than AIDS are associated with PCNSL (Table 2) but these, by virtue of their rarity, contribute few cases to the overall total.

**Table 2.** Immunodeficiency states associated with PCNSL

| |
|---|
| Primary immunodeficiency syndromes |
| Severe combined immunodeficiency |
| Wiskott-Aldrich syndrome |
| Ataxia-telangiectasia |
| X-linked lymphoproliferative syndrome |
| Secondary Immunodeficiency syndromes |
| HIV infection |
| Therapy after organ transplantation |
| Hodgkin's disease (probably therapeutic immunosuppression) |
| Auto-immune disorders – Sjögren's syndrome, systemic lupus erythematosus |

## 4.3 Clinical Aspects

PCNSL occurs throughout the neuraxis [39, 64]. Symptoms and signs reflect the location and extent of the tumour, and usually manifest as neurological deficits, such as weakness due to hemiparesis. In contrast, epilepsy may be the presenting problem. A single tumour mass is responsible for the clinical presentation in 60% of cases, but multifocal pathology, sometimes including leptomeningeal involvement, is responsible for the remainder. Spread to the subarachnoid space produces non-specific meningeal symptoms, including meningism.

Neuro-imaging, cytological examination of the lumbar cerebrospinal fluid (if not contra-indicated by raised intracranial pressure) and biopsy are central to the investigation of PCNSL. In many areas of the brain invaded by PCNSL, a computerised tomography (CT) scan shows a homogeneous enhancement with contrast [69]. Unlike the slightly irregular 'ring enhancement' shown by a glioblastoma, PCNSL usually demonstrates an extensive area of enhancement. Peritumoral oedema is generally less than with other tumours, such as metastatic carcinoma. In patients with AIDS, no imaging appearance can reliably distinguish PCNSL and encephalitis, for example due to toxoplasmosis, but bilateral altered signals in subependymal regions strongly suggest PCNSL.

A positive examination of the lumbar CSF for tumour cells confirms spread to the subarachnoid space. Cytological evaluation may allow classification of the lymphoma; immunophenotyping of tumour cells aids this process.

Careful consideration must be given to extracranial staging procedures in patients with suspected PCNSL, since some may in fact have secondary CNS involvement by lymphoma in which systemic disease is occult [94]. Recommended staging includes full clinical examination, CT of the chest, abdomen and pelvis, and bone marrow examination by both aspiration and trephine biopsy plus (in men) testicular ultrasound.

Biopsy of a PCNSL is generally undertaken using a stereotactically guided needle, because there is no indication that resection of tumour offers increased survival. Pre-operative treatment of raised intracranial pressure with steroids must be carefully managed because steroids may induce a dramatic apoptotic response in a PCNSL and seriously compromise the possibility of obtaining adequate tissue for histological diagnosis.

This response to steroids may give a misleading impression of the prognosis of PCNSL, suggesting that a relatively good outcome is to be expected. In fact, until recently, the prognosis for large B-cell PCNSL was abysmal [25, 41]. Median survival in most studies was approximately 1 year, similar to the survival with a glioblastoma. Fortunately, new chemotherapeutic regimens have improved the outlook and, with combinations of radiotherapy and different regimens of chemotherapy, median survival has been extended to about 40 months [15, 26, 40, 52, 57, 86, 95]. Age younger than 60 years, radiotherapy and radiotherapy combined with chemotherapy are favourable prognostic factors, while partial surgical resection is associated with a poor prognosis [9].

## 4.4 Macroscopic Pathology

Postmortem examination shows that PCNSL within the brain may form solitary or multifocal demarcated masses that belie the tumour cells' propensity to invade CNS tissue. The masses are associated with some swelling of adjacent tissue and are usually grey or pale yellow with a granular texture to their cut surfaces. Softening that represents necrosis and foci of haemorrhage may be present in the masses. Cerebral PCNSL is usually centred on the deep white matter and may display an invasive growth pattern in subependymal regions around lateral and third ventricles. This phenomenon is sometimes regarded as characteristic of PCNSL but may, in fact, be demonstrated by primitive neuro-ectodermal tumours (PNET). Rarely, the postmortem brain with a PCNSL may appear normal. Primary CNS lymphoma may mimic several primary CNS tumours, such as glioblastoma and PNET, both of which may contain areas of necrosis and form one or more distinct masses, despite extensive infiltration of adjacent parenchyma. When PCNSL appears as a poorly defined area of softening with patchy haemorrhage, it may look just like a subacute, haemorrhagic infarct.

In the subarachnoid space, PCNSL appears as a grey or white infiltrate that clouds the underlying brain. The appearance may be similar to the inflammatory infiltrate of infective meningitis. The neoplastic process may be extensive, surrounding the spinal cord and cauda equina as well as the brain. When it arises in the meninges, PCNSL may mimic certain meningiomas, particularly meningioma *en plaque*. Both types of tumour can form a firm mass, invade adjacent skull and brain and even extend into the extracranial subcutaneous tissues [79].

It is extremely rare for PCNSL to arise in the region of the spinal cord, a situation that is encountered in less than 1% of cases.

## 4.5 Microscopic Pathology – B-Cell Lymphoma

Large B-cell lymphomas constitute more than 80% of PCNSL [23, 54]. They are difficult to classify but generally conform to the REAL and WHO categories of diffuse large B-cell lymphoma. All show a diffuse growth pattern; follicular architecture has not been described for PCNSL. Macroscopically evident masses correspond to sheets of tumour cells, which frequently contain areas of necrosis. At the edge of these areas, lymphoma invades grey and white matter, eliciting reactive changes such as astrocytic gliosis and activation of microglia. This behaviour is exceptional for neoplasms that are not of neuro-epithelial lineage. The relationship between PCNSL and blood vessels of the CNS is characteristic and diagnostically helpful. Tumour cells pack the perivascular space, often creating a concentric pattern among layers of reticulin that surround the blood vessel. This reticulin, and the associated 'onion skin' arrangement of concentric layers of lymphoma cells, can be highlighted in silver stained sections. Perivascular infiltration may be particularly evident at the periphery of a tumour, where only small numbers of tumour cells have invaded the surrounding parenchyma.

Most B-cell PCNSL show a cytological picture dominated by polymorphous large cells (Fig. 1). Many of these cells resemble centroblasts or immunoblasts, but the histology is not identical to that of nodal diffuse large B-cell lymphomas. The nuclear:cytoplasmic ratio is high, and one or several nucleoli may be seen. Mitoses are readily found, and scattered apoptotic bodies are invariably present, sometimes in abundance. The degree of apoptosis has not been found to correlate with expression of pro- and anti-apoptotic proteins of the BCL2 family [43]. A reactive population of lymphocytes is admixed with the tumour cells.

In several series pre-dating the REAL and WHO classification schemes, diagnoses such as diffuse centroblastic lymphoma, diffuse follicle centre-cell lymphoma and diffuse immunoblastic lymphoma, have most frequently been applied to PCNSL. However, the incidence of these types has varied widely, reflecting the

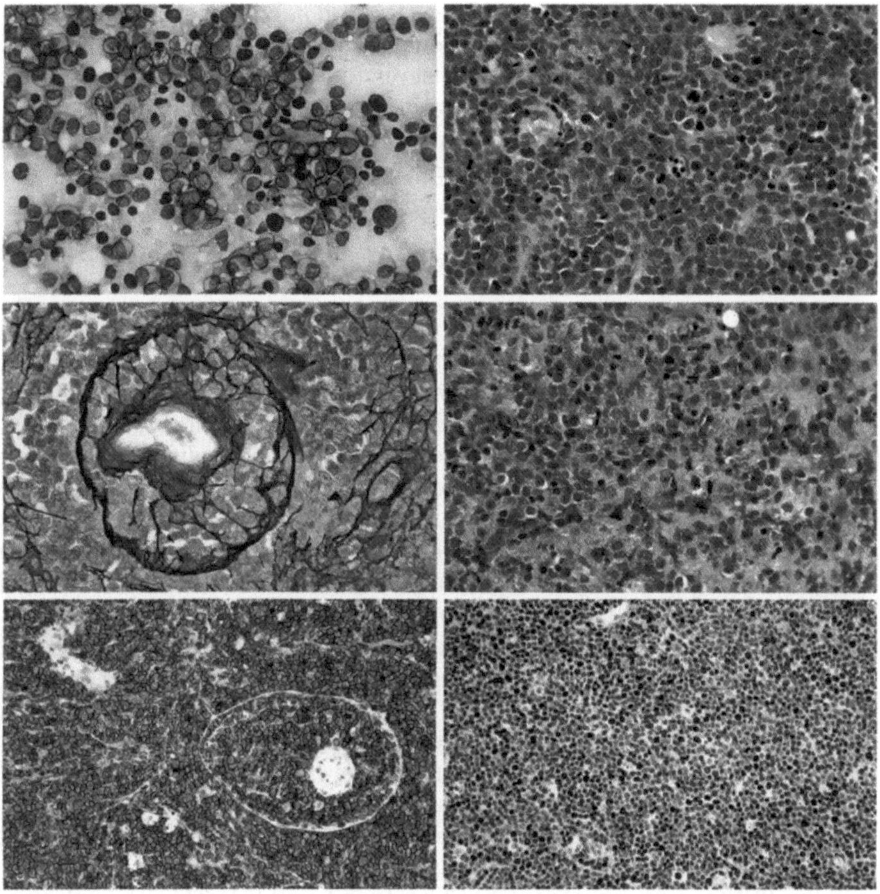


**Fig. 1a–f.** Primary central nervous system lymphoma; diffuse large B-cell lymphoma. **a** Neoplastic cells from a primary diffuse large B-cell lymphoma are admixed with small reactive lymphocytes in this smear preparation (toluidine blue, ×200), and **b** form a sheet of cells in this cerebral tumour (H&E, ×200). **c** Tumour cells crowd the perivascular space (reticulin, ×400), and **d** away from distinct tumour masses invade brain (H&E, ×200). **e** Neoplastic B cells invariably label with the anti-CD20 antibody L26. ×200. **f** The growth fraction as assessed by the Ki-67 labelling index is 30%–80%. ×100

difficulty of assessing the polymorphous population of tumour cells. The term 'polymorphous high-grade B-cell lymphoma' is possibly one of the most appropriate to have been used [121]. Primary CNS lymphoma with immunoblastic cytology is particularly associated with AIDS, and primary Burkitt-like lymphoma in the CNS has also been described in AIDS patients [77]. Rare variants, such as the so-called signet-ring follicle centre-cell lymphoma, characterised by abundant intracytoplasmic immunoglobulin accumulation, are exceptional [100].

Small B-cell lymphomas form only a minority (10%–25%) of PCNSL, and these figures are probably an over-estimate, including patients with staging that would today be considered incomplete. Cases reported as small B-cell PCNSL have been composed of lymphocytes or lymphoid cells that show some plasmacytic differentiation [22]. Such tumours have been classified as lymphocytic, lymphoplasmacytoid or lymphoplasmacytic, depending on the admixture of cell types. True primary plasmacytoma of the CNS has never, to our knowledge, been reported. Small B-cell lymphomas are over-represented among PCNSL with a leptomeningeal component [78]; some of these, in particular, may represent secondary CNS involvement by systemic low-grade lymphomas with occult disease elsewhere [90].

## 4.6 Immunohistochemistry

Immunohistochemistry readily demonstrates the B-cell origin of these tumours. Antibodies reactive with CD20 and CD79a, in a panel targeting a range of antigens, label the large cells (Fig. 1e). Immunohistochemical demonstration of $\lambda$ or $\kappa$ light chain restriction can support the diagnosis but is technically difficult and is not usually necessary in PCNSL with large cell appearances. Reactive small T lymphocytes are usually identified among the tumour cells in small to moderate numbers; it is rare for PCNSL to be extremely T cell-rich. The precise composition of the reactive T-cell population has been shown to differ between AIDS-associated tumours and those arising in immunocompetent individuals [8].

In addition to B-cell lineage, information relating PCNSL to node-based and non-CNS extranodal lymphomas can be obtained by immunostaining for CD5, CD10, CD23, cyclin D1, BCL2, BCL6 and the proliferation-associated Ki67 antigen [80, 93]. In our experience, most cases of diffuse large B-cell PCNSL lack expression of all of these, except BCL2 and Ki67 antigen. A few cases express CD10; in nodal lymphomas, expression of this antigen is associated with follicle centre cell origin. Expression of BCL2, which is generally strong and uniform in PCNSL, is associated with an adverse prognosis in nodal diffuse large B-cell lymphomas. In BCL2-negative PCNSL, over-expression of p53 has been found [93]. This is of unknown significance at present, but mutation of the p53 gene is rare in PCNSL [30]. Expression of BCL6 correlates with a good prognosis in non-CNS lymphomas, but few data exist currently regarding the expression of this antigen by PCNSL. Most PCNSL have a high Ki67 labelling index of 30%–80% (Fig. 1f), and there is some evidence that PCNSL cell-cycle kinetics differ between AIDS and non-AIDS patients [28]. This level of proliferative activity is similar to, or possibly slightly higher than, diffuse large B-cell lymphomas at other sites. Burkitt's lymphoma occurring in the CNS in the context of HIV infection has a Ki67 labelling index of 100%.

## 4.7 Intravascular Large B-Cell Lymphoma (Intravascular Lymphomatosis)

This is a rare, aggressive form of NHL, typically presenting with subcutaneous or CNS infiltration, though other organs may be affected [51, 123]. Cases presenting with CNS involvement alone are often undiagnosed until after death because of the non-specific nature of the neurological signs and the absence of any mass lesion.

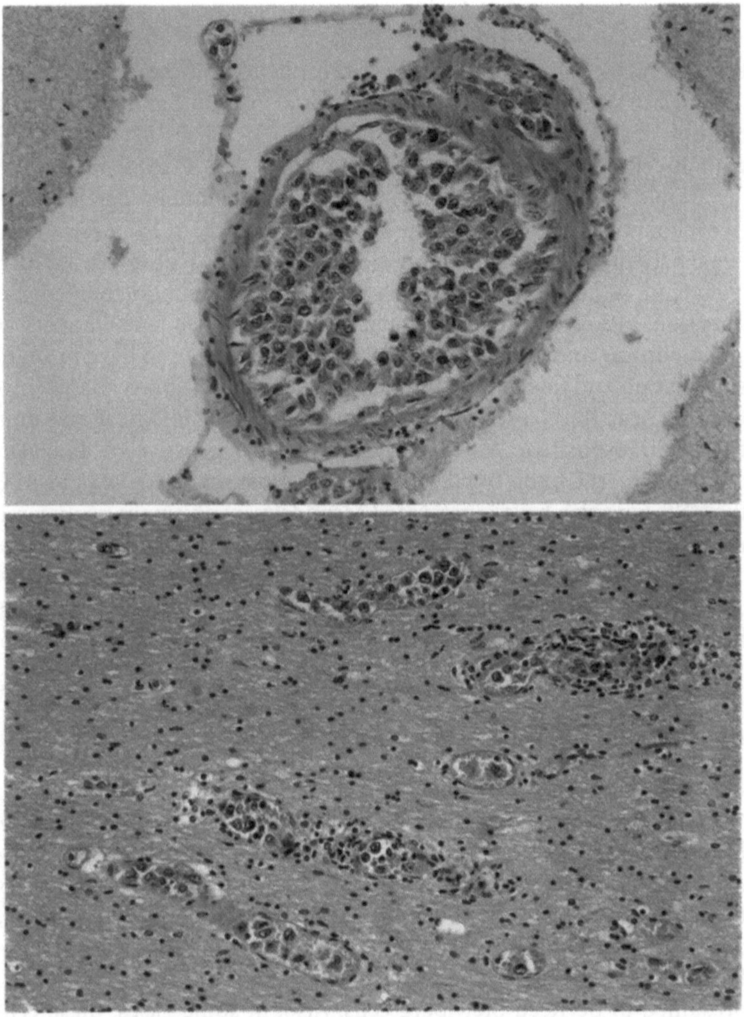

a

b

**Fig. 2 a, b.** Intravascular large B-cell lymphoma. Neoplastic cells occupy the lumina of leptomeningeal (**a**) and parenchymal (**b**) blood vessels. H & E, × 100

Affected patients may suffer a series of small strokes or present with a dementia. Large, neoplastic B cells occupy the lumina of the brain's microvasculature (Fig. 2), and in a few areas permeate the vessel wall or extend into the perivascular space and adjacent parenchyma [29, 122]. In postmortem specimens, permeation of the brain microvasculature is often widespread or multifocal, and associated with multiple small areas of infarction [128]. Absence of BCL2, p53 and EBV has been demonstrated [11, 12], by contrast with other types of PCNSL, and specific patterns of adhesion-molecule expression have been shown, which may explain the intravascular localisation of neoplastic cells [67, 107].

### 4.8 Primary CNS T-Cell Lymphomas

Primary CNS lymphomas with a T-cell phenotype are very rare but have been reported in supratentorial and infratentorial locations and, additionally, to arise in multiple intracranial sites [10, 13, 17, 21, 47, 55, 76, 84, 87, 91, 92, 133]. Compared with B-cell lymphomas, reported cases of T-cell PCNSL have had a relatively favourable prognosis and a disproportionate number has been of small cell (lymphocytic) type. Some of the latter, particularly in Far Eastern or Afro-Caribbean patients, may have been CNS manifestations of adult T-cell lymphocytic leukaemia (ATLL) associated with human T-cell lymphotropic virus-1 (HTLV-1) infection, rather than true primary CNS lymphomas [72]. Patients with ATLL of acute, chronic and lymphomatous variants are known to have profound immunosuppression and this may be the basis of their susceptibility to CNS involvement by their disease. Rare cases of PCNSL have had morphological and immunophenotypic (CD30-positive; ALK-positive) features suggestive of anaplastic large-cell lymphoma (ALCL) of T-cell type [1, 102]; most reported cases of ALCL involving the CNS, however, have represented secondary involvement by disseminated systemic disease.

In general, the architectural features of T-cell PCNSL are shared with their B-cell counterparts; tumour cells are concentrated in the perivascular spaces but also infiltrate surrounding parenchyma to a varying extent, with or without necrosis.

### 4.9 Primary Hodgkin's Lymphoma in the CNS

Very few cases of primary intracranial Hodgkin's lymphoma have been reported [42], and doubt has been expressed as to whether such cases are genuinely primary at this site. The diagnosis not only requires that no focus of Hodgkin's lymphoma be demonstrated outside the CNS, but that the tumour contains authentic Reed-Sternberg cells within the correct mixture of lymphoid cells. Some reports have failed to use immunohistochemistry to confirm the nature of large tumour cells presumed to be Reed-Sternberg cells. Also, in some cases, these cells have been admixed with an atypical cell population suggesting a different diagnosis, such as T cell-rich large B-cell lymphoma or a pleomorphic B-cell lymphoma with a small-cell component [96, 111]. One recent case report of CNS Hodgkin's disease, associated with azathioprine treatment for myasthenia gravis (and, therefore, presumed immunosuppression) seems genuinely to describe a primary tumour in the fronto-parietal region of the brain [63].

### 4.10 CNS Lymphomas and the Eye

Lymphoma within the eye is exceedingly rare [4]. Lymphomas arising in ocular adnexae which include the eyelid, lacrimal gland, conjunctiva and orbit, are encountered more frequently and make up about 8% of extranodal NHL [50]. They are mainly low-grade B-cell lymphomas and appear unrelated to PCNSL [112].

Lymphomas arising in the retina or vitreous humour are usually large B-cell lymphomas similar to intracerebral PCNSL, and at least three AIDS-associated cases have been reported [89, 114]. Ocular involvement may take the form of uveitis, retinochoroiditis, retinal vasculitis or subretinal pigment epithelial infiltration [4, 37, 85, 98]. Intra-ocular NHL either tend to be associated with PCNSL (although presentation at different sites may not be concurrent) or represent metastases from systemic lymphomas [4, 62]. One study has estimated that 15% of systemic lymphomas spread to the eye at some stage. The route of access to intra-ocular sites is currently unknown, but experimental evidence suggests the occurrence of haematogenous spread from adjacent ocular structures or extension along the optic nerve from tumour within the brain [7]. Interestingly, no evidence was found by these researchers that retrograde spread occurred from eye to brain.

### 4.11 Secondary Spread of PCNSL Beyond the Brain

Systemic dissemination from PCNSL has been estimated to occur in approximately 8% of cases [19, 62], mainly in late stages of the disease. It is far more common to find dissemination within the CNS, giving rise to multifocal involvement of the brain parenchyma, diffuse or focal meningeal involvement or lesions within the eye.

## 5 Secondary Involvement of the CNS by Systemic Nodal and Extranodal Lymphomas

Most examples of node-based or extranodal B-cell NHL involving the CNS are small-cell lymphomas with a tendency to leukaemic dissemination; B-cell chronic lymphocytic leukaemia, lymphoplasmacytic lymphoma or mantle-cell lymphoma [83, 90, 96]. In many cases, CNS involvement has occurred in association with transformation to large-cell lymphoma or, in the case of mantle-cell lymphoma, has been a component of aggressive disease with blastoid cytology. No examples of low-grade follicular lymphoma disseminating to the CNS have been reported in the absence of progression to large-cell lymphoma. Primary testicular diffuse large B-cell lymphoma has a particular propensity to involve CNS and Waldeyer's ring if it disseminates [99], and CNS involvement in a case of primary mediastinal DLC-B has also been reported [14]. Risk factors for CNS spread from node-based DLC-B have been evaluated in several large clinical series; advanced stage, involvement of at least one other extranodal site, B symptoms, high serum lactate dehydrogenase concentration and poor clinical performance status all contribute to an increased risk of CNS involvement [16, 73, 131]. Burkitt's lymphoma in childhood has been found in some cases to involve the CNS, and acute lymphoblastic leukaemia so frequently spreads to the meninges that CNS prophylaxis is a standard part of current therapy. Acute myeloid leukaemias also involve the meninges in a proportion of patients, and rare examples of solid intracranial myeloid tumours have been reported [46, 134]. Primary CNS lymphomas have also been reported as second tumours following therapy for childhood acute leukaemia [130], and it should not be forgotten that, even in the absence of direct CNS involvement, complications of acute lymphoblastic leukaemia (ALL) and its therapy may produce a spectrum of secondary CNS pathology [27].

Various peripheral T-cell lymphomas arising within lymph nodes or at non-CNS extranodal sites have been described secondarily involving the CNS. These include ATLL, ALCL, nasal-type T-cell NHL and enteropathy-associated T-cell lymphoma of the small intestine [71, 72, 103, 129, 135]; involvement of the peripheral nervous system is occasionally recorded [106, 115]. Metastasis to the CNS is a rare complication of Hodgkin's lymphoma that has mainly been reported in patients with AIDS. Involvement of the CNS by post-transplant lymphoproliferative disease arising in association with immunosuppression has also been described, in most cases as part of widespread systemic disease but occasionally as an apparently localised CNS lesion [105].

With few exceptions among these groups of patients [49], CNS involvement by lymphoma or leukaemia occurs during or after treatment, or in advanced stages of their disease, following extensive treatment. It may be speculated that alterations in the blood–brain barrier, resulting from therapy or systemic effects of widely disseminated tumour, allow neoplastic seeding into the CNS. There has been particular concern recently that treatment of acute promyelocytic leukaemia with all-trans retinoic acid (ATRA) may be associated with unusual patterns of extramedullary relapse, including relapse in the CNS [46].

## 6 The Differential Diagnosis of PCNSL

Working through the differential diagnosis of PCNSL involves three main lines of enquiry:

- Does the pathology represent a neoplastic process?
- If so, is it lymphoma?
- If so, which type of lymphoma is it?

Especially in small biopsies obtained stereotactically, lymphoma may be confused with inflammatory processes, such as occur with encephalitis or demyelination [38]. Distinguishing these entities should begin with an appraisal of relevant clinical and radiological characteristics of the disease process. However, these features are unlikely to be entirely typical, because biopsy will not be considered necessary in patients with classical clinical features of an inflammatory process or demyelination.

Histologically, an inflammatory process may be confused with lymphomas consisting of small cells without significant atypia. Attention to the composition of the infiltrating lymphoid cells is then important; an infiltrate of reactive cells is usually polymorphous, predominantly small in size and possibly admixed with plasma cells. However, the presence of reactive lymphocytes among neoplastic lymphoid cells can sometimes confuse the picture. Immunohistochemistry helps in this situation by defining distinct populations of leucocytes. In cases where doubt persists, the clonality of cells can be assessed by examining the cells for rearrangements of immunoglobulin or T-cell receptor genes. This PCR-based methodology is possible using formalin fixed, paraffin embedded tissue, with the limitations that have been described above.

Where an infective process is part of the differential diagnosis, the demonstration of organisms is crucial, so the pathologist must be prepared to undertake a range of tests in these circumstances. These may involve tinctorial methods, such as the Grocott methenamine silver stain for fungi, immunohistochemistry with, for example, toxoplasma-specific antibodies or electron microscopy for viruses. Immunohistochemistry and molecular genetic, PCR-based techniques for viruses may also be helpful in this situation. It is important to remember that dual pathology may occasionally be present. Immunocompromised patients may have a PCNSL and encephalitis, and the encephalitis may be caused by one of several pathogens, such as cytomegalovirus or toxoplasma [124].

Non-infective causes of CNS inflammation may be associated with demyelination. This is defined as the combination of loss of myelin and relative preservation of axons. This combination can be demonstrated histologically in the same section or adjacent sections. Luxol fast blue and solochrome cyanin are recommended as myelin stains. Axons can be highlighted by silver impregnation, as in the Palmgren technique, or by immunohistochemistry with an antibody reactive with neurofilament protein.

Some non-lymphomatous CNS tumours resemble PCNSL and enter into the histological differential diagnosis. For example, primitive neuro-ectodermal tumours consist of small round cells with a high nuclear:cytoplasmic ratio and high mitotic count. In practice, distinction is readily made using immunohistochemistry [45, 125]. The lymphoid nature of PCNSL can be demonstrated with antibodies reactive with CD45, CD20 and CD3. In the rare case of primary ALCL in the CNS, which may mimic a glioblastoma and not be immunoreactive for CD45, appropriate additional antibodies (particularly CD30) may be used to make the diagnosis.

## 7 Neurological Syndromes Associated with Systemic Lymphoma

Lymphoma originating outside the nervous system may be associated with neurological symptoms and signs in various ways:

1. The tumour may metastasise, affecting the nervous system either by entering the brain, spinal cord or meninges, or by compressing elements of the central or peripheral nervous system from an adjacent site, such as the vertebral column or skull.
2. Immunosuppression as a consequence of lymphoma may be associated with infection of the nervous system.
3. There may be neurological side effects of therapies for lymphoma.
4. An immunogenic paraneoplastic syndrome may arise.

A systemic lymphoma or its treatment with chemotherapeutic regimens can predispose to a range of nervous system infections. Hodgkin's disease is particularly associated with encephalitis caused by varicella-zoster virus. Progressive multifocal leukoencephalopathy is associated with diverse causes of immunosuppression and is an infection of the CNS by the JC polyomavirus. This particularly affects white matter, depleting oligodendrocytes and producing foci of demyelination. Remaining oligodendrocytes may have enlarged, pleomorphic and hyperchromatic nuclei, and contain amphophilic viral inclusions. Several opportunistic bacterial meningitides are associated with lymphoma. Listeriosis is found in this setting, and the commonest cause of fungal meningitis, *Cryptococcus neoformans*, usually occurs in immunosuppressed patients with a primary infection in the lung. Streptococcal meningitis may be seen in patients who have had a splenectomy.

A cerebellar disorder is a complication of treatment with cytosine arabinoside, while encephalopathy or myelopathy may follow radiotherapy or chemotherapy with L-asparaginase, BCNU or intrathecal methotrexate.

## 8 Paraneoplastic Neurological Syndromes and Lymphoma

Symptomatic epiphenomena linked to lymphomas and their treatment include infections, which may reflect the patient's immunocompromised status, metabolic and nutritional disorders, coagulopathies and side effects of therapy. Each of these 'non-metastatic' complications can affect the nervous system. Another group of rare immunogenic disorders associated with a variety of tumours and unrelated to invasion or compression of the affected tissue is termed 'paraneoplastic'.

Paraneoplastic neurological syndromes are uncommon, affecting about 1% of patients with cancer [36]. Most of these have an association with anti-neuronal antibodies. Antibodies generated in the course of the immunological response to antigens on neoplastic cells aberrantly target similar antigens on neurons [108]. Alternatively, the syndrome is associated with immunological dysfunction without specific paraneoplastic markers [35].

Paraneoplastic neurological syndromes may be divided into three main groups, affecting the central nervous system, the peripheral nervous system and the muscle or neuromuscular junction [35]. The principal CNS syndromes are a cerebellar degeneration and an encephalomyelitis, which may be centred on the limbic system ('limbic encephalitis'). Peripheral nerves may be damaged as part of a sensory ganglioneuropathy, and the neuromuscular junction is targeted in the Lambert-Eaton myasthenic syndrome. CNS and peripheral nervous system disorders, particularly paraneoplastic encephalomyelitis and sensory neuronopathy, may occur together [34].

Small-cell lung carcinoma is the commonest cause of paraneoplastic neurological syndromes, but Hodgkin's disease (HD) ranks third as a cause of paraneoplastic cerebellar degeneration [119]. Symptoms and signs relating to the growth or spread of tumour cells can precede or follow a paraneoplastic neurological disorder. In addition, investigation of a patient suspected of having a paraneoplastic syndrome might fail to reveal the tumour until it becomes symptomatic, typically 3–12 months later. Sometimes, a tumour is not found until autopsy. However, in HD-related paraneoplastic cerebellar degeneration, symptoms generally develop after discovery of the lymphoma, and even during remission. Its development may herald relapse [58]. Many paraneoplastic neurological syndromes bring about a fatal outcome within a few months, though recovery is recorded, notably in association with Hodgkin's disease [109].

## 8.1 Paraneoplastic Cerebellar Degeneration

Though rare, this syndrome is the commonest paraneoplastic syndrome of the CNS. It presents with a midline ataxia, and generalised incoordination and cerebellar dysarthria usually follow within a few weeks. Carcinomas of ovary, breast and lung (small cell) are responsible for the majority of cases, but lymphomas, mostly Hodgkin's disease, are implicated in 16% [24]. For patients with HD and paraneoplastic cerebellar degeneration (PCD), age at presentation can be very variable; 22–70 years in one study [58]. Most patients with HD and PCD are male. Rarely, other lymphomas may be associated with PCD. An association with T-cell lymphoma is of particular interest because of data that point to shared surface antigens on T-cells and Purkinje cells [5].

PCD is characterised histologically by cerebellar atrophy, Purkinje cell loss with relative preservation of basket cells, a decrease in the number of internal granule cells and non-specific reactive changes, such as Bergmann gliosis and activation of microglia [117]. A patchy parenchymal and perivascular lymphocytic infiltrate is evident in most cases, but may be absent. The cerebellar disorder of HD is not associated with the anti-Yo antibodies linked to ovarian and breast carcinomas, or the anti-Hu antibodies linked to small-cell lung cancer, though clinical and histological features may be identical in these PCD of different aetiology. Instead, an antibody termed anti-Tr has been discovered in some cases of HD-related PCD [56, 104]. The only patient with anti-Tr antibodies and a PCD who did not have HD had a NHL. Thus, the antibodies appear to be specific, but may not be very sensitive from a diagnostic viewpoint.

## 8.2 Paraneoplastic Encephalomyelitis and Stiff-Man Syndrome

PCD and paraneoplastic encephalomyelitis (PEM) share histological features such as loss of neurons, astrocytic gliosis and focal inflammatory infiltrates (Fig. 3). However, the distribution of their pathology differs. With PEM, the amygdala, hippocampus, insula and cingulate gyrus are typically involved in a 'limbic encephalitis', but more caudal regions, such as brain stem nuclei can be affected. PEM is usually associated with small-cell lung cancer and rarely with lymphoma. It may present as a dementia, with seizures or brain-stem dysfunction [18]. In PEM associated with small-cell lung carcinoma, anti-Hu antibodies target 35- to 40-kD proteins in neuronal nuclei [34, 35]. Both humoral and cell-mediated mechanisms are involved in its pathogenesis.

Stiff-man syndrome, which is characterised by continuous muscle spasms, is an exceptional complication of Hodgkin's disease [48]. In this case, the syndrome and lymphoma responded to chemotherapy.

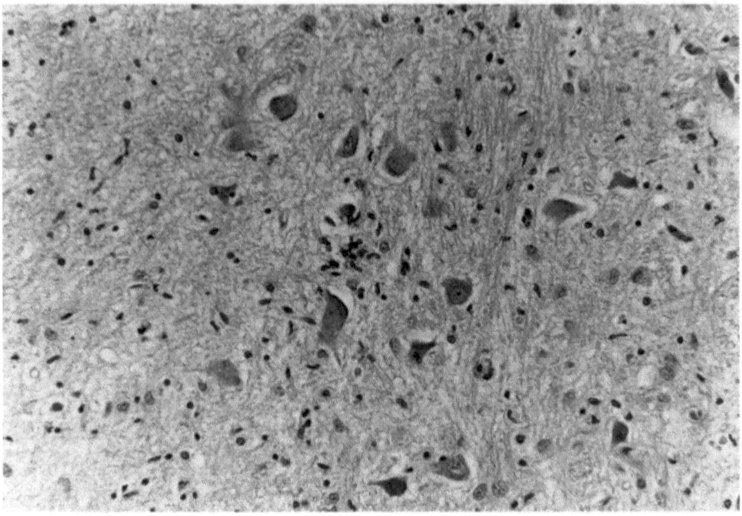

**Fig. 3.** Paraneoplastic encephalitis. A 'microglial star' marks the site of anti-Yo antibody-induced neuronal loss in the hypoglossal nucleus. The patient presented with a cerebellar syndrome, but was found to have a more widespread paraneoplastic encephalitis. H&E, ×100

## 8.3 Paraneoplastic Disorders of the Peripheral Nervous System and Lymphoma

Several paraneoplastic disorders of the peripheral nervous system are associated with lymphoreticular neoplasms. A subacute sensory or motor neuropathy has been described with lymphoma, but is rare. The sensory neuropathy is clinically and pathologically indistinguishable from the paraneoplastic disorder associated with carcinomas. The motor neuropathy involves degeneration of anterior horn cells and mild demyelination in the posterior columns [120]. HD may produce an acute or chronic relapsing Guillain-Barré syndrome [81].

Aside from compression of peripheral nerves when it produces vertebral collapse, multiple myeloma is linked to a variety of paraneoplastic neuropathies. The associated sensorimotor neuropathy with axonal degeneration is an example of a 'dying-back' neuropathy, in which the distal portions of axons are affected first. Multiple myeloma also produces a chronic demyelinating neuropathy, which principally affects motor nerves [74]. The amyloidosis associated with multiple myeloma may produce a generalised neuropathy, or carpal tunnel compression and a median nerve palsy. Waldenström's macroglobulinaemia, a chronic proliferative lymphoreticular disorder with an IgM paraproteinaemia, may produce a distal sensorimotor neuropathy [66]. This may involve either axonal degeneration or segmental demyelination. Foci of lymphocytes are found in the endoneurium, and deposits of IgM may be demonstrated immunohistochemically [110]. Ultrastructural examination usually discloses a distinctive abnormality of myelin structure, characterised by widening of lamellae (Fig. 4) [75].

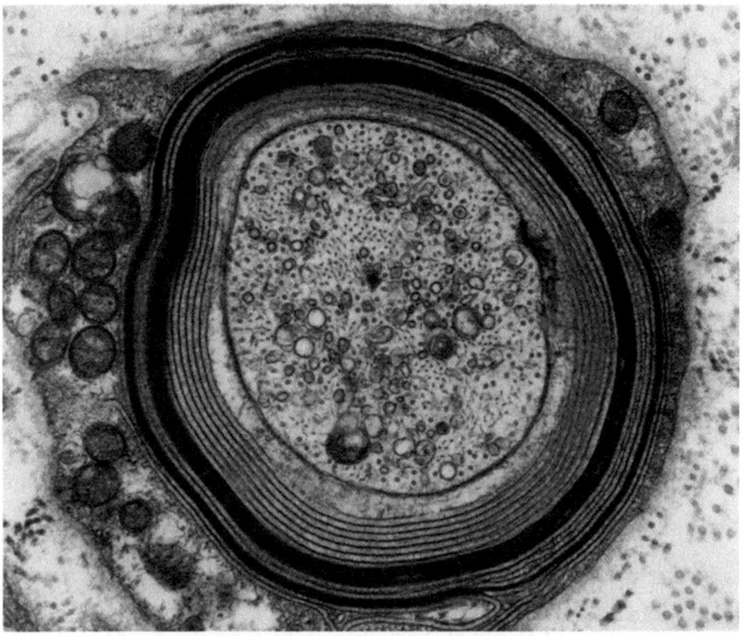

**Fig. 4.** Neuropathy associated with IgM paraproteinaemia. This transmission electron micrograph through the sural nerve of a patient with Waldenström's macroglobulinaemia shows abnormally wide periodicity of some regions in the myelin sheath. In this setting, deposition of IgM can often be demonstrated immunohistochemically. ×40,000

## References


1. Abdulkader I, Cameselle-Teijeiro J, Fraga M, Rodriguez-Nunez A et al. (1999) Primary anaplastic large cell lymphoma of the central nervous system. Hum Pathol 30:978–981
2. Agapitos E, Nanas J, Kavantzas N, Davaris P (1997) Non-Hodgkin lymphoma of brain occurring after cardiac transplantation. J Exp Clin Cancer Res 16: 441–443
3. Ahsan H, Neugut AI, Bruce JN (1995) Trends in incidence of primary malignant brain tumors in USA, 1981–1990. Int J Epidemiol 24:1078–1085
4. Akpek EK, Ahmed I, Hochberg FH, Soheilian M et al. (1999) Intraocular-central nervous system lymphoma: clinical features, diagnosis, and outcomes. Ophthalmology 106:1805–1810
5. Ang LC, Zochodne DW, Ebers GC, Kaufmann JC, Vinters HV (1986) Severe cerebellar degeneration in a patient with T-cell lymphoma. Acta Neuropathol Berl 69:171–175
6. Antinori A, Larocca LM, Fassone L, Cattani P et al. (1999) HHV-8/KSHV is not associated with AIDS-related primary central nervous system lymphoma. Brain Pathol 9:199–208
7. Assaf N, Hasson T, Hoch Marchaim H, Pe'er J et al. (1997) An experimental model for infiltration of malignant lymphoma to the eye and brain. Virchows Arch 431:459–467
8. Bashir R, Chamberlain M, Ruby E, Hochberg FH (1996) T-cell infiltration of primary CNS lymphoma. Neurology 46:440–444
9. Bataille B, Delwail V, Menet E, Vandermarcq P et al. (2000) Primary intracerebral malignant lymphoma: report of 248 cases. J Neurosurg 92:261–266
10. Bednar MM, Salerni A, Flanagan ME, Pendlebury WW (1991) Primary central nervous system T-cell lymphoma. Case report. J Neurosurg 74:668–672

11. Bergmann M, Blasius S, Bankfalvi A, Mellin W (1996) Primary non-Hodgkin lymphomas of the CNS-proliferation, oncoproteins and Epstein-Barr-virus. Gen Diagn Pathol 141: 235–242
12. Bergmann M, Terzija Wessel U, Blasius S, Kuchelmeister K et al. (1994) Intravascular lymphomatosis of the CNS: clinicopathologic study and search for expression of oncoproteins and Epstein-Barr virus. Clin Neurol Neurosurg 96:236–243
13. Bindal AK, Blisard KS, Melin Aldama H, Warnick RE (1997) Primary T-cell lymphoma of the brain in acquired immunodeficiency syndrome: case report. J Neurooncol 31:267–271
14. Bishop PC, Wilson WH, Pearson D, Janik J et al. (1999) CNS involvement in primary mediastinal large B-cell lymphoma. J Clin Oncol 17:2479–2485
15. Boiardi A, Silvani A, Pozzi A, Fariselli L et al. (1999) Chemotherapy is effective as early treatment for primary central nervous system lymphoma. J Neurol 246:31–37
16. Bollen EL, Brouwer RE, Hamers S, Hermans J et al. (1997) Central nervous system relapse in non-Hodgkin lymphoma. A single-center study of 532 patients. Arch Neurol 54: 854–859
17. Brazis PW, Menke DM, McLeish WM, Broderick DF et al. (1995) Angiocentric T-cell lymphoma presenting with multiple cranial nerve palsies and retrobulbar optic neuropathy. J Neuroophthalmol 15:152–157
18. Brierley JB, Corsellis JAN, Hierons R, Nevin S (1960) Subacute encephalitis of later adult life, mainly affecting the limbic area. Brain 83:357–368
19. Brown MT, McClendon RE, Gockerman JP (1995) Primary central nervous system lymphoma with systemic metastasis: case report and review. J Neurooncol 23:207–221
20. Burstein SD, Kernohan JW, Uihlein A (1963) Reticuloendothelial sarcomas of brain. Cancer 16:289–305
21. Buxton N, Punt J, Hewitt M (1998) Primary Ki-1-positive T-cell lymphoma of the brain in a child. Pediatr Neurosurg 29:250–252
22. Cachia AR, Theocharous C (1996) Primary intracerebral small lymphocytic non-Hodgkin's lymphoma with plasmacytoid differentiation, associated with prominent extracellular proteinaceous deposits. Pathology 28:98–101
23. Camilleri Broet S, Martin A, Moreau A, Angonin R et al. (1998) Primary central nervous system lymphomas in 72 immunocompetent patients: pathologic findings and clinical correlations. Groupe Ouest Est d'etude des Leucenies et Autres Maladies du Sang (GOELAMS). Am J Clin Pathol 110:607–612
24. Cehreli C, Payzin B, Undar B, Yilmaz U, Alakavuklar MN (1995) Paraneoplastic cerebellar degeneration in association with Hodgkin's disease: a report of two cases. Acta Haematol 94:210–213
25. Chamberlain MC, Levin VA (1990) Adjuvant chemotherapy for primary lymphoma of the central nervous system. Arch Neurol 47:1113–1116
26. Chamberlain MC, Levin VA (1992) Primary central nervous system lymphoma: a role for adjuvant chemotherapy. J Neurooncol 14:271–275
27. Chen CY, Zimmerman RA, Faro S, Bilaniuk LT et al. (1996) Childhood leukemia: central nervous system abnormalities during and after treatment. AJNR Am J Neuroradiol 17:295–310
28. Christov C, Adle-Biassette H, Lechapt E, Poron F et al. (1999) Primary brain lymphoma cell turnover differs in patients with and without AIDS: relationships to bcl-2 expression and host cell reaction. J Neuropathol Exp Neurol 58:1069–1077
29. Clark WC, Dohan FC, Jr., Moss T, Schweitzer JB (1991) Immunocytochemical evidence of lymphocytic derivation of neoplastic cells in malignant angioendotheliomatosis. J Neurosurg 74:757–762
30. Cobbers JM, Wolter M, Reifenberger J, Ring GU et al. (1998) Frequent inactivation of CDKN2 A and rare mutation of TP53 in PCNSL. Brain Pathol 8:263–276
31. Corboy JR, Garl PJ, Kleinschmidt DeMasters BK (1998) Human herpesvirus 8 DNA in CNS lymphomas from patients with and without AIDS [see comments]. Neurology 50: 335–340
32. Corn BW, Marcus SM, Topham A, Hauck W, Curran WJ Jr (1997) Will primary central nervous system lymphoma be the most frequent brain tumor diagnosed in the year 2000? Cancer 79:2409–2413

33. Cote TR, Manns A, Hardy CR, Yellin FJ, Hartge P (1996) Epidemiology of brain lymphoma among people with or without acquired immunodeficiency syndrome. AIDS/Cancer Study Group. J Natl Cancer Inst 88:675–679
34. Dalmau J, Graus F, Rosenblum MK, Posner JB (1992) Anti-Hu–associated paraneoplastic encephalomyelitis/sensory neuronopathy. A clinical study of 71 patients. Medicine Baltimore 71:59–72
35. Dalmau J, Gultekin HS, Posner JB (1999) Paraneoplastic neurologic syndromes: pathogenesis and physiopathology. Brain Pathol 9:275–284
36. Dalmau JO, Posner JB (1999) Paraneoplastic syndromes. Arch Neurol 56:405–408
37. Dean JM, Novak MA, Chan CC, Green WR (1996) Tumor detachments of the retinal pigment epithelium in ocular/central nervous system lymphoma. Retina 16:47–56
38. DeAngelis LM (1990) Primary central nervous system lymphoma imitates multiple sclerosis. Journal of Neuro-Oncology 9:177–181
39. DeAngelis LM (1999) Primary central nervous system lymphoma. Curr Opin Neurol 12:687–691
40. DeAngelis LM (1999) Primary CNS lymphoma: treatment with combined chemotherapy and radiotherapy. J Neurooncol 43:249–257
41. DeAngelis LM, Yahalom J, Thaler HT, Kher U (1992) Combined modality therapy for primary CNS lymphoma. J Clin Oncol 10:635–643
42. Deckert Schluter M, Marek J, Setlik M, Markova J et al. (1998) Primary manifestation of Hodgkin's disease in the central nervous system. Virchows Arch 432:477–481
43. Deckert Schluter M, Rang A, Wiestler OD (1998) Apoptosis and apoptosis-related gene products in primary non-Hodgkin's lymphoma of the central nervous system. Acta Neuropathol Berl 96:157–162
44. DeMario MD, Liebowitz DN (1998) Lymphomas in the immunocompromised patient. Semin Oncol 25:492–502
45. Ellison DW (2000) Primary CNS lymphomas. In: Ellison D, Love S, eds. Neuropathology. A reference text of CNS pathology. London: Mosby,
46. Evans GD, Grimwade DJ (1999) Extramedullary disease in acute promyelocytic leukemia. Leuk Lymphoma 33:219–229
47. Ferracini R, Bergmann M, Pileri S, Rigobello L et al. (1995) Primary T-cell lymphoma of the central nervous system. Clin Neuropathol 14:125–129
48. Ferrari P, Federico M, Grimaldi LM, Silingardi V (1990) Stiff-man syndrome in a patient with Hodgkin's disease. An unusual paraneoplastic syndrome. Haematologica 75:570–572
49. Ferreri AJ, Reni M, Zoldan MC, Terreni MR, Villa E (1996) Importance of complete staging in non-Hodgkin's lymphoma presenting as a cerebral mass lesion. Cancer 77:827–833
50. Freeman C, Berg JW, Cutler SJ (1972) Occurrence and prognosis of extranodal lymphomas. Cancer 29:252–260
51. Glass J, Hochberg FH, Miller DC (1993) Intravascular lymphomatosis. A systemic disease with neurologic manifestations. Cancer 71:3156–3164
52. Glass J, Shustik C, Hochberg FH, Cher L, Gruber ML (1996) Therapy of primary central nervous system lymphoma with pre-irradiation methotrexate, cyclophosphamide, doxorubicin, vincristine, and dexamethasone (MCHOD). J Neurooncol 30:257–265
53. Goplen AK, Dunlop O, Liestol K, Lingjaerde OC et al. (1997) The impact of primary central nervous system lymphoma in AIDS patients: a population-based autopsy study from Oslo. J Acquir Immune Defic Syndr Hum Retrovirol 14:351–354
54. Grant JW, Isaacson PG (1992) Primary Central Nervous System Lymphoma. Brain Pathol 2:97–109
55. Grant JW, von Deimling A (1990) Primary T-cell lymphoma of the central nervous system. Arch Pathol Lab Med 114:24–27
56. Graus F, Dalmau J, Valldeoriola F, Ferrer I et al. (1997) Immunological characterization of a neuronal antibody (anti-Tr) associated with paraneoplastic cerebellar degeneration and Hodgkin's disease. J Neuroimmunol 74:55–61
57. Guha Thakurta N, Damek D, Pollack C, Hochberg FH (1999) Intravenous methotrexate as initial treatment for primary central nervous system lymphoma: response to therapy and quality of life of patients. J Neurooncol 43:259–268

58. Hammack J, Kotanides H, Rosenblum MK, Posner JB (1992) Paraneoplastic cerebellar degeneration. II. Clinical and immunologic findings in 21 patients with Hodgkin's disease. Neurology 42:1938–1943
59. Hanson MN, Morrison VA, Peterson BA, Stieglbauer KT et al. (1996) Posttransplant T-cell lymphoproliferative disorders–an aggressive, late complication of solid-organ transplantation [see comments]. Blood 88:3626–3633
60. Harris NL, Jaffe ES, Diebold J, Flandrin G et al. (2000) The World Health Organization classification of neoplastic diseases of the haematopoietic and lymphoid tissues: Report of the Clinical Advisory Committee Meeting, Airlie House, Virginia, November 1997. Histopathology 36:69–86
61. Harris NL, Jaffe ES, Stein H, Banks PM et al. (1994) A revised European-American classification of lymphoid neoplasms: a proposal from the International Lymphoma Study Group [see comments]. Blood 84:1361–1392
62. Herrlinger U (1999) Primary CNS lymphoma: findings outside the brain. J Neurooncol 43:227–230
63. Herrlinger U, Klingel K, Meyermann R, Kandolf R et al. (2000) Central nervous system Hodgkin's lymphoma without systemic manifestation: case report and review of the literature. Acta Neuropathologica 99:709–714
64. Herrlinger U, Schabet M, Bitzer M, Petersen D, Krauseneck P (1999) Primary central nervous system lymphoma: from clinical presentation to diagnosis. J Neurooncol 43:219–226
65. Hochberg FH, Miller DC (1988) Primary central nervous system lymphoma. J Neurosurg 68:835–853
66. Iwashita H, Argyrakis A, Lowitzsch K, Spaar FW (1974) Polyneuropathy in Waldenstrom's macroglobulinaemia. J Neurol Sci 21:341–354
67. Jalkanen S, Aho R, Kallajoki M, Ekfors T et al. (1989) Lymphocyte homing receptors and adhesion molecules in intravascular malignant lymphomatosis. Int J Cancer 44:777–782
68. Jellinger KA, Paulus W (1995) Primary central nervous system lymphomas–new pathological developments. J Neurooncol 24:33–36
69. Jenkins CN, Colquhoun IR (1998) Characterization of primary intracranial lymphoma by computed tomography: an analysis of 36 cases and a review of the literature with particular reference to calcification haemorrhage and cyst formation. Clin Radiol 53:428–434
70. Julien S, Radosavljevic M, Labouret N, Camilleri Broet S et al. (1999) AIDS primary central nervous system lymphoma: molecular analysis of the expressed VH genes and possible implications for lymphomagenesis. J Immunol 162:1551–1558
71. Kaplinsky C, Toren A, Neumann Y, Mandel M et al. (1997) Central nervous system involvement at diagnosis in a case of pediatric CD30+ anaplastic large cell lymphoma. Med Pediatr Oncol 28:132–135
72. Kawasaki C, Ikeda H, Fukumoto T (1995) Cerebral mass lesions associated with adult T-cell leukemia/lymphoma. Int J Hematol 61:97–102
73. Keldsen N, Michalski W, Bentzen SM, Hansen KB, Thorling K (1996) Risk factors for central nervous system involvement in non-Hodgkins-lymphoma–a multivariate analysis. Acta Oncol 35:703–708
74. Kelly JJ, Jr, Kyle RA, Miles JM, Dyck PJ (1983) Osteosclerotic myeloma and peripheral neuropathy. Neurology 33:202–210
75. King RH, Thomas PK (1984) The occurrence and significance of myelin with unusually large periodicity. Acta Neuropathol Berl 63:319–329
76. Kleopa K, Becker G, Roggendorf W, Reichmann H (1996) Primary T-cell lymphoma of the cerebellum. A case report. J Neurooncol 27:225–230
77. Knowles DM (1999) Immunodeficiency-associated lymphoproliferative disorders. Mod Pathol 12:200–217
78. Lachance DH, O'Neill BP, Macdonald DR, Jaeckle KA et al. (1991) Primary leptomeningeal lymphoma: report of 9 cases, diagnosis with immunocytochemical analysis, and review of the literature. Neurology 41:95–100
79. Landys KE, Berg GE, Torgerson JS, Klingenstierna HA et al. (1995) Bulky centroblastic non-Hodgkin's lymphoma of the cranium vault mimicking brain involvement managed with chemotherapy: a case report. Cancer 76:1261–1267

80. Larocca LM, Capello D, Rinelli A, Nori S et al. (1998) The molecular and phenotypic profile of primary central nervous system lymphoma identifies distinct categories of the disease and is consistent with histogenetic derivation from germinal center-related B cells. Blood 92:1011-1019
81. Lisak RP, Mitchell M, Zweiman B, Orrechio E, Asbury AK (1977) Guillain-Barre syndrome and Hodgkin's disease: three cases with immunological studies. Ann Neurol 1:72-78
82. Lutz JM, Coleman MP (1994) Trends in primary cerebral lymphoma. Br J Cancer 70:716-718
83. Majumdar G (1998) Chronic lymphocytic leukaemia with cerebral infiltration. Leuk Lymphoma 28:603-605
84. Marsh WL, Jr, Stevenson DR, Long HJd (1983) Primary leptomeningeal presentation of T-cell lymphoma. Report of a patient and review of the literature. Cancer 51:1125-1131
85. Matsuo T, Yamaoka A, Shiraga F, Matsuo N (1998) Two types of initial ocular manifestations in intraocular-central nervous system lymphoma. Retina 18:301-307
86. McAllister LD, Doolittle ND, Guastadisegni PE, Kraemer DF et al. (2000) Cognitive outcomes and long-term follow-up results after enhanced chemotherapy delivery for primary central nervous system lymphoma. Neurosurgery 46:51-60
87. McCue MP, Sandrock AW, Lee JM, Harris NL, Hedley Whyte ET (1993) Primary T-cell lymphoma of the brainstem. Neurology 43:377-381
88. Miller DC, Hochberg FH, Harris NL, Gruber ML et al. (1994) Pathology with clinical correlations of primary central nervous system non-Hodgkin's lymphoma. The Massachusetts General Hospital experience 1958-1989. Cancer 74:1383-1397
89. Mittra RA, Pulido JS, Hanson GA, Kajdacsy Balla A, Brummitt CF (1999) Primary ocular Epstein-Barr virus-associated non-Hodgkin's lymphoma in a patient with AIDS: a clinicopathologic report. Retina 19:45-50
90. Montserrat E, Bosch F, Lopez Guillermo A, Graus F et al. (1996) CNS involvement in mantle-cell lymphoma. J Clin Oncol 14:941-944
91. Morgello S, Maiese K, Petito CK (1989) T-cell lymphoma in the CNS: clinical and pathologic features. Neurology 39:1190-1196
92. Novak JA, Katzin WE (1995) Primary central nervous system T-cell lymphoma with a predominant CD8 immunophenotype. Cancer 75:2180-2185
93. Nozaki M, Tada M, Mizugaki Y, Takada K et al. (1998) Expression of oncogenic molecules in primary central nervous system lymphomas in immunocompetent patients. Acta Neuropathol Berl 95:505-510
94. O'Neill BP, Dinapoli RP, Kurtin PJ, Habermann TM (1995) Occult systemic non-Hodgkin's lymphoma (NHL) in patients initially diagnosed as primary central nervous system lymphoma (PCNSL): how much staging is enough? J Neurooncol 25:67-71
95. O'Neill BP, Wang CH, O'Fallon JR, Colgan JD et al. (1999) Primary central nervous system non-Hodgkin's lymphoma (PCNSL): survival advantages with combined initial therapy? A final report of the North Central Cancer Treatment Group (NCCTG) Study 86-72-52. Int J Radiat Oncol Biol Phys 43:559-563
96. Oinonen R, Franssila K, Elonen E (1999) Central nervous system involvement in patients with mantle cell lymphoma. Ann Hematol 78:145-149
97. Onda K, Wakabayashi K, Tanaka R, Takahashi H (1999) Intracranial malignant lymphomas: clinicopathological study of 26 autopsy cases. Brain Tumor Pathol 16:29-35
98. Ormerod LD, Puklin JE (1997) AIDS-associated intraocular lymphoma causing primary retinal vasculitis. Ocul Immunol Inflamm 5:271-278
99. Ostronoff M, Soussain C, Zambon E, Moran A et al. (1995) Localized stage non-Hodgkin's lymphoma of the testis: a retrospective study of 16 cases. Nouv Rev Fr Hematol 37:267-272
100. Pappas CT, Johnson PC, Sonntag VK (1988) Signet-ring cell lymphoma of the central nervous system. Case report. Journal of Neurosurgery 69:789-792
101. Paulus W (1999) Classification, pathogenesis and molecular pathology of primary CNS lymphomas. J Neurooncol 43:203-208
102. Paulus W, Ott MM, Strik H, Keil V, Muller Hermelink HK (1994) Large cell anaplastic (KI-1) brain lymphoma of T-cell genotype. Hum Pathol 25:1253-1256

103. Pawson R, Richardson DS, Pagliuca A, Kelsey SM et al. (1998) Adult T-cell leukemia/lymphoma in London: clinical experience of 21 cases. Leuk Lymphoma 31:177–185
104. Peltola J, Hietaharju A, Rantala I, Lehtinen T, Haapasalo H (1998) A reversible neuronal antibody (anti-Tr) associated paraneoplastic cerebellar degeneration in Hodgkin's disease. Acta Neurol Scand 98:360–363
105. Penn I, Porat G (1995) Central nervous system lymphomas in organ allograft recipients. Transplantation 59:240–244
106. Peris K, Fargnoli MC, Berardelli A, Crecco M et al. (1998) Peripheral nervous system involvement in a patient with large T-cell lymphoma arising from a pre-existing mycosis fungoides. Br J Dermatol 139:299–301
107. Ponzoni M, Arrigoni G, Gould VE, Del Curto B et al. (2000) Lack of CD 29 (beta1 integrin) and CD 54 (ICAM-1) adhesion molecules in intravascular lymphomatosis. Hum Pathol 31:220–226
108. Posner JB (1992) Pathogenesis of central nervous system paraneoplastic syndromes. Rev Neurol Paris 148:502–512
109. Posner JB, Dalmau J (1995) Clinical enigmas of paraneoplastic neurologic disorders. Clin Neurol Neurosurg 97:61–70
110. Propp RP, Means E, Deibel R, Sherer G, Barron K (1975) Waldenstrom's macroglobulinemia and neuropathy. Deposition of M-component on myelin sheaths. Neurology 25:980–988
111. Ramsay AD, Smith WJ, Isaacson PG (1988) T-cell-rich B-cell lymphoma. Am J Surg Pathol 12:433–443
112. Restrepo A, Raez LE, Byrne GE, Jr., Johnson T et al. (1998) Is central nervous system prophylaxis necessary in ocular adnexal lymphoma? Crit Rev Oncog 9:269–273
113. Rickert CH, Dockhorn Dworniczak B, Simon R, Paulus W (1999) Chromosomal imbalances in primary lymphomas of the central nervous system. Am J Pathol 155:1445–1451
114. Rivero ME, Kuppermann BD, Wiley CA, Garcia CR et al. (1999) Acquired immunodeficiency syndrome-related intraocular B-cell lymphoma. Arch Ophthalmol 117:616–622
115. Roncaroli F, Poppi M, Riccioni L, Frank F (1997) Primary non-Hodgkin's lymphoma of the sciatic nerve followed by localization in the central nervous system: case report and review of the literature. Neurosurgery 40:618–621
116. Russell DS, Rubinstein LJ, *Pathology of tumours of the nervous system* (Edward Arnold, London, ed. Fifth, 1989).
117. Scaravilli F, An SF, Groves M, Thom M (1999) The neuropathology of paraneoplastic syndromes. Brain Pathology 9:251–260
118. Schabet M (1999) Epidemiology of primary CNS lymphoma. J Neurooncol 43:199–201
119. Schlake HP, Husstedt IW, Grotemeyer KH, Potter R (1989) Paraneoplastic subacute cerebellar degeneration in Hodgkin's disease. Report of three cases and review of the literature. Clin Neurol Neurosurg 91:329–35
120. Schold SC, Cho ES, Somasundaram M, Posner JB (1979) Subacute motor neuronopathy: a remote effect of lymphoma. Ann Neurol 5:271–287
121. Schwechheimer K, Braus DF, Schwarzkopf G, Feller AC et al. (1994) Polymorphous high-grade B-cell lymphoma is the predominant type of spontaneous primary cerebral malignant lymphomas. American Journal of Surgical Pathology 18:931–937
122. Sheibani K, Battifora H, Winberg CD, Burke JS et al. (1986) Further evidence that "malignant angioendotheliomatosis" is an angiotropic large-cell lymphoma. N Engl J Med 314:943–948
123. Stroup RM, Sheibani K, Moncada A, Purdy LJ, Battifora H (1990) Angiotropic (intravascular) large cell lymphoma. A clinicopathologic study of seven cases with unique clinical presentations. Cancer 66:1781–1788
124. Tachikawa N, Goto M, Hoshino Y, Gatanaga H et al. (1999) Detection of Toxoplasma gondii, Epstein-Barr virus, and JC virus DNAs in the cerebrospinal fluid in acquired immunodeficiency syndrome patients with focal central nervous system complications [see comments]. Intern Med 38:556–562
125. Tani E, Costa I, Svedmyr E, Skoog L (1995) Diagnosis of lymphoma, leukemia, and metastatic tumor involvement of the cerebrospinal fluid by cytology and immunocytochemistry. Diagn Cytopathol 12:14–22

126. Thompsett AR, Ellison DW, Stevenson FK, Zhu D (1999) V(H) gene sequences from primary central nervous system lymphomas indicate derivation from highly mutated germinal center B cells with ongoing mutational activity. Blood 94:1738–1746
127. Tomlinson FH, Kurtin PJ, Suman VJ, Scheithauer BW et al. (1995) Primary intracerebral malignant lymphoma: a clinicopathological study of 89 patients. Journal of Neurosurgery 82:558–566
128. Torenbeek R, Scheltens P, Strack van Schijindel RJ, Algra PR et al. (1993) Angiotropic intravascular large-cell lymphoma with massive cerebral extension. J Neurol Neurosurg Psychiatry 56:914–916
129. Tutt AN, Brada M, Sampson SA (1997) Enteropathy associated T cell lymphoma presenting as an isolated CNS lymphoma three years after diagnosis of coeliac disease: T cell receptor polymerase chain reaction studies failed to show the original enteropathy to be a clonal disorder. Gut 40:801–3
130. Uetsuka S, Kajiwara K, Suehiro E, Nishizaki T et al. (1999) T cell malignant lymphoma in the central nervous system after acute lymphoblastic leukemia in a child. Childs Nerv Syst 15:486–489
131. van Besien K, Ha CS, Murphy S, McLaughlin P et al. (1998) Risk factors, treatment, and outcome of central nervous system recurrence in adults with intermediate-grade and immunoblastic lymphoma. Blood 91:1178–1184
132. van Dongen JJ, Wolvers-Tettero IL (1991) Analysis of immunoglobulin and T cell receptor genes. Part II: possibilities and limitations in the diagnosis and management of lymphoproliferative diseases and related disorders. Clinica Chimica Acta 198:93–174
133. Villegas E, Villa S, Lopez Guillermo A, Petit J et al. (1997) Primary central nervous system lymphoma of T-cell origin: description of two cases and review of the literature. J Neurooncol 34:157–161
134. Vinters HV, Gilbert JJ (1982) Multifocal chloromas of the brain. Surg Neurol 17:47–51
135. Yeh KH, Lien HC, Hsu SM, Cheng AL (1999) Quiescent nasal T/NK cell lymphoma manifested as primary central nervous system lymphoma. Am J Hematol 60:161–163

# Appendix

## Sampling of Brains at Autopsy

Optimum preservation of the brain for macroscopic and microscopic examination is achieved by suspending and fixing it intact for 2–3 weeks in formalin. However, circumstances may arise in which detailed neuropathological examination is desirable but consent is limited to the retention of only a few samples of brain for histology. The following guidelines may help in the selection of appropriate samples in different clinical contexts.

### Some General Points

1. Do not place the samples directly into cassettes for tissue processing. The samples will be of inadequate size and the sections will be of poor quality. The quality of the neurohistology is immeasurably improved by taking larger samples and fixing them for a week or so before trimming them to a size suitable for processing.
2. Take samples that are at least 1.5 cm in thickness. The reason for this is twofold. First, the process of slicing through unfixed brain introduces artefactual changes in the tissue immediately adjacent to the cut surface, and these can interfere with histological assessment. Second, the cut surface develops irregular convolutions during fixation. However, if the samples are thick enough, the artefactually disrupted and convoluted tissue at the cut surface is readily trimmed away after fixation, facilitating detailed macroscopic and microscopic examination.
   An exception to this general advice is the postmortem sampling of brain tissue for genetic or detailed immunophenotypic studies (e.g. to characterize tumour). In this case, in addition to prolonged fixation of large blocks of brain, cryostorage of tissue and formalin-fixation of multiple small tissue blocks over 12–24 h should be considered. The latter will allow the detection of some antigens that are difficult to detect after longer fixation.
3. Allow the sliced samples to fix flat. If they are crammed into a container and allowed to fix in a distorted shape they will be difficult later to orientate and trim.

The diagrams in this section indicate sampling strategies that are appropriate in most cases of dementia, problematic head injury (e.g. if the gross abnormalities

Current Topics in Pathology, Vol. 95
S. Love (Ed.): Neuropathology

appear too mild to account for the clinical findings) and miscellaneous neurodegenerative disorders. Once fixed, the tissue can be sliced and subdivided into multiple blocks. The suggested samples should be supplemented by blocks of macroscopically visible lesions noted when the brain is sliced at autopsy.

The appendix concludes with brief guidelines for taking samples of cerebrospinal fluid, brain tissue and other material for microbiological studies in suspected CNS infection.

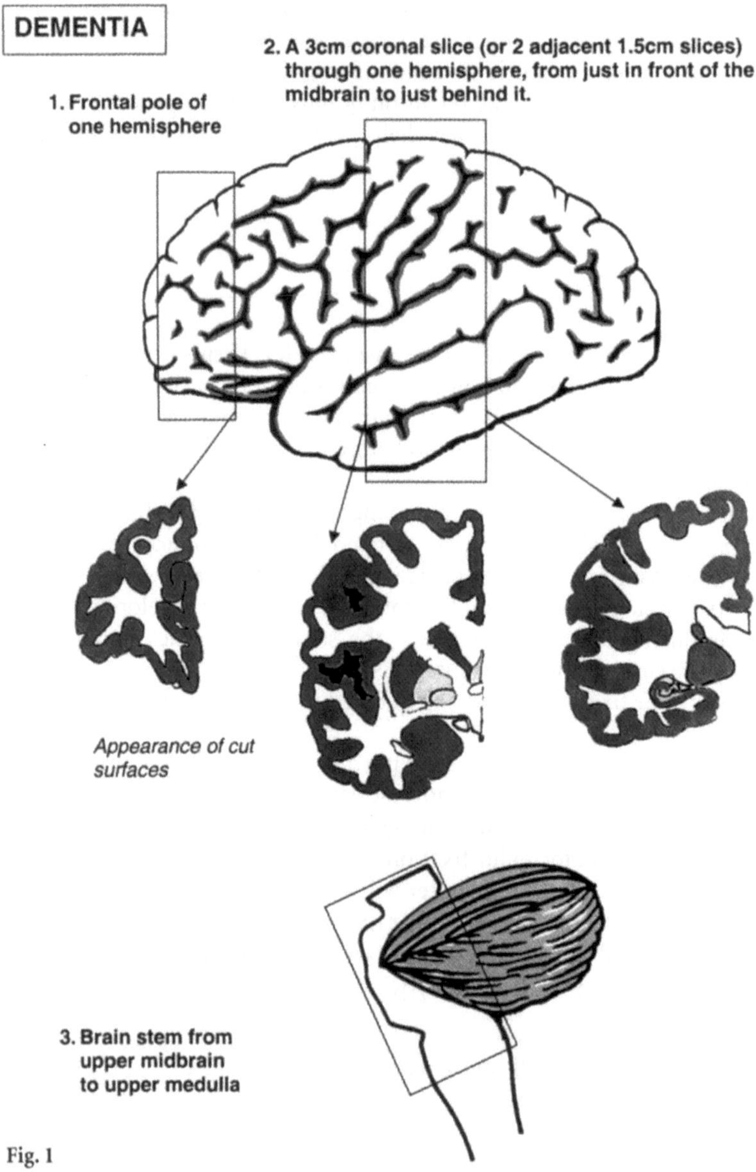


Fig. 1

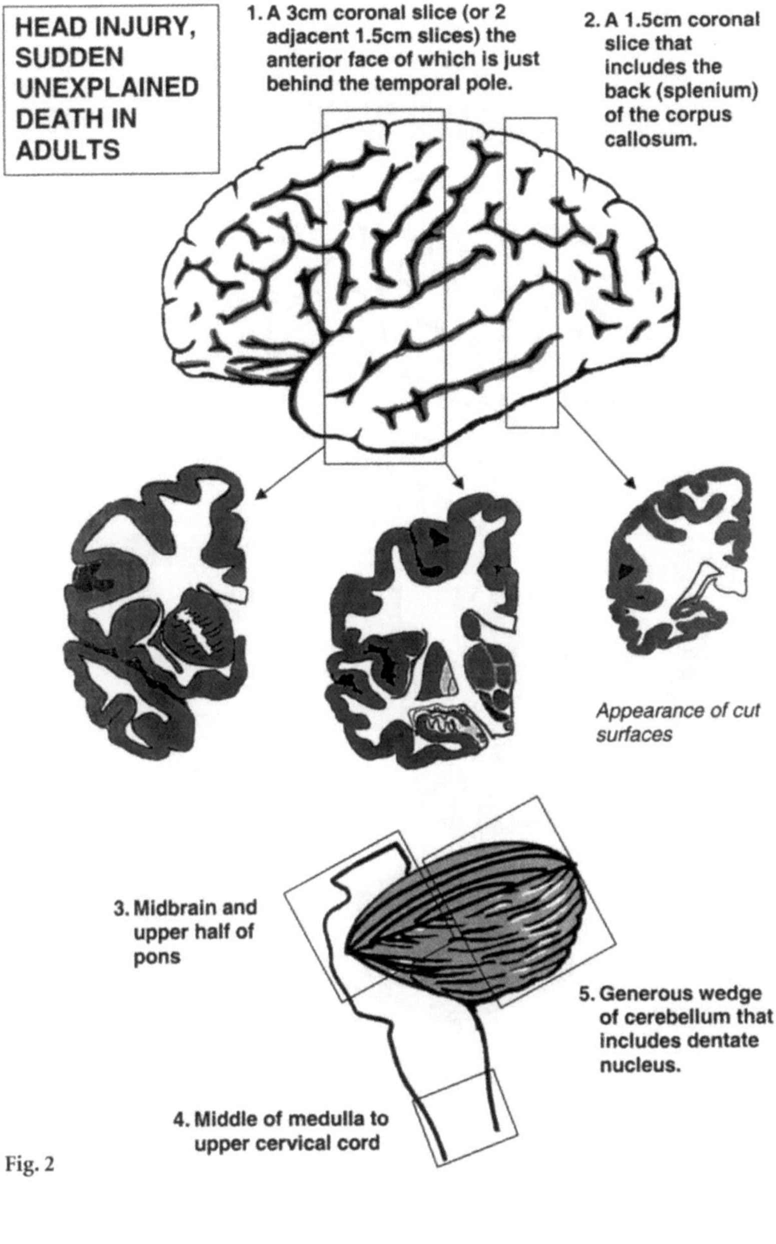
HEAD INJURY, SUDDEN UNEXPLAINED DEATH IN ADULTS
1. A 3cm coronal slice (or 2 adjacent 1.5cm slices) the anterior face of which is just behind the temporal pole.
2. A 1.5cm coronal slice that includes the back (splenium) of the corpus callosum.
Appearance of cut surfaces
3. Midbrain and upper half of pons
5. Generous wedge of cerebellum that includes dentate nucleus.
4. Middle of medulla to upper cervical cord

Fig. 2

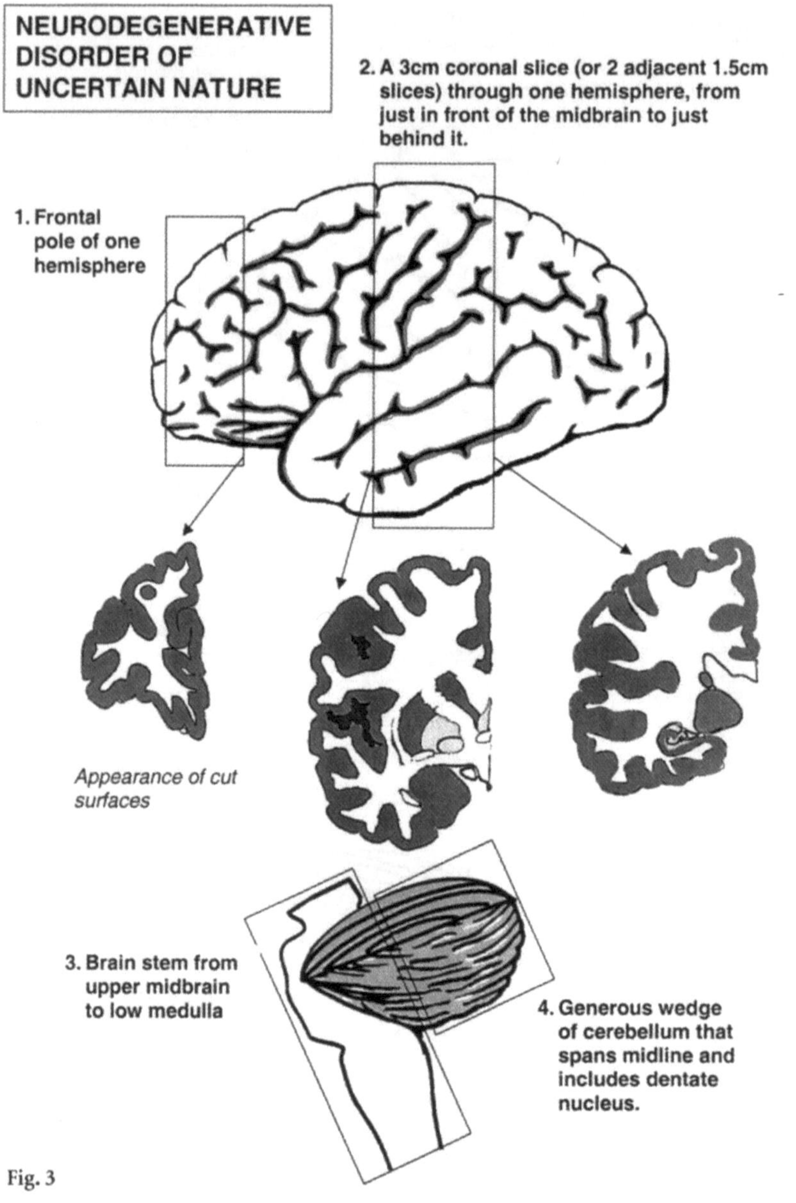


Fig. 3

If there is clinical evidence of spinal or neuromuscular involvement, take cord and samples of peripheral nerve and muscle, as well as the blocks shown in Fig. 3.

If the clinical history raises the possibility of Creutzfeldt-Jakob disease (and permission to keep the whole brain is not given), the following steps should be added to the above protocol:

- Sample the occipital pole of one cerebral hemisphere for paraffin histology.

- Freeze one frontal pole (i.e. contralateral to that sampled for paraffin histology) and, if possible, one cerebellar hemisphere at -70 °C (for Western blotting, transmission studies, DNA sequencing, etc).
- Ideally, also take samples of tonsil, spleen, appendix and lymph nodes, pituitary, trigeminal ganglia, spinal cord and dorsal root ganglia for paraffin histology, and freeze one tonsil at -70 °C for Western blot analysis.

## Specimens for Microbiological Investigation

### Cerebrospinal Fluid

Reflect the dura with the brain in situ, gently part the cerebral hemispheres and insert the needle of a sterile syringe about 30° to the vertical through the corpus callosum and into the lateral ventricle. Slight negative pressure should then be applied to the plunger of the syringe whilst slowly withdrawing the needle. When the tip of the needle enters the lateral ventricle, the fluid will be drawn into the syringe. In addition, swabs should be taken from the subarachnoid space, particularly in the region of any exudates - to do so use fine forceps to elevate the leptomeninges, make a small cut into the meninges with a sterile blade and insert the swab into the subarachnoid space.

If viral infection is suspected, samples of cerebrospinal fluid, brain (see below) and serum or clotted blood should be frozen, ideally at -70 °C. The frozen samples can later be used for viral culture, polymerase chain reaction (PCR) studies and serology, as needed.

### Abscess or Empyema

In most cases, the nature of the infection will not be in doubt. However, if identification of the responsible micro-organisms is needed, the purulent material should be cultured, in which case it should be aspirated into a sterile syringe, expelled into a sterile universal container and taken to a microbiology laboratory with as little delay as possible. The likelihood of recovering the responsible micro-organisms is greater if the contents of the abscess are aspirated than if only swabs are taken.

### Brain or Spinal Tissue

Samples of abnormal tissue for bacterial or fungal culture should be removed with a sterile scalpel, placed in a sterile universal container and taken to a microbiology laboratory as soon as possible.

In suspected viral infection, several small blocks of tissue (1-2 g is ample) should be taken from regions showing macroscopic abnormalities and, together with samples of CSF and serum or clotted blood (see above), frozen at -70 °C for later culture or PCR studies. The regions sampled in suspected herpes encephalitis should include the anterior part of the temporal lobes and the inferior part of the frontal lobes.

# Subject Index

## Index of Volumes 92–94 Current Topics in Pathology

**Volume 94: Dermatopathology.** Edited by R. Cerio

MIX
Papier aus verantwortungsvollen Quellen
Paper from responsible sources
FSC® C105338

If you have any concerns about our products,
you can contact us on
**ProductSafety@springernature.com**

In case Publisher is established outside the EU,
the EU authorized representative is:
**Springer Nature Customer Service Center GmbH**
**Europaplatz 3, 69115 Heidelberg, Germany**

Printed by Libri Plureos GmbH
in Hamburg, Germany